Basics of the U.S. Health Care System

Nancy J. Niles MS, MPH, PhD

Assistant Professor
Lander University
Greenwood, South Carolina

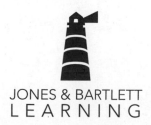

JONES & BARTLETT
LEARNING

World Headquarters
Jones & Bartlett Learning
5 Wall Street
Burlington, MA 01803
978-443-5000
info@jblearning.com
www.jblearning.com

Jones & Bartlett Learning books and products are available through most bookstores and online booksellers. To contact Jones & Bartlett Learning directly, call 800-832-0034, fax 978-443-8000, or visit our website, www.jblearning.com.

Substantial discounts on bulk quantities of Jones & Bartlett Learning publications are available to corporations, professional associations, and other qualified organizations. For details and specific discount information, contact the special sales department at Jones & Bartlett Learning via the above contact information or send an email to specialsales@jblearning.com.

Production Credits
Publisher: Michael Brown
Editorial Assistant: Catie Heverling
Editorial Assistant: Teresa Reilly
Production Manager: Tracey Chapman
Senior Marketing Manager: Sophie Fleck
Manufacturing and Inventory Control Supervisor: Amy Bacus
Composition: DSCS, LLC/Absolute Services, Inc.
Cover Design: Scott Moden
Cover Image: © Zorik Galstyan/ShutterStock, Inc.
Printing and Binding: Edwards Brothers Malloy
Cover Printing: Edwards Brothers Malloy

6048

To order this product, use ISBN: 978-1-4496-1519-2

978-0-7637-6984-0
Printed in the United States of America
17 16 15 14   10 9 8

About the Author

Nancy J. Niles is in her seventh year of full-time undergraduate teaching. She is in her third year of teaching undergraduate business and healthcare management classes in the AACSB-accredited Department of Business Administration at Lander University in Greenwood, South Carolina, having spent four years teaching in the Department of Business Administration at Concord University in Athens, West Virginia. She became very interested in health issues as a result of spending two tours with the US Peace Corps in Senegal, West Africa. She focused on community assessment and development, obtaining funding for business and health-related projects. Her professional experience also includes managing the New York State lead poisoning prevention program and managing a small business development center in Myrtle Beach, South Carolina.

Her graduate education has focused on health policy and management. She received a master of public health from the Tulane School of Public Health in New Orleans, Louisiana, a master of management with a healthcare administration emphasis from the University of Maryland University College, and a doctorate from University of Illinois at Urbana–Champaign in health policy. She is completing her master of business administration at the University of Maryland University College.

Acknowledgments

I would like to thank my mother, Joyce Robinson, who is a tremendous role model to me and who has always encouraged me to pursue my goals.

I would like to thank my husband, Donnie Niles, the love of my life, for his continued love and support. How lucky that I have my sister, Donna Berger, her husband, Vin, my brother, Greg, and my nephew and nieces, Coby, Emily, and Jenna, in my life . . . and of course, my loyal and dear friend, Richard Gibney and our constant canine companion, Maisy McNabb.

On a professional note, I would like to also thank Dr. Kendra Boggess, who gave me my first opportunity to teach full-time and my first boss, Dr. Taimi Carnahan, who gave me my first job in health care. I would also like to thank Mike Brown at Jones and Bartlett Publishers who provided me with this opportunity to write my first textbook. Ms. Catie Heverling, Editorial Assistant at Jones and Bartlett, and Katy Whipple of Absolute Services were very helpful to me in making this a reality.

Reviewers

Mary Agnes (Aggie) Garrison MS, RRT
Director of Clinical Education, Respiratory Care Program
Daytona State College
Daytona Beach, Florida

Justine Tutuska, MPH
Chair, Health Care Studies Department
Daemen College
Amherst, New York

Cathy Dolan, PhDc, MEd, MA, RN
Instructor
Chandler-Gilbert Community College
Gilbert, Arizona

Preface

I am writing this textbook because I would like to increase students' awareness of healthcare issues that impact them as US citizens.

Here are just two examples of how the US healthcare system currently operates. One of my undergraduate students is no longer qualified under her parents' healthcare coverage because she is over 25 years of age. She has asthma, a respiratory condition that could cause her to stop breathing, but because she can't afford the medicine for her condition, she goes without. She feels she has no choice. A friend of mine is undergoing chemotherapy and radiation for breast cancer treatment. Her doctor suggested she take a shot prior to her treatment that would alleviate her nausea so she could continue to work and take care of her family. The shot costs $2000. Her insurance company would not pay for it, and she could not afford to pay for it herself. So, she suffered while continuing to work and take care of her family. We are the most powerful country in the world and have been lauded internationally for our state-of-the-art medical technology and our advances in research to prevent disease. Yet unfortunate examples like this occur and will continue to occur until there is some type of healthcare system reform that will focus on affordable and accessible health care.

Table of Contents

Contents

Contents

Contents

Chapter 1

Overview of the US Healthcare Delivery System

LEARNING OBJECTIVES

The student will be able to:

- Identify 10 milestones of medicine and medical education and their importance to health care.
- Identify 10 milestones of the hospital system and their importance to health care.
- Identify 10 milestones of public health and their importance to health care.
- Identify 10 milestones of health insurance and their importance to health care.
- Explain the difference between primary, secondary, and tertiary prevention.
- Explain the concept of the iron triangle as it applies to health care.

DID YOU KNOW THAT?

- When the practice of medicine first began, tradesmen such as barbers practiced medicine. They often used the same razor to cut hair as to perform surgery.
- As of May 2009, the number of unemployed persons increased to 14.5 million. According to estimates, over 50% lost their health insurance benefits.

- In 2006, the United States spent over $2 trillion on healthcare spending, which is the highest in the world.
- In 2007, there were over 47 million uninsured US citizens.
- The Centers for Medicare and Medicaid Services (CMS) predicts annual healthcare costs will be $4.1 trillion by 2016, which represents nearly 20% of the US gross domestic product.
- The United States is one of only a few developed countries that do not have universal healthcare coverage.

INTRODUCTION

It is important as a healthcare consumer to understand the history of the US healthcare delivery system, how it operates today, who participates in the system, what legal and ethical issues arise as a result of the system, and what problems continue to plague the healthcare system. We are all consumers of health care. Yet, in many instances, we are ignorant of what we are actually purchasing. If we were going to spend $1000 on an appliance or a flat screen television, many of us would research the product to determine if what we are purchasing is the best product for us. This same concept should be applied to purchasing healthcare services.

Increasing healthcare consumer awareness will protect you in both the personal and professional aspects of your life. You may decide to pursue a career in health care either as a provider or as an administrator. You may also decide to manage a business where you will have the responsibility of providing health care to your employees. And lastly, from a personal standpoint, you should have the knowledge from a consumer point of view so you can make informed decisions about what matters most—your health.

As the US population's life expectancy continues to increase—increasing the "graying" of the population—the US will be confronted with more chronic health issues because, as we age, more chronic health conditions develop. The US healthcare system is one of the most expensive systems in the world. According to 2006 statistics, the US spent over $2 trillion on healthcare expenditures (CMS, 2006), or 16% of its gross domestic product. The **gross domestic product** is the total finished products or services that are produced in a country within a year. These statistics mean that over 15% of all of the products made within the borders of the United States within a year are healthcare related. Estimates indicate that healthcare spending will exceed $4 trillion by 2016, which represents nearly 20% of the gross domestic product (Brownlee, 2007; Kaiser Family Foundation, 2007). In 2007, there were over 47 million uninsured US citizens (Centers for Disease Control and Prevention [CDC], 2008). The Institute of Medicine's (IOM) 1999 report indicated that nearly 100,000 citizens die each year as a result of medical errors (Kohn, Corrigan, & Donaldson, 1999). Department of Labor (DOL) statistics reported in 2009 indicated that the number of unemployed persons increased to 14.5 million. Estimates indicate that more than 50% have lost their health insurance because the unemployed could not pay the premiums without employer contributions to their health care (DOL, 2009).

These rates are some of the highest in the world but, unlike most developed countries, the US does not offer healthcare coverage as a right of citizenship. Most developed countries have a **universal healthcare program,** which means access to all citizens. Many of these systems are typically run by the federal government, have centralized health policy agencies, are financed through different forms of taxation, and **payment of healthcare services are by a single payer—the government** (Shi & Singh, 2008). France and the United Kingdom have been discussed as possible models for the United States to follow to improve access to health care, but these programs have problems and may not be the ultimate solution for the United States. However, because the United States does not offer any type of universal healthcare coverage, many citizens, who are not eligible for government-sponsored programs, are expected to provide the service for themselves through the purchase of health insurance or the purchase of actual services. Many citizens cannot afford this option. Chapter 13, the last chapter of the book, will discuss the different types of universal healthcare systems in depth and offer possible solutions to US healthcare services issues.

In order to understand the current healthcare delivery system and its issues, it is important to learn the history of the development of the US healthcare system. There are four major sectors of our healthcare system that will be discussed in this chapter that have impacted our current system of operations: (1) the history of practicing medicine and the development of medical education, (2) the development of the hospital system, (3) the history of public health, and (4) the history of health insurance. In Tables 1-1 to 1-4, several important milestones are listed by date and illustrate historic highlights of each system component. The list is by no means exhaustive but provides an introduction to how each sector has evolved as part of the US healthcare system. Several of these highlights will be integrated and discussed in more depth in other chapters.

ORGANIZATION OF THE BOOK

Chapter 2 focuses on the current systems of operation in the United States. Chapter 3 discusses the government's role in health care and Chapter 4 specifically discusses the role of public health. Chapter 5 details the role of the different types of US healthcare institutions and Chapter 6 outlines the role of healthcare professionals in the US delivery system. Chapter 7 discusses public and private financing of US healthcare services and Chapter 8 outlines the impact of managed care on the delivery of these services. Chapter 9 discusses the impact of technology on healthcare services. Chapters 10 and 11 focus on the legal and ethical aspects of US health care. Chapter 12 discusses a major challenge in our system—mental health issues. Finally, Chapter 13 analyzes the healthcare system, compares it internationally with other countries' systems, and discusses possible solutions to problems. At the end of each chapter, a brief overview is given for the next chapter. This is an opportunity for you to understand the links between

TABLE 1-1 Milestones of Medicine and Medical Education 1700–2005

- 1700s: Training and apprenticeship under one physician was common until hospitals were founded in the mid-1700s. In 1765, the first medical school was established at the University of Pennsylvania.

- 1800s: Medical training was provided through internships with existing physicians who often were poorly trained themselves. There were only four medical schools in the United States that graduated only a handful of students. There was no formal tuition with no mandatory testing.

- 1847: The **American Medical Association (AMA)** was established as a membership organization for physicians to protect the interests of its providers. It did not become powerful until the 1900s when it organized its physician members by county and state medical societies. The AMA wanted to ensure they were protecting their financial well-being. It also began to focus on standardizing medical education.

- 1900s to 1930s: The medical profession was represented by general or family practitioners who operated in solitary practices. A small percentage of physicians were women. Total expenditures for medical care were less than 4% of the gross domestic product.

- 1904: The AMA created the Council on Medical Education to establish standards for medical education.

- 1928: Formal medical education was attributed to Abraham Flexner, who wrote an evaluation of medical schools in the United States and Canada indicating many schools were substandard. He made recommendations to close several schools, enact admission requirements, and set a standard curriculum. The Flexner Report led to standardized admissions testing for students called the Medical College Admission Test (MCAT).

- 1930s: The healthcare industry was dominated by male physicians and hospitals. Relationships between patient and physicians were sacred. Payments for physician care were personal.

- 1940s to 1960s: When group health insurance was offered, the relationship between patient and physician changed because of third-party payers (insurance). In the 1950s, federal grants supported medical school operations and teaching hospital. In the 1960s, the Regional Medical Programs provided research grants and emphasized service innovation and provider networking.

- 2000: There are 125 medical schools that still follow the Flexner curriculum. All require the MCAT for admission. Approximately 30% of physicians are women, many operate in multispecialty groups, and nearly two thirds are specialty physicians.

- 2005: Approximately 38,000 applied to medical school; 17,000 were admitted. The average annual cost for a public medical school for an in-state resident is $20,000. The annual cost for a private medical school is $40,000.

each chapter. Hopefully, by the end of the text, you will understand the connections between each component of health care. At the end of each chapter, there are several activities for you to complete that reinforce chapter concepts.

MILESTONES OF MEDICINE AND MEDICAL EDUCATION

The early practice of medicine did not require a major course of study, training, board exams, and licensing as is required today. During this period, anyone who

had the inclination to set up a physician practice could do so; oftentimes, clergy were also medical providers. Tradesmen such as barbers also practiced medicine. The red and white striped poles outside barber shops represented blood and bandages because the barbers were often also surgeons. They used the same blades to cut hair and to perform surgery (Starr, 1982). Because there were no restrictions, competition was very intense. In most cases, physicians did not possess any technical expertise, they relied mainly on common sense to make diagnoses (Stevens, 1971). During this period, there was no health insurance so consumers decided when they would visit a physician and paid for their visits out of their own pockets. Often, physicians treated their patients in the patients' homes. During the late 1800s, the medical profession became more cohesive as more technically advanced services were delivered to patients. The establishment of the **American Medical Association (AMA)** in 1847 as a professional membership organization for providers was a driving force for the concept of private practice in medicine. The AMA was also responsible for standardizing medical education (AMA, 2007; Goodman & Mugrave, 1992).

In the early history of medical education, physicians gradually established large numbers of medical schools because they were inexpensive to operate, increased their prestige, and enhanced their income. Medical schools only required four or more physicians, a classroom, some discussion rooms, and legal authority to confer degrees. Physicians received the students' tuitions directly and operated the school from this influx of money. Many physicians would affiliate with established colleges to confer degrees. Because there were no entry restrictions, as more students entered into medical schools, the existing internship program with physicians was dissolved and the Doctor of Medicine became the standard (Vault Career Intelligence, 2008). Although there were major issues with the quality of education provided because of the lack of educational requirements, medical school education became the gold standard for practicing medicine (Sultz & Young, 2006). The publication of the **Flexner Report** in 1910, which evaluated medical schools in Canada and the United States, was responsible for forcing medical schools to develop curriculums and admission testing. The curriculum and admission testing is still in existence today. In 2000, there were 125 medical schools that still followed the Flexner curriculum and all required admission testing. As of 2005, approximately 30% of physicians were women, many operated in multispecialty groups, and nearly two thirds were specialty physicians. In 2005, the average annual cost for a public medical school for an in-state resident was $20,000. The annual cost for a private medical school was $40,000 (Association of American Medical Colleges [AAMC], 2008).

MILESTONES OF THE HOSPITAL SYSTEM

In the early 19th century, **almshouses** or **poorhouses** were established to serve the indigent. They provided shelter to them while treating illness. Government-operated **pesthouses** segregated those who could spread

their disease. The framework of these institutions set up the conception of the hospital. Initially, wealthy people did not want to go to hospitals because the conditions were deplorable and the providers were not skilled, so hospitals, which were first built in urban areas, were used by the poor. During this period, many of the hospitals were owned by the physicians who practiced in them (Rosen, 1983).

In the early 20th century, with the establishment of more standardized medical education, hospitals became more accepted across socioeconomic classes and became the symbol of medicine. With the establishment of the AMA, who protected the interests of providers, the reputation of providers became more prestigious. During the 1930s and 1940s, the ownership of the hospitals changed from physician owned to church related and government operated (Starr, 1982).

In 1973, the first **Patient Bill of Rights** was established to protect healthcare consumers in the hospitals. In 1974, a federal law was passed that required all states to have **Certificate of Need (CON)** laws to ensure the state approved any capital expenditures associated with hospital/medical facilities' construction and expansion. The Act was repealed in 1987 but 36 states still have some type of CON mechanism (National Conference of State Legislatures [NCSL], 2008). The concept of CON was important but it encouraged state planning to ensure their medical system was based on need.

In 1985, the **Emergency Medical Treatment and Active Labor Act (EMTALA)** was enacted to ensure that consumers were not refused treatment for emergency treatment. During this period, inpatient hospital use was typical; however, by the 1980s, many hospitals were offering outpatient or ambulatory surgery that continues into the 21st century. The Balanced Budget Act of 1997 authorized outpatient Medicare reimbursement to support these cost-saving measures (CDC, 2008). In 2002, the **Joint Commission on the Accreditation of Healthcare Organizations** (now **The Joint Commission**) issued standards to increase consumer awareness by requiring hospitals to inform patients if their results were not consistent with typical results (American Hospital Association [AHA], 2008).

Hospitals are the foundation of our healthcare system. As our health insurance system evolved, the first type of health insurance was hospital insurance. As society's health needs increased, expansion of different medical facilities increased. There was more of a focus on ambulatory or outpatient services because we, as

TABLE 1-2	Milestones of the Hospital System 1820–2000

- 1820s: **Almshouses or poorhouses**, the precursor of hospitals, were developed to serve the poor primarily. They provided food and shelter to the poor and consequently treated the ill. **Pesthouses**, operated by local governments, were used to quarantine people who had contagious diseases such as cholera. The first hospitals were built around urban areas in New York City, Philadelphia, and Boston and were used often as a refuge for the poor. Dispensaries or pharmacies were established to provide free care to those who could not afford to pay and to dispense drugs to ambulatory patients.

- 1850s: A hospital system was finally developed but their conditions were deplorable because there were unskilled providers. Hospitals were owned primarily by the physicians who practiced in them.

- 1890s: Patients went to hospitals because they had no choice. There became more cohesiveness among providers because they had to rely on each other for referrals and access to hospitals, which gave them more professional power.

- 1920s: The development of medical technological advances increased quality of medical training and specialization and the economic development of the United States. The establishment of hospitals became the symbol of the institutionalization of health care. In 1929, President Coolidge signs the Narcotic Control Act, which provides funding for hospital construction for drug addicts.

- 1930s to 1940s: Once physician-owned hospitals were now owned by church groups, larger facilities, and government at all levels.

- 1970 to 1980: The first **Patient Bill of Rights** was introduced to protect healthcare consumer representation in hospital care. In 1974, National Health Planning and Resources Development Act required states to have **CON** laws to qualify for federal funding.

- 1980 to 1990: According to the AHA, 87% of hospitals were offering ambulatory surgery. In 1985, the **EMTALA** was enacted, which required hospitals to provide screening and stabilizing treatment regardless of the ability to pay by the consumer.

- 1990 to 2000: As a result of the Balanced Budget Act cuts of 1997, the federal government authorized an outpatient Medicare reimbursement system.

consumers, prefer outpatient services and, secondly, it is more cost-effective. In 1980, the AHA estimated that 87% of hospitals offered outpatient surgery. Although hospitals are still an integral part of our healthcare delivery system, the method of their delivery has changed. **Hospitalists**, created in 1996, are providers that focus specifically on the care of a patient when they are hospitalized. This new type of provider recognized the need of providing quality hospital care (AHA, 2008; Sultz & Young, 2006). More hospitals have recognized the trend of outpatient services and have integrated those types of services in their delivery.

MILESTONES OF PUBLIC HEALTH

The development of public health is important to note because its development was separate from the development of private medicine practices. Physicians were worried that government health departments could regulate how they practiced medicine, which could limit their income. Public health specialists also approached health from a collectivistic and preventive care viewpoint—to protect as many citizens as possible from health issues and to provide strategies to prevent health issues from occurring. Private practitioners held an individualistic viewpoint—citizens more often would be paying for physician services from their health insurance or from their own pockets and physicians would be providing them guidance on how to cure their diseases, not prevent them. The two contrasting viewpoints still exist today, but there have been efforts to coordinate and collaborate more of the traditional and public health activities.

TABLE 1-3	Milestones in Public Health 1700–2003

- 1700 to 1800: The United States was experiencing strong industrial growth. Long work hours in unsanitary conditions resulted in massive disease outbreaks. US public health practices targeted reducing **epidemics**, or **large patterns of disease in a population**, that impacted the population. Some of the first public health departments were established in the urban areas as a result of these epidemics.

- 1800 to 1900: Three very important events occurred. In 1942, Britain's Edwin Chadwick produced the *General Report on the Sanitary Condition of the Labouring Population of Great Britain*, which is considered one of the most important documents of public health. This report stimulated a similar US survey. In 1854, Britain's John Snow performed an analysis that determined contaminated water in London was the cause of the cholera epidemic in London. This discovery established a link between the environment and disease. In 1850, Lemeuel Shattuck, based on Chadwick's report and Snow's activities, developed state public health law that became the foundation for public health activities.

- By 1900 to 1950: In 1920, Charles Winslow defined **public health** as a focus of preventing disease, prolonging life, and promoting physical health and efficiency through organized community efforts.
- During this period, most states had public health departments that focused on sanitary inspections, disease control, and health education. Throughout the years, **public health functions** included child immunization programs, health screenings in schools, community health services, substance abuse programs, and sexually transmitted disease control.
- In 1923, a vaccine for diphtheria and whooping cough was developed. In 1928, Alexander Fleming discovered penicillin. In 1933, initial polio vaccine research was developed with mixed results. In 1946, the **National Mental Health Act** provided funding for research, prevention, and treatment of mental illness.

- 1950 to 1980: In 1950, cigarette smoke is identified as a cause of lung cancer.
- In 1952, Dr. Jonas Salk successfully developed the polio vaccine.
- The **Poison Prevention Packaging Act of 1970** was enacted to prevent children from accidentally ingesting substances. Childproof caps were developed for use on all drugs. In 1980, the eradication of smallpox was announced.

- 1980 to 1990: The first recognized cases of AIDS occurred in the United States in the early 1980s.
- 1988: The *Institute of Medicine Report* defined public health as organized community efforts to address the public interest in health by applying scientific and technical knowledge and promote health.

- 1990 to 2000: In 1997, Oregon voters approved a referendum that allowed physicians to assist terminally ill, mentally competent patients to commit suicide. From 1998 to 2006, 292 patients exercised their rights under the law.

- 2000s: The terrorist attack on United States on September 11, 2001, impacted and expanded the role of public health. The **Public Health Security and Bioterrorism Preparedness and Response Act of 2002** provided grants to hospitals and public health organizations to prepare for bioterrorism as a result of September 11, 2001. In 2008, the state of Washington passed legislation for physician-assisted suicide.

- 2003: International outbreak of severe acute respiratory syndrome (SARS).

During the 1700s to 1800s, the concept of public health was born. In their reports, Edwin Chadwick, Dr. John Snow, and Lemuel Shattuck demonstrated a relationship between the environment and disease (Chadwick, 1842; Turnock, 1997). As a result of their work, public health law was enacted and, by the 1900s, public health departments were focused on the environment and its relationship to disease outbreaks. Disease control and health education were also integral components of public health departments. In 1916, the Johns Hopkins University, one of the most prestigious universities in the world, established the first public health school (Duke

University Library, 2008). Winslow's definition of **public health** focuses on the prevention of disease, while the IOM defines public health as the organized community effort to protect the public by applying scientific knowledge (IOM, 1988; Winslow, 1920). These definitions are exemplified by the development of several vaccines for whooping cough, polio, smallpox, diphtheria, and the discovery of penicillin. All of these efforts focus on the protection of the public from disease.

The three most important public health achievements are (1) the recognition by the Surgeon General that tobacco use is a health hazard; (2) the number of vaccines that have been developed that have eradicated some diseases and controlled the number of childhood diseases that exist; and (3) early detection programs for blood pressure and heart attacks and smoking cessation programs, which have dramatically reduced the number of deaths in this country (Novick, Morrow, & Mays, 2008).

Assessment, policy development, and assurance were developed based on the 1988 report, *The Future of Public Health*, which indicated there was an attrition of public health activities in protecting the community (IOM, 1988). There was poor collaboration between public health and private medicine, no strong mission statement and weak leadership, and politicized decision making. **Assessment** was recommended because it focused on the systematic continuous data collection of health issues, which would ensure that public health agencies were vigilant in protecting the public (IOM, 1988; Turnock, 1997). **Policy development** should also include planning at all health levels, not just federally. Federal agencies should support local health planning (IOM, 1988).

Assurance focuses on evaluating any processes that have been put in place to assure that the programs are being implemented appropriately. These core functions will ensure that public health remains focus on the community, has programs in place that are effective, and has an evaluation process in place to ensure that the programs do work (Turnock, 1997).

The **Healthy People 2000** report, which started in 1987, was created to implement a new national prevention strategy with three goals: increase life expectancy, reduce health disparities, and increase access to preventive services. Also, three categories of health promotion, health prevention, and preventive services were identified and surveillance activities were emphasized. **Healthy People** provided a vision to reduce preventable disabilities and

death. Target objectives were set throughout the years to measure progress (CDC, 2009a).

The **Healthy People 2010** report was released in 2000. The report contained a health promotion and disease prevention focus to identify preventable threats to public health and to set goals to reduce the threats. Nearly 500 objectives were developed according to 28 focus areas. Focus areas ranged from access to care, food safety, education, environmental health, to tobacco and substance abuse. An important component of the Healthy People 2010 is the development of an infrastructure to ensure public health services are provided. Infrastructure includes skilled labor, information technology, organizations, and research (CDC, 2009a; Novick, Morrow, & Mays, 2008). Its major goals were to increase quality and life expectancy and to reduce health disparities. The goals for both reports are consistent with the definitions of public health in both Winslow's and the IOM's reports.

It is important to mention the impact the terrorist attack on the United States on September 11, 2001, the anthrax attacks, the outbreak of global diseases such as severe acute respiratory syndrome (SARS), and the US natural disaster of Hurricane Katrina had on the scope of public health responsibilities. As a result of these major events, public health has expanded their area of responsibility. The terms "bioterrorism" and disaster preparedness have more frequently appeared in public health literature and have become part of strategic planning. The **Public Health Security and Bioterrorism Preparedness and Response Act of 2002** provided grants to hospitals and public health organizations to prepare for bioterrorism as a result of September 11, 2001 (CDC, 2008).

Public health is challenged by its very success because the public now takes public health measures for granted: there are several successful vaccines that targeted almost all childhood diseases, tobacco use has decreased significantly, accident prevention has increased, there are safer workplaces because of Occupational Safety and Health Administration (OSHA), fluoride is added to the public water supply, there is decreased mortality because of heart attacks, etc. (Turnock, 1997). When some major event occurs like anthrax poisoning or a SARS outbreak, people immediately think that public health will automatically control these problems. The public may not realize how much effort and dedication and research takes place to protect the public.

TABLE 1-4	Milestones of the US Health Insurance System 1800–2009

- 1800 to 1900: Insurance was purchased by individuals like one would purchase car insurance. In 1847, the Massachusetts Health Insurance Co. of Boston was the first insurer to issue "sickness insurance." In 1853, a French mutual aid society established a prepaid hospital care plan in San Francisco, California. This plan resembles the modern Health Maintenance Organization (HMO).

- 1900 to 1920: In 1913, the International Ladies Garment Workers began the first union-provided medical services. The National Convention of Insurance Commissioners drafted the first model for regulation of the health insurance industry.

- 1920s: The blueprint for health insurance was established in 1929 when J. F. Kimball began a hospital insurance plan for school teachers at the Baylor University Hospital in Texas. This initiative became the model for Blue Cross plans nationally. The Blue Cross plans were nonprofit and covered only hospital charges so as not to infringe on private physicians' income.

- 1930s: There were discussions regarding the development of a national health insurance program. However, the AMA opposed the move (Raffel & Raffel, 1994). With the Depression and the US participation in World War II, the funding required for this type of program was not available. In 1935, President Roosevelt signed the Social Security Act which created "old age insurance" to help those of retirement age. In 1936, Vassar College, in New York, was the first college to establish a medical insurance group policy for students.

- 1940s to 1950s: The War Labor Board freezes wages, forcing employers to offer health insurance to attract potential employees. In 1947, the Blue Cross Commission was established to create a national doctors network. By 1950, 57% of the population had hospital insurance.

- 1965: President Johnson signs Medicare and Medicaid programs into law.

- 1970s to 1980s: President Nixon signs the Health Maintenance Organization (HMO) Act, which was the predecessor of managed care. In 1982, Medicare proposed paying for hospice or end-of-life care. In 1982, diagnosis related groups (DRGs) and prospective payment guidelines were developed to control insurance reimbursement costs. In 1985, the **Consolidated Omnibus Budget Reconciliation Act (COBRA)** requires employers to offer partially subsidized health coverage to terminated employees.

- 1990 to 2000: President Clinton's Health Security Act proposes a universal healthcare coverage plan, which was never passed. In 1993, the **Family Medical Leave Act (FMLA)** was enacted, which allowed employees up to 12 weeks of unpaid leave because of family illness. In 1996, the **Health Insurance Portability and Accountability Act (HIPAA)** was enacted, making it easier to carry health insurance when changing employment. It also increased the confidentiality of patient information. In 1997, the Balanced Budget Act (BBA) of 1997 was enacted to control the growth of Medicare spending. It also established the State-based Children's Insurance Program (SCHIP).

- 2000: The SCHIP, now the Children's Health Insurance Program, was implemented.

- 2000: The Medicare, Medicaid, and SCHIP Benefits Improvement and Modernization Act provided some relief from the BBA by providing across-the-board program increases.

- 2003: The Medicare Prescription Drug, Improvement and Modernization Act was passed, which created Medicare Part D, prescription plans for the elderly.

- 2006: Massachusetts mandated all residents have health insurance by 2009.

- In 2009, President Obama signed the **American Recovery and Reinvestment Act**, which protected health coverage for the unemployed by providing a 65% subsidy for COBRA coverage to make the premiums more affordable.

MILESTONES OF THE HEALTH INSURANCE SYSTEM

There are two key concepts in **group insurance**: "risk is transferred from the individual to the group and the group shares the cost of any covered losses incurred by its member" (Buchbinder & Shanks, 2007, p. 158). Like life insurance or homeowner's insurance, **health insurance** was developed to provide protection should a covered individual experience an event that required health care. In 1847, a Boston insurance company offered sickness insurance to consumers (Starr, 1982).

During the 19th century, large employers such as coal mining and railroad companies offered medical services to their employees by providing company doctors. Fees were taken from their pay to cover the service. In 1913, a union-provided health insurance was provided by the International Ladies Garment Workers where health insurance was negotiated as part of their contract (Duke University Library, 2008). During this period, there were several proposals for a national health insurance program but the efforts failed. The AMA was worried that any national health insurance would impact the financial security of their providers. The AMA persuaded the federal government to support private insurance efforts (Raffel & Raffel, 1994).

In 1929, a group hospital insurance plan was offered to teachers at a hospital in Texas. This became the foundation of the nonprofit Blue Cross plans. In order to placate the AMA, Blue Cross initially offered only hospital insurance in order to avoid infringement of physicians' incomes (Blue Cross Blue Shield Association, 2007; Starr, 1982). In 1935, the **Social Security Act** was created and was considered "old age" insurance. During this period, there was continued discussion of a national health insurance program. But, with the impact of World War II and the Depression, there was no funding for this program. The government felt that the Social Security Act was a sufficient program to protect consumers. These events were a catalyst for the development of a health insurance program that included private participation. Although a universal health coverage program was proposed during President Clinton's administration in the 1990s, it was never passed. In 2009, there has been a major public outcry at regional town hall meetings opposing any type of government universal healthcare coverage. In 2006, Massachusetts proposed mandatory health coverage for all citizens so it may be that universal health coverage may be a state-level initiative (Kaiser Family Foundation, 2007).

By the 1950s, nearly 60% of the population had hospital insurance (AHA, 2008). Disability insurance was attached to Social Security. In the 1960s, President Johnson signed Medicare and Medicaid into law, which protect the elderly, disabled, and indigent. President Nixon established the Health Maintenance Organization (HMO), which focused on effective cost measures for health delivery. Also, in the 1980s, diagnostic related groups (DRGs) and prospective payment guidelines were established to provide guidelines for treatment. These DRGs were attached to appropriate insurance reimbursement categories for treatment. The **Consolidated Omnibus Budget Reconciliation Act (COBRA)** was passed to provide health insurance protection if an individual changes jobs. In 1993, the **Family Medical Leave Act** (FMLA) was passed to protect an employee if there is a family illness. An employee can receive up to 12 weeks of unpaid leave and their health insurance during this period. Also, in 1996, the **Health Insurance Portability and Accountability Act (HIPAA)** was passed to provide stricter confidentiality regarding the health information of individuals. In 1997, the Balanced Budget Act (BBA) was passed that required massive program reductions for Medicare and authorized Medicare reimbursement for outpatient services (CMS, 2008).

At the start of the 21st century, cost, access, and quality continue to be issues for US health care. Employers continue to play an integral role in health insurance coverage. In 2004, nearly 60% of the population was covered by employer insurance (AMA, 2008). The largest public coverage program is Medicare —14% of the population. The Children's Health Insurance Program (CHIP) was implemented to ensure that children, who are not Medicaid eligible, receive health care. The Medicare, Medicaid, and SCHIP Benefits Improvement and Modernization Act provided some relief from the BBA of 1997 by restoring some funding to these consumer programs. In 2003, a consumer law, the Medicare Prescription Drug, Improvement, and Modernization Act, created a major overhaul of the Medicare system (CMS, 2008). The Act created Medicare Part D, a prescription plan that became effective in 2006 that provided different prescription programs to the elderly, based on their prescription needs. It has been criticized because it is so complex. The elderly had a difficult time understanding which plan to select. It also has not been cost effective; the cost of the program has been estimated at $550 billion. The 10-year estimated cost of this program is $1.2 trillion (Brownlee, 2007). In 2005, nearly 5 million citizens lost their health insurance in part because they lost their jobs (Blumenthal, 2006). Health insurance coverage continues to be an issue for the United States.

CURRENT SYSTEM OPERATIONS

Government's Participation in Health Care

The US government plays an important role in healthcare delivery. The United States has three governmental levels participating in the healthcare system: federal, state, and local. The federal government provides a range of regulatory and funding mechanisms including **Medicare** and **Medicaid**, established in 1965 as federally funded programs to provide health access to the elderly (65 years or older) and the poor, respectively. Over the years, these programs have expanded to include the disabled. They also have developed programs for military personnel, veterans, and their dependents.

Federal law does ensure access to emergency services regardless of ability to pay as a result of EMTALA (Regenstein, Mead, & Lara, 2007). The federal government determines a national healthcare budget, sets reimbursement rates, and also formulates standards for providers for eligible Medicare and Medicaid patients (Barton, 2003). The state level is also responsible for regulatory and funding mechanisms but also provides healthcare programs as dictated by the federal government. The local or county level of government is responsible for implementing programs dictated by both the federal and state level.

The US healthcare system is not a true system because of its fragmentation and lack of centralized decision making (Shi & Singh, 2008). The United States has several federal health regulatory agencies including the **CDC** for public health, the **Food and Drug Administration** (FDA) for pharmaceutical controls, and **CMS** for indigent, disabled, and the elderly. There is also **The Joint Commission**, a private organization that focuses on healthcare organizations' oversight and the **Agency for Healthcare Research and Quality** is the primary federal source for quality delivery of health services. The **Center for Mental Health Services**, in partnership with state health departments, leads national efforts to assess mental health delivery services. Although the federal government is to be commended because of the many agencies that focus on major healthcare issues, with

multiple organizations there is often duplication of effort and miscommunication which results in inefficiencies (Kaiser Family Foundation, 2007). However, there are several regulations in place that protect patient rights and privacy. Regulations such as HIPAA protects patient information, COBRA gives workers and families the right to continue healthcare coverage if they lose their job, the **Newborn and Mothers' Health Protection Act** prevents health insurance companies from discharging a mother and child too early from the hospital, the **Women's Health and Cancer Rights Act** prevents discrimination of women who have cancer, the **Mental Health Parity Act** requires health insurance companies to provide fair coverage for mental health conditions, and the **Sherman Antitrust Act** ensures fair competition in the marketplace for patients by prohibiting monopolies (Barton, 2003; DOL, 2009). All of these regulations are considered social regulations because they were enacted to protect the healthcare consumer.

Private Participation in Health Care

The private sector focuses on the financial and delivery aspects of the system. Approximately 36% of the 2005 healthcare expenditures were paid from private health insurance, insurance offered by a private insurance company such as Blue Cross; private **out-of-pocket payments**, funds paid by the individual were 15%; and federal, state, and local governments paid 44% (National Center for Health Statistics, 2006). Approximately 55% of private healthcare financing is through **employer health insurance**, a type of **voluntary or private health insurance** set up by an individual's employer. The delivery of the services provided is through legal entities such as hospitals, clinics, physicians, and other medical providers (Barton, 2003). The different providers are an integral part of the medical care system and need to coordinate their care with the layers of the US government. In order to ensure access to health care, communication is vital between the public and private components of healthcare delivery.

CONSUMER PERSPECTIVE ON HEALTH CARE

Basic Concepts of Health

Prior to discussing this complex system, it is important to identify three major concepts of healthcare delivery: primary, secondary, and tertiary prevention. These concepts are vital to understanding the US healthcare system because different components of the healthcare system focus on these different areas of health, which often results in lack of coordination between the different components.

Primary, Secondary, and Tertiary Prevention

According to the American Heritage Dictionary (2001, p. 666), prevention is defined as "slowing down or stopping the course of an event." **Primary prevention** avoids the development of a disease. Promotion activities such as health education are primary prevention. Other examples include smoking cessation programs, immunization programs, and educational programs for pregnancy and employee safety. State health departments often develop targeted, large education campaigns regarding a specific health issue in their area. **Secondary prevention** activities are focused on early disease detection, which prevents progression of the disease. Screening programs, such as high blood pressure testing, are examples of secondary prevention activities. Colonoscopies and mammograms are also examples of secondary prevention activities. Many local health departments implement secondary prevention activities. **Tertiary prevention** reduces the impact of an already established disease by reducing disease-related complications. Tertiary prevention focuses on rehabilitation and monitoring of diseased individuals. A person with high blood pressure who is taking blood pressure medicine is an example of tertiary prevention. A physician that writes a prescription for that blood pressure medication to control high blood pressure is an example of tertiary prevention. Traditional medicine focuses on tertiary prevention (CDC, 2009b).

We, as healthcare consumers, would like to receive primary prevention to prevent disease. We would like to participate in secondary prevention activities such as screening for cholesterol or blood pressure because it helps us manage any health problems we may be experiencing and reduces the potential impact of a disease. And, we would like to also visit our physicians for tertiary measures so, if we do have a disease, it can be managed by taking a prescribed drug, etc. From our perspective, these three areas of health should be better coordinated for the healthcare consumer so the United States will have a healthier population.

ASSESSING YOUR HEALTHCARE SYSTEM USING THE IRON TRIANGLE

Many healthcare systems are evaluated using the **Iron Triangle**—a concept that focuses on the balance of three factors: quality, cost, and accessibility to health care (Smolensky, 2003). If one factor is emphasized, such as cost reduction, it may create an inequality of quality and access because costs are being cut. Because lack of access is a problem in the United States, healthcare systems may focus on increasing access, which could increase costs. In order to assess the success of a healthcare delivery, it is vital that consumers assess their health care by analyzing the balance between cost, access, and quality. Are you receiving quality care from your provider? Do you have easy access to your healthcare system? Is it costly to receive health care? Although the Iron Triangle is used by many experts in analyzing large healthcare delivery systems, as a healthcare consumer, you can also evaluate your healthcare delivery system by using the Iron Triangle. An effective healthcare system should have a balance between the three components.

CONCLUSION

Despite US healthcare expenditures, the US disease rates remain higher than many developed countries because the United States has an expensive system that is available to only those who can afford it (Regenstein, Mead, & Lara, 2007). Because the United States does not have universal health coverage, there are more health disparities across the nation. Persons living in poverty are more likely to be in poor health and less likely to use the healthcare system compared to those with incomes above the poverty line (CDC, 2008). If the United States offered universal health coverage, the per capita expenditures would be more evenly distributed and likely more effective. The major problem for the United States is that healthcare insurance is a major determinant of access to health care. With 47 million uninsured in the United States, the disease rates and mortality rates will not improve. Based on the fragmented development of US health care, the system is based on individualism and self-determination and focusing on the individual rather than collectivistic needs of the population (Shi & Singh, 2008). For example, there are over 20 million citizens who have type 2 diabetes, a chronic and serious disease that impacts how your body breaks down food to obtain energy. This chronic disease has severe complications if not treated appropriately. Unless something is done to prevent this insidious disease, there will be 35 million heart attacks, 13 million strokes, 8 million instances of blindness, 2 million amputations, and 62 million deaths over the next 30 years (Rizza, 2006). In 2002, infant mortality rates increased because of low birth weight babies. Racial disparities in disease and death rates are a concern (CDC, 2005). Both private and public participants in the US health delivery system need to increase their collaboration to reduce these disease rates. Leaders need to continue to assess our healthcare system using the Iron Triangle to ensure there is a balance between access, cost, and quality.

PREVIEW OF CHAPTER TWO

Chapter 2 will discuss the different stakeholders or participants of the US healthcare system and their roles in the system, so as a consumer, you will have an understanding of how they all participate. A comparison of the general health status of the United States will be compared to several industrialized countries because it is important to assess how the US health status compares to other parts of the world.

VOCABULARY

Agency for Healthcare Research and Quality (AHRQ)

Almshouses

American Medical Association (AMA)

American Recovery and Reinvestment Act (ARRA)

Assessment

Assurance

Centers for Disease Control and Prevention (CDC)

Centers for Medicare and Medicaid Services (CMS)

Center for Mental Health Services (CMHS)

Certificate of Need (CON)

Consolidated Omnibus Budget Reconciliation Act (COBRA)

Emergency Medical Treatment and Active Labor Act (EMTALA)

Employer health insurance

Epidemics

Family Medical Leave Act (FMLA)

Flexner Report

Graying of the population

Gross domestic product (GDP)

Group insurance

Health

Health insurance

Health Insurance Portability and Accountability Act (HIPAA)

Healthy People reports

Hospitalists

Iron Triangle

Joint Commission

Medicaid

Medicare

Mental Health Parity Act (MHPA)

National Mental Health Act (NMHA)

Newborn and Mothers' Health Protection Act (NMHPA)

Out-of-pocket payments

Patient Bill of Rights

Pesthouses

Poison Prevention Packaging Act (PPPA)

Primary prevention

Public health

Public health functions

Public Health Security and Bioterrorism Preparedness and Response Act (Bioterrorism Act)

Secondary prevention

Sherman Antitrust Act

Social Security Act (SSA)

Tertiary prevention

Universal healthcare coverage

Voluntary health insurance

Women's Health and Cancer Rights Act (WHCRA)

REFERENCES

American Heritage Dictionary. (4th ed.). (2001). New York: Bantam Dell.

American Hospital Association. (2008). Community accountability and transparency: Helping hospitals better serve their communities. Retrieved June 1, 2008, from http://www.aha.org/aha/content/2007/pdf/07accountability.pdf.

American Medical Association. (2007). Our history. Retrieved May 1, 2007, from http://www.ama-assn.org/ama/pub/about-ama/our-history.shtml.

American Medical Association. (2008). Reports of council on medical service. Retrieved May 29, 2008, from http://www.ama-assn.org/ama1/pub/upload/mm/38/i05cmspdf.pdf.

Association of American Medical Colleges. (2008). Tuition and student fees, first-year medical school students 2004–2005. Retrieved May 31, 2008, from https://services.aamc.org/tsfreports/select.cfm?year_of_study=2005.

Barton, P. (2003). *Understanding the U.S. health services system*. Chicago: Health Administration Press.

BlueCross BlueShield Assocation. (2007). Blue beginnings. Retrieved May 1, 2007, from http://www.bcbs.com/about/history/blue-beginnings.html.

Blumenthal, D. (2006). Employer-sponsored health insurance in the United States-Riding the health care tiger. *New England Journal of Medicine, 355*, 195-202.

Brownlee, S. (2007). *Overtreated: Why too much medicine is making us sicker and poorer* (pp. 1–12). New York: Holzbrinck Publishers.

Buchbinder, S., & Shanks, N. (2007) *Introduction to health care management*. Sudbury, MA: Jones and Bartlett.

Centers for Disease Control and Prevention. (2005). Quickstats: Infant mortality rates by selected racial/ethnic populations-United States, 2002. *MMWR Morbidity and Mortality Weekly Report, 51*, 126.

Centers for Disease Control and Prevention. (2008). Retrieved May 29, 2008, from www.cdc.gov/nchs/data/series/sr_13/sr13_150.pdf.

Centers for Disease Control and Prevention. (2009a). Retrieved October 18, 2009, from http://www.cdc.gov/osi/goals/.

Centers for Disease Control and Prevention. (2009b). Retrieved June 12, 2009, from http://www.cdc.gov/excite/skincancer/mod13.htm.

Centers for Medicare and Medicaid Services. (2006). *National health care expenditures projections: 2000–2015*. Baltimore, MD: Centers for Medicare and Medicaid Services, Office of the Actuary.

Centers for Medicare and Medicaid Services. (2008). Retrieved May 29, 2008, from http://www.cms.hhs.gov/HIPAAGenInfo/01_Overview.asp.

Chadwick, E. (1842). *The sanitary conditions of the labouring class*. London: W. Clowes.

Department of Labor. (2009). Retrieved October 18, 2009, from http://www.bls.gov/cps/.

Duke University Library. (2008). Medicine and Madison Avenue. Timeline. Retrieved June 2, 2008, from http://library.duke.edu/digitalcollections/mma/timeline.html.

Goodman, J. C., & Mugrave, G. L. (1992). *Patient power: Solving America's health care crisis*. Washington, DC: CATO Institute.

Institute of Medicine. (1988). *The future of public health* (pp. 1–5). Washington, DC: National Academies Press.

Kaiser Family Foundation. (2007). Health care spending in the United States and OECD countries. Retrieved February 10, 2007, from http://www.kff.org/insurance/snapshot/chcm010307oth.cfm.

Kohn, L. T., Corrigan, J. M., & Donaldson, M. S. (1999). *To err is human: Building a safer health system*. Washington, DC: Institute of Medicine. Retrieved June 10, 2008, from http://www.iom.edu/CMS/8089/5575.aspx.

National Center for Health Statistics. (2006). *Health, United States, 2006: With chartbook on trends in the health of Americans*. Washington, DC: US Government Printing Office.

National Conference of State Legislatures. (2008). *Certificate of need: State health laws and programs*. Retrieved May 31, 2008, from http://www.ncsl.org/progams/health/cert-need.htm.

Novick, L., Morrow, C., & Mays, G. (2008). *Public health administration* (2nd ed., pp. 1–68). Sudbury, MA: Jones and Bartlett.

Raffel, M. W., & Raffel, N. K. (1994). *The U.S. health system: Origins and functions* (4th ed.). Albany, NY: Delmar Publishers.

Regenstein, M., Mead, M., & Lara, A. (2007). The heart of the matter: The relationship between communities, cardiovascular services and racial and ethnic gaps in care. *Managed Care Interface, 20*, 22–28.

Rizza, R. (2006). *Call for a new commitment to diabetes care in America*. Washington, DC: American Diabetes Organization.

Rosen, G. (1983). *The structure of American medical practice 1875–1941*. Philadelphia: University of Pennsylvania Press.

Shi, L., & Singh, D. (2008). *Delivering health care in America*. Sudbury, MA: Jones and Bartlett.

Smolensky, K. (2003). Telemedicine reimbursement: Raising the iron triangle to a new plateau. *Journal of Law Medicine, 13*, 371–413.

Starr, P. (1982). *The social transformation of American medicine*. Cambridge, MA: Basic Books.

Stevens, R. (1971). *American medicine and the public interest*. New Haven, CT: Yale University Press.

Sultz, H., & Young, K. (2006). *Health care USA: Understanding its organization and delivery* (5th ed.). Sudbury, MA: Jones and Bartlett.

Turnock, J. (1997). *Public health and how it works*. Gaithersburg, MD: Aspen Publishers, Inc.

Vault Career Intelligence. (2008). Home page. Retrieved May 31, 2008, from http://www.vault.com/wps/portal/usa/.

Winslow, C. E. A. (1920). *The untilled fields of public health* (pp. 30–35). New York: Health Service, New York Chapter of the American Red Cross.

NOTES

CROSSWORD PUZZLE

Instructions: Please complete the puzzle using the vocabulary words found in the chapter. There may be multiple-word answers. The number in the parenthesis indicates the number of words in the answer.

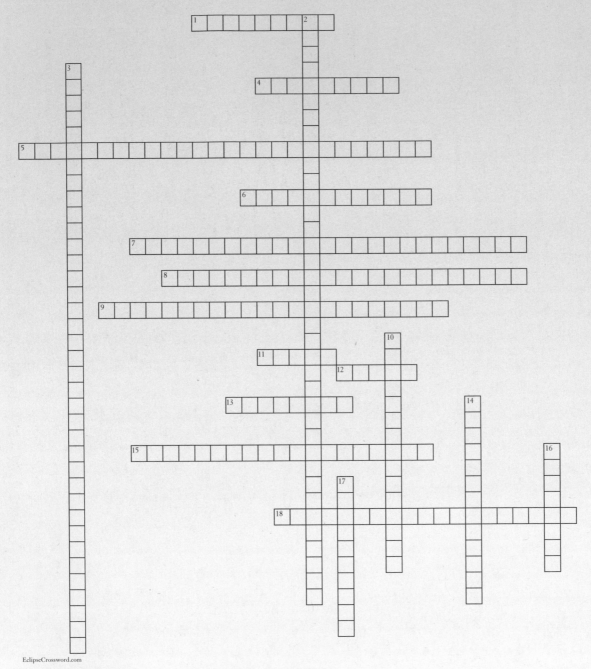

EclipseCrossword.com
Created with EclipseCrossword © 1999–2009 Green Eclipse

STUDENT ACTIVITY 1-1

Across

1. Large patterns of disease that affect a population and can be devastating. (1 word)

4. This health insurance program was the first to start a group health insurance program nationally. (2 words)

5. Established in 1847, this professional membership organization was created to protect physician rights. (3 words)

6. Science and art of preventing disease. (2 words)

7. This federal government agency is responsible for pharmaceutical controls. (4 words)

8. This type of health insurance represents 55% of US health insurance coverage. (3 words)

9. The US population is living longer, which taxes the healthcare system. This phrase characterizes the fact that we are living longer. (4 words)

11. This acronym is a law that focuses on balancing cost, access, and quality of a healthcare system. (1 acronym)

12. This acronym is a law that increases patient confidentiality restrictions. (1 acronym)

13. Government sponsored program that provides services to the elderly and disabled. (1 word)

15. These payments for health services are paid by the individual. They are a type of cost sharing of health insurance. (4 words)

18. This law enables consumers to choose their hospitals because it provides competition. (3 words)

Down

2. This federal agency is responsible for public health policy. (6 words)

3. This federal agency oversees public programs for the elderly, poor, and disabled. (6 words)

10. The concept provides a system that financially assists those individuals who need health care. Many employers provide this benefit to their employees. They both share the cost. (2 words)

14. This document was responsible for improving medical education in this country by recommending a curriculum and admissions testing. (2 words)

16. This government program focuses on providing services to the indigent. (1 word)

17. These institutions, which provided services to the poor, were the basis for the development of hospitals. (1 word)

STUDENT ACTIVITY 1-2

IN YOUR OWN WORDS

Based on Chapter 1, please provide a definition of the following vocabulary words in your own words. DO NOT RECITE the text definition.

Group insurance: _____

_____

_____

Gross domestic product (GDP): _____

_____

_____

Pesthouses: _____

_____

_____

Voluntary health insurance: _____

_____

_____

Public health functions: _____

_____

_____

Primary prevention: _____

_____

_____

Secondary prevention: _____

_____

_____

Tertiary prevention: _____

_____

_____

Universal healthcare coverage: _____

_____

_____

Epidemics: _____

_____

_____

STUDENT ACTIVITY 1-3

REAL LIFE APPLICATIONS: CASE STUDY

As the human resource manager of a large multinational corporation, you are responsible for providing an orientation to health insurance in the United States. You recently hired an international employee from a country that offers a universal health program. She is totally unfamiliar with the US healthcare system and has asked you to describe it to her.

ACTIVITY

(1) Briefly describe the history of healthcare delivery and health insurance, (2) describe who participates in the system, and (3) discuss the strengths and weaknesses of the US healthcare system. Your responses should be based on the information in the text and your own opinion.

RESPONSES

_____

_____

_____

_____

_____

_____

_____

_____

_____

_____

STUDENT ACTIVITY 1-4

INTERNET EXERCISES

Write your answers in the space provided.

- Visit each of the Web sites listed here.
- Name the organization.
- Locate their mission statement or statement of purpose on their Web site.
- Provide a brief overview of the activities of the organization.
- How do these organizations participate in the US healthcare system?

Web Sites

http://www.ama-assn.org

Organization Name: _____

Mission Statement:

_____

_____

_____

Overview of Activities:

_____

_____

_____

Importance of organization to US health care:

_____

_____

_____

http://www.cdc.gov

Organization Name: _____

Mission Statement:

_____

_____

Overview of Activities:

_____

_____

_____

Importance of organization to US health care:

_____

_____

_____

http://www.cms.hhs.gov

Organization Name: _____

Mission Statement:

_____

_____

Overview of Activities:

_____

_____

Importance of organization to US health care:

_____

_____

_____

http://www.hhs.gov

Organization Name: _____

Mission Statement:

_____

_____

_____

Overview of Activities:

_____

_____

Importance of organization to US health care:

_____

_____

_____

STUDENT ACTIVITY 1-4

http://www.jointcommission.org

Organization Name: _____

Mission Statement:

_____

_____

_____

Overview of Activities:

_____

_____

_____

Importance of organization to US health care:

_____

_____

_____

http://www.ahrq.gov

Organization Name: _____

Mission Statement:

_____

_____

_____

Overview of Activities:

_____

_____

_____

Importance of organization to US health care:

_____

_____

_____

Chapter 2

Current Operations of the Healthcare System

LEARNING OBJECTIVES

The student will be able to:

- Identify and discuss at least five major stakeholders and their roles in the healthcare industry.
- Discuss an overview of the US healthcare system operations.
- Discuss the importance of healthcare statistics.
- Compare the United States to five other countries using different health statistics.
- List at least five current statistics regarding the US healthcare system.
- Discuss complementary and alternative medicine and its role in health care.
- Define OECD and its importance to international health care.

DID YOU KNOW THAT?

- The healthcare industry employs 14 million individuals with a projected 3 million new jobs by 2016.
- Most healthcare workers have jobs that do not require a 4-year college degree but health diagnostic and treatment providers are the most educated workers in the United States.

- Healthcare employment is found predominantly in large states such as New York, Pennsylvania, Texas, and Florida.
- The working middle class adults group has experienced the most recent increase in the number of uninsured.
- The South has the highest uninsured rate nationally; the Midwest has the lowest overall uninsured rate.

INTRODUCTION

The one commonality with all of the world's healthcare systems is that they all have consumers or users of their systems. Systems were developed to provide a service to their citizens. The US healthcare system, unlike other systems in the world, does not provide healthcare access to all of its citizens. It is a very complex system which is comprised of many public and private components. Healthcare expenditures comprise approximately 16% of the gross domestic product (GDP). Healthcare costs are very expensive and most citizens cannot afford it if they had to pay for it themselves. Individuals rely on health insurance to pay a large portion of their healthcare costs. Healthcare insurance is predominantly offered by employers. There are nearly 47 million uninsured in the United States with a high percentage of people who are underinsured. This statistic may increase because of the dramatic increase in US unemployment rates in 2009.

In the United States, in order to provide healthcare services, there are several **stakeholders** or interested entities that participate in the industry. There are providers, of course, that consist of trained professionals such as physicians, nurses, dentists, and other nonphysician providers, which are discussed in Chapter 6. There are also inpatient and outpatient facilities, which are discussed in Chapter 5; the payers such as the insurance companies, the government, and self pay individuals, which are discussed in Chapter 7; and the suppliers of products such as pharmaceutical companies, medical equipment companies, and the research and educational facilities, which are discussed throughout the textbook (Sultz & Young, 2006). Each component plays an integral role in the healthcare industry. These different components further emphasize the complexity of the US system. The current operations of the delivery system and utilization statistics will be discussed in depth in this chapter. An international comparison of the US healthcare system and select country systems will also be discussed in this chapter, which provides another aspect of analyzing the US healthcare system.

OVERVIEW OF THE CURRENT SYSTEM

As of 2008, the healthcare industry provided 14.3 million jobs and is expected to generate over 3 million wage and salary jobs by 2018 (US Bureau of Labor Statistics [BLS], 2010). Currently, the United States does not have complete access to health care services. Approximately 1 in 5 citizens do not have health insurance coverage (Pointer, Williams, Isaacs, & Knickman, 2007).

The United States spends the highest proportion of its GDP on healthcare expenditures. The system is a combination of private and public resources. Since World War II, the United States has had a private, fee-for-service system that has produced generous incomes for physicians and has been profitable for many participants in the healthcare industry (Jonas, 2003). The healthcare industry operates like traditional business industries. For those organizations designated as for profit, they need to make money in order to operate. For those entities that are designated as not for profit, their main goal is based on a particular social goal, but they also have to make money in order to continue their operations.

There are several major stakeholders that participate or have an interest in the industry. The stakeholders identified as participants in the healthcare industry include: consumers, employers, healthcare providers, healthcare facilities, government (federal, state, local), insurance companies, educational and training institutions, professional associations that represent the different stakeholders, pharmaceutical companies, and research institutions. It is also important to mention the increasing prominence of alternative therapy medicine. Each role will be discussed briefly.

MAJOR STAKEHOLDERS IN THE HEALTHCARE INDUSTRY

Consumers

The main group of consumers is the patients who need healthcare services either from a physician, hospital, or outpatient facility. The healthcare industry operates like a business. If a consumer has the means to pay out of pocket, from government sources, or from health insurance, the services will be provided. If an individual does not have the means to pay from any of these sources of funding, a service may not be provided. There is a principle of the US health care system, **duty to treat**, that means that any person deserves basic care (Pointer et al., 2007). In some instances, healthcare providers will give care to someone who has no funding source and designate the care provided as a **charitable care** or **bad debt**, which means the provider either does not expect payment after the person's inability to pay has been determined or efforts to secure the payment have failed (Smith, 2008). Businesses also take the same action. Many of them provide a community service or donate funds to a charitable cause, yet both traditional business and healthcare organizations need to charge for their services in order to continue their operations.

There are also other consumer relationships in the healthcare industry. Consumers purchase drugs either from their provider or over the counter from pharmacies. The pharmaceutical companies market their products to physicians who in turn prescribe their products to their patients. The pharmaceutical companies also market their products to hospitals and outpatient facilities to encourage the use of their drugs in these facilities. Medical equipment companies also sell their products to facilities and individual providers.

Employers

Employers consist of both private and public employers. As stated previously, the healthcare industry is the largest US employer. According to the 2006 BLS, there are several segments of employers including hospitals, nursing and residential care facilities, physicians and other healthcare practitioners, home health care, outpatient and ambulatory care centers, and laboratories. Of the 580,000 healthcare establishments, nearly 77% are physicians, dentists, or other types of healthcare practitioner offices such as chiropractors, optometrists, psychologists, etc. Hospitals only constitute 1% of all healthcare establishments but employ 35% of all workers. Although healthcare employment is found throughout the United States, healthcare employment opportunities can be more easily found in large states such as Florida, New York, Pennsylvania, Texas, and California. The following information is a summary from the BLS (BLS, 2009).

Hospitals

Hospitals provide total medical care that ranges from diagnostic services to surgery and continuous nursing care. They can provide both outpatient and inpatient care. Some hospitals specialize in treatments for cancer, children's health, and mental health. Although hospitals represent only 1% of all healthcare establishments, in 2006, 7 out of 10 hospital employees were in facilities with more than 1,000 workers. It is important to note that hospitals are an integral component of the healthcare system (American Hospital Association, 2009; BLS, 2009).

Nursing and Residential Care Facilities

These types of facilities provide nursing, rehabilitation, and health-related personal care to those who need ongoing care. These facilities represent 11.5% of all healthcare establishments. Nursing aides provide the majority of care. **Residential care facilities** provide around-the-clock social and personal care to the elderly, children, and others who cannot take care of themselves. Examples of residential care facilities are drug rehabilitation centers, group homes, and assisted living facilities (BLS, 2009).

Physicians and Other Healthcare Practitioners

Approximately 37% of all healthcare establishments are physician offices. Physicians traditionally practice as a solo practice but more often physicians are practicing in a group practice to reduce administrative costs. One of five healthcare establishments are dentists and they comprise 21% of all healthcare establishments. Dentists usually employ few workers. Other healthcare practitioners include chiropractors, optometrists, psychologists, therapists, and alternative medicine practitioners. They comprise 19% of all healthcare establishments (BLS, 2009).

It is important to note that alternative health or **complementaryand alternative medicine (CAM)** practitioners who practice unconventional health therapies such as yoga, vitamin therapy, and spiritual healing are being sought out by consumers who have to pay out of pocket for these services because they are currently not covered by health insurance companies. However, chiropractors and acupuncturists who are also considered alternative medicine practitioners are more likely to be covered by health insurance companies. Recognizing consumer interest in this type of medicine, in 1998, as part of the National Institute of Health, the **National Center for Complementary and Alternative Medicine (NCCAM)** was established. Its purpose was to explore these types of practices in the context of rigorous science, train complementary and alternative researchers, and disseminate information. More medical schools are now offering some courses in alternative medicine. In the United States, nearly 40% of adults (about 4 in 10) and over 10% of children (about 1 in 9) are using some form of CAM. Adults are most likely to use CAM for musculoskeletal problems such as back, neck, or joint pain (National Center for Health Statistics, 2008).

Home Healthcare Services

Mobile medical technology allows for more home healthcare for medical problems. These services are provided primarily to the elderly. As discussed in other chapters, more consumers prefer to remain at home for treatment. Although it only represents 3% of all healthcare establishments, this is one of the fastest growing components of the industry as a form of employment because of consumer preference and the cost effectiveness of home medical care (BLS, 2009).

Outpatient Care Centers and Ambulatory Healthcare Services

Representing 3% of all healthcare establishments, **outpatientcare centers** include kidney dialysis centers, mental health and substance abuse clinics, surgical, and emergency centers. Ambulatory health care services, which represent 1.5% of all healthcare establishments, includes transport services, blood and organ banks, and smoking cessation programs (BLS, 2009).

Laboratories

Medical and diagnostic laboratories, which represent 2.3% of all healthcare establishments, provide support services to the medical profession. Workers may take blood, take scans or x-rays, or perform other medical tests. This segment provides the fewest number of jobs in the industry (BLS, 2009).

Government

As a result of Medicare and Medicaid, the federal and state governments are the largest stakeholders in the US healthcare system. The government at both levels is responsible for financing health care through these programs as well as playing the public provider role through state and local health departments. Veterans' Affairs medical facilities also provide services to those in the armed forces (Sultz & Young, 2006).

Insurance Companies

The insurance industry is also a major stakeholder in the healthcare industry. They often are blamed for the problems with the healthcare system because of the millions that are underinsured and uninsured. There have been many news reports highlighting the number of medical procedures that have been disproved for insurance coverage, the cost of health insurance coverage, etc. There are traditional indemnity plans such as **Blue Cross and Blue Shield** but managed care, which is also considered an insurance plan, has become more popular for cost control.

Educational and Training Organizations

Educational and training facilities such as medical schools, nursing schools, public health schools, and allied health programs play an important role in the US healthcare industry because they are responsible for the education and training of healthcare employees. These institutions help formulate behaviors of the healthcare workforce.

Research Organizations

Government research organizations such as the National Institute for Health (NIH) and the Centers for Disease Control and Prevention (CDC) are discussed in Chapter 3. They not only provide regulatory guidance but perform research activities to improve health care. However, there are also private research organizations such as **Robert Wood Johnson Foundation**, the **Pew Charitable Trust**, and the **Commonwealth Fund** that support research efforts through grants.

Professional Associations

Professional associations play an important role in healthcare policy. There are associations that represent physicians, nurses, hospitals, long term care facilities, etc. Most healthcare stakeholders are represented by a professional organization that guides them regarding their role in the healthcare industry. They also play a large role in government regulations because they often lobby at all government levels to protect their constituents. The following are examples of professional associations that represent some of the major stakeholder organizations in this industry.

- **American Hospital Association (AHA)**: The AHA is the most prominent association for all types of hospitals and healthcare networks. Founded in 1898, the AHA, which is a membership organization, provides education and lobbies for hospital representation in the political process at all governmental levels (AHA, 2009).

- **American Health Care Association (AHCA)**: Founded in 1949, the AHCA is a membership organization that represents not for profit and for profit nursing, assisted living, developmentally disabled, and subacute providers. Their focus is to monitor and improve standards of nursing home facilities (AHCA, 2009).

- **American Association of Homes and Services for the Aging (AAHSA)**: The AAHSA, which is a membership organization, represents not-for-profit adult day care services, home healthcare services, community services, senior housing, assisted living facilities, continuous care retirement communities, and nursing homes. It lobbies all government levels regarding legislation that can impact their industry and provides technical assistance for these organizations (AAHSA, 2009).

Pharmaceutical Companies

A functioning healthcare system needs medicine that is prescribed by a provider or is purchased as an over-the-counter medicine from a pharmacy. The pharmaceutical industry is integral to the success of a healthcare system. Innovative drugs have improved people's quality of life.

There are currently 200 major pharmaceutical companies that are part of one of the most profitable industries in the world. From 1995 to 2006, in the United States, prescriptions have increased to 3.4 billion annually; a 61% increase. Retail sales of prescription drugs jumped 250% from $72 billion to $250 billion, while the average price of prescriptions has more than doubled from $30 to $68 (US Census Bureau, 2009). Like health insurance companies, the pharmaceutical industry is often villainized because of the cost of some prescribed medicines that often preclude any consumers from purchasing these medications themselves without health insurance assistance. The industry's response is that it takes millions of dollars and years of research to develop an effective medicine and that is a major reason why some medicines cost so much. The pharmaceutical industry is represented by the **Pharmaceutical Research and Manufacturers of America (PhRMA)**. According to PhRMA, the industry invested an estimated $65.2 billion in 2008 to discover and develop new medicines (PhRMA, 2009).

STAKEHOLDERS' ENVIRONMENT

Working Conditions

Many healthcare workers work part-time and comprise 19% of the healthcare workforce. Approximately 40% of part-time workers were employed by dentists and 30% were employed by other healthcare practitioners. The incidence of occupational and injury in hospitals were 8 cases per 100 full-time workers compared to 4.4 in private industry. Nursing care facilities have a rate of 9.8 per 100 full-time (BLS, 2009).

Projected Outlook for Employment

The healthcare industry's employment outlook is positive, despite the economic conditions. It is anticipated that there will be over 3 million new wage and salary jobs generated by 2018 which is more than any other industry (BLS, 2010). Growth will most likely be outside the inpatient hospital centers because cost containment is the major priority for health care. Health care will continue to grow for three major reasons: the aging of our population, advances in medical technology, and the increased focus on outpatient care.

HEALTHCARE STATISTICS

US Healthcare Utilization Statistics

The National Center for Health Statistics, which is part of the CDC, produces an annual report on the health status of the United States. This publication, *Health, United States, 2007*, provides an overview of healthcare utilization, resources, and expenditures. This publication examines all different aspects of the US healthcare delivery system as well as assessing the health status of US citizens. The following information was summarized from this publication.

US Demographics and Healthcare

In the United States, the number of people over 75 years of age will increase from 6% in 2005 to 12% by 2050. With people living longer, there will be an increase in chronic disease and disability. In 2005, 44% of those people over 75 years of age reported a chronic disease which limited activity. This age group will continue to access the healthcare system. In 2005, 15% of Americans were Hispanic, 12% were African American, 4% were Asian, and 1% were American Indian or Alaska Native. The different ethnic groups have different access to health care because of cultural and language differences. Hispanic or American Indians are more likely to be uninsured than other ethnic groups (CDC, 2007) Unfortunately, racial and ethnic minorities have higher disease rates including cancer, obesity, and diabetes. Seven out of 10 African Americans, ages 18 to 64 are overweight. African American males are 50% more likely than Caucasian males to have prostate cancer. Hispanic and Vietnamese women have higher rates of cervical cancer than Caucasian women (HealthReform.gov, 2009).

Access to Health Care

In 2005, more than 40 million adults did not receive healthcare services because they could not afford them. Nearly 15 million did not obtain eye glasses, 25 million did not receive dental care, 19 million did not receive their prescriptions, and 15 million did not receive any services because they could not afford them. Many rural areas have inadequate access to health care. Rural inhabitants must travel to receive services and may not receive timely emergency care. The percentage of people under 65 years of age who have no health insurance coverage is approximately 16 to 17% (CDC, 2007).

Healthcare Resources

The United States spends more on health per capita than any other country worldwide. In 2006, the total expenditure on health per capita was $6714. In 2005, national healthcare expenditures totaled $2 trillion. Hospital spending accounts for nearly 31% of healthcare expenditures. Prescription drugs account for 10% national health expenditures. In 2005, private health insurance paid 36% of total personal health care, the federal government 34%, state and local governments 11%, and out of pocket payments were 15% (CDC, 2007).

US and International Comparison of Health Statistics

Established in 1961, the Organisation for Economic Co-operation and Development (OECD) is a membership organization that provides comparable statistics of economic and social data worldwide and monitors trends of economic development. There are currently 30 countries, including the United States, that are members of this organization. Their budget is derived from the member countries of which the United States contributes 25% of the budget. The OECD produces, on a continual basis, a health data set of the 30 member countries (OECD, 2009). The following are highlights from the 2005–2008 US health data.

Health indicators such as infant mortality rates, average life expectancy, chronic disease rates, etc., are used to evaluate the health status of a population. Other surveys conduct information regarding access to healthcare services, financing, and responsiveness to patient needs (Pointer et al., 2007). Because the United States spends the highest per capita on health care in the world, it is expected that United States health indicators would rank superior to all other countries' healthcare indicators.

2000–2006 Health Expenditures as a Percentage of the Gross Domestic Product (Tables 2-1 and 2-2, pages 29–32)

In 2006, the United States spent 15.3% of its GDP on health care, which is the highest of the 30 OECD members. The US percentage has increased from 13.2% in 2000. The average of the member countries was 8.9%. Switzerland, France, and Germany were the next three highest percentages. Korea and Turkey spend the least amount of their GDP of the 30 countries. In 2000, they spent 4.5 and 4.9%, respectively; in 2006, Korea had increased to 6.4%. Turkey did not report data in 2006 but, in 2005, the percentage was 5.7%.

The United States also spends per capita the most in relation to their member countries. In 2000, the United States spent $4570—a difference of $2144 over the 6-year period. In 2000, Switzerland was second

with $3256 and Norway was third with $3039. Mexico and Turkey were last in spending per capita at $508 and $432, respectively. In 2006, Switzerland and Norway increased spending per capita by $1055 and $1481, respectively. Mexico increased its spending in 2006 by $286. Turkey did not report in 2006 but, in 2005, it had increased spending by $161. The average of the member countries was $2824. These data are important because they should reflect the health status of a country. For example, US health indicators should be at the top of the rankings because of their spending and Turkey, Mexico, and Korea would have less healthy indicators because they spend less money. These data represented in the remaining tables will indicate the health status of these countries.

Public Expenditures on Health (Table 2-3, pages 33–34)

The public sector is the main source of healthcare funding in all of the OECD countries except for the United States and Mexico, which is logical because they all have some form of universal health coverage. The Czech Republic has the highest public expenditures for health with 88%, which is a slight decrease from 2000. There were nine countries that have over 80% of their health expenditures derived from public funding. The average of public health sector funding for all OECD countries is 73% with the United States spending only 46%. Mexico was second to last with only 44% in public funding. In the United States, 36% of healthcare spending is from private insurance. These percentages represent the fact that all of these countries have a form of national health care although Canada and France both have 12% of health funding from private insurance.

2000–2006 Pharmaceutical Expenditures (Tables 2-4 and 2-5, pages 35–38)

In 2006, the United States spent 12.6% of total health expenditures on pharmaceuticals. The Slovak Republic, Korea, and Turkey spent the most with 29.7%, 25.95, and 23.1%, respectively. The US percentage was less than the average of OECD countries of 15.3%. There was a minimal increase over the 6-year period. However, in 2006, the United States was the top spender in 2006 of pharmaceuticals per capita at $843 followed by Canada, Belgium, and France. In 2000, the United States spent $534 on pharmaceuticals. The increase over the 6-year period was over $300. These statistics reflect the culture of US traditional medicine that provides drugs to resolve medical issues.

TABLE 2-1   Current Operations of US Healthcare System: Total Expenditure on Health per Gross Domestic Product

Countries	2000 Total expendit. on health, % GDP	2001 Total expendit. on health, % GDP	2002 Total expendit. on health, % GDP	2003 Total expendit. on health, % GDP	2004 Total expendit. on health, % GDP	2005 Total expendit. on health, % GDP	2006 Total expendit. on health, % GDP
United States	13.2	13.9	14.7	15.1	15.2	15.2	15.3
Germany	10.3	10.4	10.6	10.8	10.6	10.7	10.6
Switzerland	10.3	10.7	11.0	11.4	11.4	11.4	11.3 e
France	10.1	10.2	10.5	10.9	11.0	11.1	11.0
Austria	9.9	10.0	10.1	10.2	10.3	10.3	10.1
Iceland	9.5	9.3	10.2	10.4	9.9	9.4	9.1
Canada	8.8	9.3	9.6	9.8	9.8	9.9	10.0
Portugal	8.8 b	8.8	9.0	9.7	10.0	10.2	10.2
Belgium	8.6	8.7	9.0	10.5 b	10.7	10.6 b	10.3
Norway	8.4	8.8	9.8	10.0	9.7	9.1	8.7
Australia	8.3	8.4	8.6	8.6	8.8	8.8	8.7
Denmark	8.3	8.6	8.8	9.3 b	9.5	9.5	9.5
Sweden	8.2	9.0 b	9.3	9.4	9.2	9.2	9.2
Italy	8.1	8.2	8.3	8.3	8.7	8.9	9.0
Netherlands	8.0	8.3	8.9	9.4 b	9.5		
Greece	7.8 b	8.4	8.2	8.5	8.3	9.0	9.1
Japan	7.7	7.9	8.0	8.1	8.0	8.2	8.1

continues

TABLE 2-1 Current Operations of US Healthcare System: Total Expenditure on Health per Gross Domestic Product (*Continued*)

Countries	2000 Total expendit. on health, % GDP	2001 Total expendit. on health, % GDP	2002 Total expendit. on health, % GDP	2003 Total expendit. on health, % GDP	2004 Total expendit. on health, % GDP	2005 Total expendit. on health, % GDP	2006 Total expendit. on health, % GDP
New Zealand	7.7	7.8	8.2	8.0			
Spain	7.2	7.2	7.3	8.1 b	8.2	8.3	8.4
United Kingdom	7.2	7.5	7.6	7.7 b	8.0 d	8.2 d	8.4 d
Finland	7.0	7.2	7.6	8.0	8.1	8.3	8.2
Hungary	6.9	7.2	7.6	8.4	8.2	8.5	8.3
Czech Republic	6.5 b	6.7	7.1	7.4 b	7.2	7.1	6.8
Ireland	6.3	6.9	7.1	7.3	7.5	8.2	7.5
Luxembourg	5.8	6.4	6.8	7.6 b	8.1	7.8	7.3 e
Mexico	5.6	6.0	6.2	6.3	6.5	6.4	6.6
Poland	5.5	5.9	6.3 b	6.2	6.2	6.2	6.2
Slovak Republic	5.5	5.5	5.6	5.9	7.2 b	7.1	7.4
Turkey	4.9	5.6	5.9	6.0	5.9	5.7	
Korea	4.5	5.2	5.1	5.4	5.4	5.9	6.4

b, break in series; d, differences in methodology; e, estimate; expendit., expenditure; GDP, gross domestic product.

Source: From OECD Health Data 2008. Retrieved October 12, 2009, from http://www.ecosante.org/index2.php?base=OCDE&langs=ENG&langh=ENG.

TABLE 2-2   Current Operations of US Healthcare System: Total Expenditure on Health

Countries	2000 Total expendit. on health/ capita, US$ purchasing power parity	2001 Total expendit. on health/ capita, US$ purchasing power parity	2002 Total expendit. on health/ capita, US$ purchasing power parity	2003 Total expendit. on health/ capita, US$ purchasing power parity	2004 Total expendit. on health/ capita, US$ purchasing power parity	2005 Total expendit. on health/ capita, US$ purchasing power parity	2006 Total expendit. on health/ capita, US$ purchasing power parity
United States	4570	4915	5305	5682	6014	6347	6714
Switzerland	3256	3471	3719	3829	3990	4069	4311
Norway	3039	3266	3629	3840	4082	4328	4520
Austria	2859	2890	3068	3206	3397	3507	3606
Iceland	2736	2846	3156	3198	3338	3373	3340
Germany	2671	2809	2937	3090	3162	3251	3371
Luxembourg	2554	2738	3081	3582 b	4083	4153	4303
France	2542	2719	2922	2988	3117	3306	3449
Canada	2513	2731	2874	3058	3218	3460	3678
Denmark	2379	2521	2696	2834 b	3057	3179	3362
Belgium	2377	2484	2685	3153 b	3311	3385 b	3462
Netherlands	2337	2556	2833	2988 b	3156		
Sweden	2284	2511 b	2707	2841	2964	3012	3202
Australia	2265	2397	2566	2686	2885	2999	3141
Italy	2053	2215	2223	2272	2401	2496	2614
Japan	1967	2080	2137	2224	2337	2474	2578

continues

TABLE 2-2 Current Operations of US Healthcare System: Total Expenditure on Health *(Continued)*

Countries	2000 Total expendit. on health/capita, US$ purchasing power parity	2001 Total expendit. on health/capita, US$ purchasing power parity	2002 Total expendit. on health/capita, US$ purchasing power parity	2003 Total expendit. on health/capita, US$ purchasing power parity	2004 Total expendit. on health/capita, US$ purchasing power parity	2005 Total expendit. on health/capita, US$ purchasing power parity	2006 Total expendit. on health/capita, US$ purchasing power parity
United Kingdom	1847	2021	2165	2259 b	2509 d	2580 d	2760
Ireland	1801	2128	2360	2515	2724	3126	3082
Finland	1794	1913	2089	2210	2412	2523	2668
New Zealand	1604	1707	1846	1856			
Spain	1536	1636	1745	2019 b	2128	2260	2458
Portugal	1509 b	1569	1657	1824	1913	2029	2120
Greece	1429 b	1669	1792	1928	1991	2283	2483
Czech Republic	980 b	1082	1195	1340 b	1388	1447	1509
Hungary	852	971	1114	1302	1327	1440	1504
Korea	747	900	945	1026	1110	1263	1464
Slovak Republic	603	665	730	792	1058 b	1130	1308
Poland	583	642	733 b	749	808	843	910
Mexico	508	551	584	628	679	724	794
Turkey	432	456	483	502	576	591	

b, break in series; d, differences in methodology; expendit., expenditure.

Source: From OECD Health Data 2008. Retrieved October 12, 2009, from http://www.ecosante.org/index2.php?base=OCDE&langs=ENG&langh=ENG.

TABLE 2-3 Current Operations of US Healthcare System: Public Expenditure on Health

Countries	2000 Public expendit. on health, TEH	2001 Public expendit. on health, TEH	2002 Public expendit. on health, TEH	2003 Public expendit. on health, TEH	2004 Public expendit. on health, TEH	2005 Public expendit. on health, TEH	2006 Public expendit. on health, TEH
Czech Republic	90.3 b	89.8	90.5	89.8 b	89.2	88.6	88.0
Slovak Republic	89.4	89.3	89.1	88.3	73.8 b	74.4	68.3
Luxembourg	89.3	87.9	90.3	89.8 b	90.1	90.2	90.9 e
Sweden	84.9	81.8 b	82.1	82.5	81.8	81.7	81.7
Norway	82.5	83.6	83.5	83.7	83.6	83.5	83.6
Denmark	82.4	82.7	82.9	83.9 b	83.8	83.7	84.1
Japan	81.3	81.7	81.5	81.5	81.7	82.7	81.3
Iceland	81.1	81.0	81.9	81.7	81.2	81.4	82.0
United Kingdom	80.9	83.0	83.4	85.5 b	86.3 d	86.9 d	87.3 d
Germany	79.7	79.3	79.2	78.7	77.0	77.0	76.9
France	79.4	79.4	79.7	79.9	79.8	79.9	79.7
New Zealand	78.0	76.4	77.9	78.3			
Austria	75.8	75.6	75.4	75.2	75.6	76.5	76.2
Ireland	73.5	74.1	76.0	77.2	78.6	79.5	78.3
Finland	73.4	71.9	74.2	73.9	74.4	75.0	76.0
Italy	72.5	74.6	74.5	74.5	76.0	76.7	77.2
Portugal	72.5 b	71.5	72.2	73.3	72.0	71.8	70.6
Spain	71.6	71.2	71.3	70.4 b	70.5	70.6	71.2

continues

33

TABLE 2-3 Current Operations of US Healthcare System: Public Expenditure on Health (*Continued*)

Countries	2000 Public expendit. on health, TEH	2001 Public expendit. on health, TEH	2002 Public expendit. on health, TEH	2003 Public expendit. on health, TEH	2004 Public expendit. on health, TEH	2005 Public expendit. on health, TEH	2006 Public expendit. on health, TEH
Hungary	70.7	69.0	70.2	71.9	71.3	70.9	70.9
Canada	70.4	70.0	69.6	70.3	70.3	70.2	70.4
Poland	70.0	71.9	71.2 b	69.9	68.6	69.3	69.9
Australia	67.0	65.9	66.6	66.5	66.9	67.0	67.7
Netherlands	63.1	62.8	62.5				
Turkey	62.9	68.2	70.4	71.6	72.3	71.4	
Greece	60.9 b	63.8	63.5	62.8	61.8	62.8	61.6
Switzerland	55.6	57.1	57.9	58.5	58.5	59.6	60.3
Korea	48.8	54.8	53.5	51.9	52.9	53.7	55.7
Mexico	46.6	44.9	43.9	44.1	46.4	45.5	44.2
United States	43.7	44.6	44.6	44.5	44.8	45.1	45.8
Belgium							

b, break in series; d, differences in methodology; e, estimate; expendit., expenditure; TEH, % total expenditure on health.

Source: From OECD Health Data 2008. Retrieved October 12, 2009, from http://www.ecosante.org/index2.php?base=OCDE&langs=ENG&langh=ENG.

TABLE 2-4 Current Operations of US Healthcare System: Pharmaceuticals and Other Medical Nondurables Total Expenditures

Countries	2000 Total expendit. on pharm. & other, TEH	2001 Total expendit. on pharm. & other, TEH	2002 Total expendit. on pharm. & other, TEH	2003 Total expendit. on pharm. & other, TEH	2004 Total expendit. on pharm. & other, TEH	2005 Total expendit. on pharm. & other, TEH	2006 Total expendit. on pharm. & other, TEH
Slovak Republic	34.0	34.0	37.3	38.5	31.4 b	31.9	29.7
Korea	27.3	26.2	26.6	27.3	27.5	26.4	25.9
Turkey	24.8						
Czech Republic	23.4 b	24.0	23.9	24.2	24.8	25.1	23.1
Portugal	22.4 b	23.0	23.3	21.4	21.8	21.6	21.3
Italy	22.0	22.5	22.5	21.8	21.2	20.3	20.0
Spain	21.3	21.1	21.8	23.2 b	22.7	22.4	21.7
Mexico	19.4 d	19.6 d	21.2 b	21.5	20.9	21.3	22.9
Japan	18.7	18.8	18.4	19.2	19.0	19.8	19.6
Greece	17.8 b	16.3	16.8	17.8	19.7	18.5	17.6
France	16.5	16.9	16.8	16.7	16.8	16.7	16.4
Canada	15.9	16.2	16.7	17.0	17.3	17.2	17.4
Finland	15.2	15.4	15.6	15.6	15.8	15.8	14.6
Australia	14.7	15.1	14.5	14.8	14.7	14.2	13.7
Iceland	14.5	14.1	14.0	14.5	14.6	13.4	13.1

continues

TABLE 2-4 Current Operations of US Healthcare System: Pharmaceuticals and Other Medical Nondurables Total Expenditures *(Continued)*

Countries	2000 Total expendit. on pharm. & other, TEH	2001 Total expendit. on pharm. & other, TEH	2002 Total expendit. on pharm. & other, TEH	2003 Total expendit. on pharm. & other, TEH	2004 Total expendit. on pharm. & other, TEH	2005 Total expendit. on pharm. & other, TEH	2006 Total expendit. on pharm. & other, TEH
Sweden	13.8	13.9 b	14.0	13.7	13.8	13.7	13.3
Germany	13.6	14.2	14.4	14.5	13.9	15.1	14.8
Austria	11.9	11.6	12.2	12.6	12.2	12.0	12.4
Netherlands	11.7	11.7	11.5				
United States	11.7	12.0	12.3	12.5	12.6	12.4	12.6
Luxembourg	11.0	11.5	10.3	9.7 b	8.9	8.4	
Switzerland	10.7	10.6	10.3	10.5	10.4	10.5	
Norway	9.5	9.3	9.4	9.2	9.4	9.1	8.5
Denmark	8.8	9.2	9.8	9.1 b	8.7	8.6	8.5
Belgium						17.1 b	16.9
Hungary		28.5	27.6	27.1	28.3	30.5	31.0
New Zealand			28.4				
Poland				30.3	29.6	28.0	27.2

b, break in series; d, differences in methodology; expendit., expenditure; TEH, % total expenditure on health.
Source: From OECD Health Data 2008. Retrieved October 12, 2009, from http://www.ecosante.org/index2.php?base=OCDE&langs=ENG&langh=ENG.

TABLE 2-5 Current Operations of US Healthcare System: Pharmaceuticals and Other Medical Nondurables Expenditures, Power Parity

Countries	2000 Total expendit. on pharm. & other/ capita, US$ purchasing power parity	2001 Total expendit. on pharm. & other/ capita, US$ purchasing power parity	2002 Total expendit. on pharm. & other/ capita, US$ purchasing power parity	2003 Total expendit. on pharm. & other/ capita, US$ purchasing power parity	2004 Total expendit. on pharm. & other/ capita, US$ purchasing power parity	2005 Total expendit. on pharm. & other/ capita, US$ purchasing power parity	2006 Total expendit. on pharm. & other/ capita, US$ purchasing power parity
United States	534	591	654	710	756	790	843
Italy	452	499	499	495	510	506	524
France	419	461	491	499	524	553	564
Canada	399	441	479	519	556	595	639
Iceland	396	400	442	463	487	452	439
Japan	367	391	392	428	445	489	506
Germany	363	399	423	447	440	492	500
Switzerland	349	368	382	401	416	427	
Austria	339	336	373	405	413	421	449
Portugal	337 b	361	386	390	418	439	451
Australia	334	362	372	398	424	426	432
Spain	327	346	381	469 b	484	505	533
Sweden	316	350 b	379	389	410	412	426
Norway	289	303	342	355	384	392	384
Luxembourg	280	315	318	346 b	364	349	
Finland	273	295	325	345	382	399	389

continues

TABLE 2-5 Current Operations of US Healthcare System: Pharmaceuticals and Other Medical Nondurables Expenditures, Power Parity *(Continued)*

Countries	2000 Total expendit. on pharm. & other/ capita, US$ purchasing power parity	2001 Total expendit. on pharm. & other/ capita, US$ purchasing power parity	2002 Total expendit. on pharm. & other/ capita, US$ purchasing power parity	2003 Tot. expendit. on pharm. & other/ capita, US$ purchasing power parity	2004 Total expendit. on pharm. & other/ capita, US$ purchasing power parity	2005 Total expendit. on pharm. & other/ capita, US$ purchasing power parity	2006 Total expendit. on pharm. & other/ capita, US$ purchasing power parity
Netherlands	273	298	325				
Greece	254 b	272	301	344	393	423	438
Czech Republic	229 b	260	285	324	345	364	349
Denmark	209	232	264	257 b	266	272	286
Slovak Republic	205	226	272	305	332 b	360	389
Korea	204	236	252	280	305	333	380
Turkey	107						
Mexico	99 d	108 d	124 b	135	142	154	182
Belgium						577 b	584
Hungary		277	308	353	376	440	466
New Zealand					249	278	303
Poland			208	227	239	236	248

b, break in series; d, differences in methodology; expendit., expenditure.

Source: From OECD Health Data 2008. Retrieved October 12, 2009, from http://www.ecosante.org/index2.php?base=OCDE&langs=ENG&langh=ENG.

Healthcare Resources: Physician Resources (Table 2-6, pages 40–41)

In the United States, there are fewer physicians per capita than in most other OECD countries. In 2006, the United States had 2.4 practicing physicians per 1000, which is below the OECD average of 3.1. The United States ranked 20th of the 30 OECD countries. In 2000, there were only 2.3 practicing physicians per 1000 populations. This statistic, coupled with the facts that there are not enough primary physicians in the United States and there is a shortage of physicians in rural areas, this continues to present issues for the healthcare system. In 2006, Italy, Belgium, and Switzerland had the most physicians per 1000. Mexico, Turkey, and Korea have the fewest physicians per 1000 at 3.7, 4.0, and 3.8, respectively.

2000–2005 Medical Graduates (Table 2-7, pages 42–43)

From 2000 to 2005, there was a drop in medical graduates from 27.8 per 1000 practicing physicians to 25.7 per 1000 in the United States. The United States has one of the lowest graduate rates compared to the rest of the OECD countries. The United States ranks 23rd of OECD countries. In 2006, Portugal had 20.8 and France had 16.7, which are the other two countries with low medical graduate rates. Portugal increased slightly from 19 per 1000 practicing physicians. In 2000, Ireland had the highest rate at 64.7, which dropped to 51.9 by 2006. Austria was 59.9 in 2000 and dropped to 58.1 by 2006. Turkey was the third highest in 2000 for medical graduate rates of 59.4. They also dropped to 41.1. This lower rate of medical graduates could be reflective of the difficult curriculum followed in US medical schools.

2000–2006 Hospital Beds (Table 2-8, pages 44–45)

In 2000, the United States ranked in the bottom five of the OECD countries with 3.5 hospital beds per 1000 populations. The highest during 2000 was Japan at 14.7. In 2006, the rates were 3.2 and 14, respectively, for each country. These rates may address that fact that the United States has increased their outpatient services as have other countries. The lowest hospital bed ratio is Mexico with 1.8 in 2000, which decreased to 1.7 in 2006.

2000–2005 Female and Male Life Expectancy at Birth (Tables 2-9 and 2-10, pages 46–49)

According to OECD, **life expectancy at birth and age 65 and by gender** is the average number of years that a person at that age and by gender can be expected to live, assuming that age-specific mortality levels remain constant. In 2000 in the United States, the female life expectancy at birth was 79.5 years of age, which ranked 22nd out of the 30 countries. By 2006, it had increased to 80.4, which is nearly another year of life. The number one nation was Japan at 84.6 in 2000; that country increased its rate to 85.5 in year 2005. The second country was France with 83 in 2000, which increased to 83.7 by 2005. These are interesting statistics for the United States because it spends so much of GDP on healthcare expenditures. The statistics could also reflect the sedentary lifestyle and poor diet in the United States.

US males' life expectancy at birth was lower than females but ranked slightly higher—20th out of the 30 countries. In 2000, the male expectancy was 74.1 with an increase of nearly 12 months to 75.2. The highest life expectancy of males was in Iceland at 78.4, which increased to 79.2 by 2006. These gender projections are typical of other data analyses from the CDC, the World Health Organization (WHO), and others.

2000–2005 Total Life Expectancy at Birth (Table 2-11, pages 50–51)

Japan continues to lead the life expectancy at birth with 81.2 in 2000, which increased to 82.0 by 2005. Iceland was second with 80.1 in 2000 with an increase to 81.2 by 2005. The United States remained in 10th place with 76.8 in 2000 with an increase to 77.8 by 2005. These statistics are a reflection of the gender life expectancy statistics. These statistics are often used as a comparison of countries worldwide to assess their health status.

2000–2005 Life Expectancy of Females and Males at Age 65 (Tables 2-12 and 2-13, pages 52–55)

These statistics address the quality of health care for the elderly. Although there is statistics that address life expectancy at birth and by gender, this statistic focuses on life expectancy after age 65. In 2000, Japan was the top country at 22.4 years of life expectancy for females age 65, which increased to 23.2 years in 2006. In 2000, the top nine countries included Japan, France, Switzerland, Spain, Italy, Austria, Canada, and Luxembourg and they had life expectancies of 20 years or greater for women at 65 years old. All of them increased their life expectancy by 2006. The bottom country was Turkey with an expectancy rate of 14.6 in 2000 which did marginally increase to 15 years by 2006. The United States was ranked higher than previous statistics at 18th with a life expectancy of 19.2, which did increase to 20 by 2006.

TABLE 2-6 Current Operations of US Healthcare System: Practicing Physicians

Countries	2000 Practicing physicians, density per 1000 population (head counts)	2001 Practicing physicians, density per 1000 population (head counts)	2002 Practicing physicians, density per 1000 population (head counts)	2003 Practicing physicians, density per 1000 population (head counts)	2004 Practicing physicians, density per 1000 population (head counts)	2005 Practicing physicians, density per 1000 population (head counts)	2006 Practicing physicians, density per 1000 population (head counts)
Greece	4.3	4.4	4.6	4.7	4.9	5.0	
Italy	4.1	4.3	4.4	4.1	4.2	3.8	3.7
Belgium	3.9	3.9	3.9	4.0	4.0	4.0	4.0
Switzerland	3.5	3.5	3.6	3.7 b	3.8	3.8	3.8
Czech Republic	3.4 b	3.4	3.5	3.5	3.5	3.6	3.6
Iceland	3.4	3.5	3.6	3.6	3.6	3.7	3.7
France	3.3	3.3	3.3	3.3	3.4	3.4	3.4
Germany	3.3	3.3	3.3	3.4	3.4	3.4	3.5
Netherlands	3.2 d	3.3 d	3.4 d	3.5 d	3.6 d	3.7 d	3.8 d
Spain	3.2	3.1	2.9	3.2	3.4	3.8	3.6
Austria	3.1	3.2	3.3	3.4	3.5	3.5	3.6
Hungary	3.1 e	3.2 e	3.2	3.2	3.3	2.8 b	3.0
Portugal	3.1 d	3.2 d	3.2 d	3.2 d	3.3 d	3.4 d	
Slovak Republic	3.1	3.1	3.1	3.1	3.1		
Sweden	3.1	3.2	3.3	3.4	3.4	3.5	
Denmark	2.9	2.9	3.0	3.0	3.2	3.3	

Norway	2.9	3.0	3.4 b	3.4	3.5	3.7	3.7
Finland	2.8	2.3	2.6 b	2.6	2.7	2.7	2.7
Australia	2.5	2.5	2.5	2.6	2.7	2.8	
United States	2.3	2.3	2.3	2.4	2.4	2.4	2.4
Ireland	2.2	2.4	2.4	2.6	2.8	2.8	2.9
New Zealand	2.2	2.2	2.1	2.2	2.2	2.1	2.3
Poland	2.2	2.3	2.3	2.5 b	2.3 b	2.1 b	2.2
Canada	2.1	2.1	2.1	2.1	2.1	2.1	2.1
Luxembourg	2.1 b	2.2	2.3	2.4	2.4	2.5	2.8 b
Japan	1.9		2.0		2.0		2.1
United Kingdom	1.9	2.0	2.1	2.2	2.3	2.4	2.5
Mexico	1.6	1.5	1.5	1.6	1.7	1.8	1.9
Korea	1.3	1.4	1.5	1.6	1.6	1.6	1.7
Turkey	1.3	1.3	1.4	1.4	1.5	1.5	1.6

b, break in series; d, differences in methodology; e, estimate

Source: From OECD Health Data 2008. Retrieved October 12, 2009, from http://www.ecosante.org/index2.php?base=OCDE&langs=ENG&langh=ENG.

TABLE 2-7 Current Operations of US Healthcare System: Medical Graduates

Countries	2000 Medical graduates per 1000 practicing physicians	2001 Medical graduates per 1000 practicing physicians	2002 Medical graduates per 1000 practicing physicians	2003 Medical graduates per 1000 practicing physicians	2004 Medical graduates per 1000 practicing physicians	2005 Medical graduates per 1000 practicing physicians
Ireland	64.7	60.2	60.1	59.2	57.3	51.9
Austria	59.9	43.7	72.7	58.3	61.4	58.1
Turkey	59.4	53.6	49.0	43.9	42.2	41.1
Korea	58.0	57.2	56.6	59.5	55.6	55.7
Belgium	45.1	52.3	47.9	51.0	43.8	
United Kingdom	38.6	36.1	36.1	35.9	34.7	35.9
New Zealand	37.5	35.0	36.7	37.4	38.0	36.4
Slovak Republic	34.3	31.4	31.9	34.8	34.6	
Iceland	34.1	34.3	36.9	28.7	33.1	39.9
Spain	33.2	32.8	34.1	29.6	28.8	24.5
Norway	31.8	30.9	24.6	29.8	28.9	27.4
Finland	31.2	34.0	33.9	32.5	24.9	24.1
Germany	30.7	25.8				
Japan	30.5		30.8		29.1	
Switzerland	30.0	30.9	27.0	22.9	24.3	22.0
Australia	29.6	27.4 b	28.4	31.7	32.1	31.9
Hungary	29.5	31.5	32.0	29.7	33.3	41.0
Sweden	29.4	28.7	26.5	27.8	25.9	25.5

Denmark	28.8	35.1	39.4	43.0	44.7	45.6
Netherlands	27.8	27.0	28.8	29.2	29.1	28.8
United States	27.8	27.4	27.0	26.2	26.5	25.7
Italy	27.6	25.8	27.7	30.7	27.4	28.9
Canada	25.0	24.0	23.6	25.1	25.9	27.1
Czech Republic	23.3	21.6	20.0	24.3	23.4	22.8
France	20.3	18.5 e	16.3	19.0	17.5	16.7
Portugal	19.0	18.3	16.7	17.9	20.1	20.8
Greece		29.0				26.5
Poland						28.8

b, break in series; e, estimate.

Source: From OECD Health Data 2008. Retrieved October 12, 2009, from http://www.ecosante.org/index2.php?base=OCDE&langs=ENG&langh=ENG.

TABLE 2-8 Current Operations of US Healthcare System: Hospital Beds

Country	2000 Total hospital beds per 1000 population	2001 Total hospital beds per 1000 population	2002 Total hospital beds per 1000 population	2003 Total hospital beds per 1000 population	2004 Total hospital beds per 1000 population	2005 Total hospital beds per 1000 population	2006 Total hospital beds per 1000 population
Japan	14.7	14.6	14.4	14.3	14.2	14.1	14.0
Germany	9.1	9.0	8.9	8.7	8.6	8.5	8.3
Austria	8.6	8.5	8.4	8.3	7.7 b	7.7	7.6
Czech Republic	8.5 b	8.5	8.5	8.5	8.4	8.3	8.2
France	8.1	7.9	7.8	7.6	7.5	7.5	7.2
Hungary	8.1	7.9	7.9	7.8	7.8	7.9	7.9
Belgium	7.8	7.7	7.6	7.5	7.5	7.4	6.7 b
Slovak Republic	7.8	7.7	7.6	7.2	6.9	6.8	6.7
Finland	7.5	7.4	7.5	7.3	7.1	7.0	6.9
Ireland	6.3	6.0	5.9	5.8	5.7	5.6	
Korea	6.1	6.1	6.6	7.1	7.4	7.9	8.5
Netherlands	5.2	5.0	4.6 b	4.5	4.5	4.5	4.5
Greece	4.7	4.8	4.7	4.7	4.7	4.7	
Italy	4.7	4.6	4.4	4.2	4.0	4.0	4.0
Denmark	4.3	4.2	4.1	4.0	3.8	3.7	3.6
Switzerland	4.1	4.0	3.9	3.9	3.8	3.6	3.5
United Kingdom	4.1	4.0	4.0	3.9	3.9	3.7	3.6

Australia	4.0	3.9	3.9	3.9	4.0	3.9
Portugal	3.9	3.9	3.8	3.8	3.7	3.6
Canada	3.8	3.7	3.6	3.5	3.4	3.4
Norway	3.8	3.3	3.8	3.8	3.7	3.6
Spain	3.7	3.5	3.5	3.4	3.4	3.4
United States	3.5	3.5	3.4	3.3	3.3	3.2
Turkey	2.6	2.5	2.6	2.6	2.6	2.7
Mexico	1.8	1.8	1.8	1.7	1.8	1.7
Luxembourg				6.5	5.9	5.8
Poland		6.7	6.7	6.7	6.5	6.5

b, break in series.

Source: From OECD Health Data 2008. Retrieved October 12, 2009, from http://www.ecosante.org/ird=x2.php?base=OCDE&langs=ENG&langh=ENG.

TABLE 2-9 Current Operations of US Healthcare System: Life Expectancy, Females at Birth

Countries	2000 Females at birth (years)	2001 Females at birth (years)	2002 Females at birth (years)	2003 Females at birth (years)	2004 Females at birth (years)	2005 Females at birth (years)
Japan	84.6	84.9	85.2	85.3	85.6	85.5
France	83.0	83.0	83.0	82.7	83.8	83.7
Italy	82.9	83.2	83.2	82.8	83.8	83.7
Spain	82.9	83.2	83.2	83.0	83.7	83.7
Switzerland	82.8	83.2	83.2	83.2	83.8	84.0
Australia	82.0	82.4	82.6	82.8	83.0	83.3
Sweden	82.0	82.1	82.1	82.5	82.7	82.8
Canada	81.9	82.1	82.1	82.4	82.6	82.7
Iceland	81.8	82.2	82.5	82.7	82.7	83.1
Norway	81.5	81.6	81.6	82.1	82.6	82.7
Luxembourg	81.3	80.7	81.5	80.8	82.3	82.3
Finland	81.2	81.7	81.6	81.9	82.5	82.5
Germany	81.2	81.4	81.3	81.3	81.9	82.0
Austria	81.1	81.5	81.7	81.6	82.1	82.2
Belgium	81.0	81.2	81.2	81.1	81.8	81.9
New Zealand	80.8 e	81.1	81.2	81.3	81.7	81.9
Greece	80.5	81.0	81.1	81.3	81.5	81.7
Netherlands	80.5	80.7	80.7	80.9	81.4	81.6
United Kingdom	80.3	80.5	80.6	80.5	81.0	81.1
Portugal	80.2	80.5	80.6	80.6	81.5	81.3

Korea	79.6	80.0	80.5	80.8	81.4	81.9
United States	79.5	79.8	79.9	80.1	80.4	80.4
Denmark	79.2	79.3	79.4	79.8	80.2	80.5
Ireland	79.2	79.9	80.5	80.8	81.4	81.7
Czech Republic	78.5	78.6	78.7	78.6	79.2	79.2
Poland	78.0	78.3	78.7	78.8	79.2	79.4
Slovak Republic	77.4	77.7	77.7	77.8	77.8	77.9
Mexico	76.5	76.8	77.1	77.4	77.6	77.9
Hungary	75.9	76.4	76.7	76.7	76.9	76.9
Turkey	72.8	73.0	73.2	73.4	73.6	73.8

e, estimate.

Source: From OECD Health Data 2008. Retrieved October 12, 2009, from http://www.ecosante.org/index2.php?base=OCDE&langs=ENG&langh=ENG.

TABLE 2-10 Current Operations of US Healthcare System: Life Expectancy, Males at Birth

Countries	2000 Males at birth (years)	2001 Males at birth (years)	2002 Males at birth (years)	2003 Males at birth (years)	2004 Males at birth (years)	2005 Males at birth (years)
Iceland	78.4	78.1	78.7	79.7	79.2	79.2
Japan	77.7	78.1	78.3	78.4	78.6	78.6
Sweden	77.4	77.6	77.7	77.9	78.4	78.4
Italy	77.0	77.2	77.4	77.1	77.9	78.7
Switzerland	77.0	77.5	77.9	78.0	78.6	78.0
Canada	76.7	77.0	77.2	77.4	77.8	78.5
Australia	76.6	77.0	77.4	77.8	78.1	77.8
Norway	76.0	76.2	76.4	77.1	77.6	77.9
New Zealand	75.9 e	76.3	76.7	77.0	77.5	77.0
Spain	75.8	76.2	76.3	76.3	76.9	76.8
Greece	75.5	75.9	76.2	76.5	76.6	77.2
Netherlands	75.5	75.8	76.0	76.2	76.9	77.1
United Kingdom	75.5	75.8	76.0	76.2	76.8	76.7
France	75.3	75.5	75.7	75.8	76.7	76.7
Austria	75.1	75.6	75.8	75.9	76.4	76.7
Germany	75.1	75.6	75.7	75.8	76.5	76.2
Belgium	74.6	75.0	75.1	75.3	76.0	76.7
Luxembourg	74.6	75.1	74.6	74.8	75.9	76.0
Denmark	74.5	74.7	74.8	75.0	75.4	75.6
Finland	74.2	74.6	74.9	75.1	75.4	

United States	74.1	74.4	74.5	74.8	75.2	75.2
Ireland	74.0	74.5	75.2	75.9	76.4	77.3
Portugal	73.2	73.5	73.8	74.2	75.0	74.9
Korea	72.3	72.8	73.4	73.9	74.5	75.1
Czech Republic	71.7	72.1	72.1	72.0	72.6	72.9
Mexico	71.6	71.9	72.1	72.4	72.7	73.0
Poland	69.7	70.2	70.4	70.5	70.7	70.8
Slovak Republic	69.1	59.5	69.8	69.9	70.3	70.1
Turkey	68.1	58.2	68.4	68.6	68.8	68.9
Hungary	67.4	68.1	68.4	68.4	68.6	68.6

e, estimate.

Source: From OECD Health Data 2008. Retrieved October 12, 2009, from http://www.ecosante.org/index2.php?base=OCDE&langs=ENG&langh=ENG.

TABLE 2-11 Current Operations of US Healthcare System: Life Expectancy, Total Population at Birth

Countries	2000 Total population at birth (years)	2001 Total population at birth (years)	2002 Total population at birth (years)	2003 Total population at birth (years)	2004 Total population at birth (years)	2005 Total population at birth (years)	2006 Total population at birth (years)
Japan	81.2	81.5	81.8	81.9	82.1	82.0	82.4
Iceland	80.1	80.2	80.6	81.2	81.0	81.2	81.2
Italy	80.0	80.2	80.3	80.0	80.9		
Switzerland	79.9	80.4	80.6	80.6	81.2	81.4	81.7
Sweden	79.7	79.9	79.9	80.2	80.6	80.6	80.8
Spain	79.4	79.7	79.8	79.7	80.3	80.4	81.1
Australia	79.3	79.7	80.0	80.3	80.6	80.9	81.1
Canada	79.3	79.6	79.7	79.9	80.2	80.4	
France	79.2	79.3	79.4	79.3	80.3	80.2	80.9
Norway	78.8	78.9	79.0	79.6	80.1	80.3	80.6
New Zealand	78.4 e	78.7	79.0	79.2	79.6	79.9	80.2
Germany	78.2	78.5	78.5	78.6	79.2	79.4	79.8
Austria	78.1	78.6	78.8	78.8	79.3	79.5	79.9
Greece	78.0	78.5	78.7	78.9	79.1	79.3	79.6
Luxembourg	78.0	77.9	78.1	77.8	79.1	79.5	79.4
Netherlands	78.0	78.3	78.4	78.6	79.2	79.4	79.8
United Kingdom	77.9	78.2	78.3	78.4	78.9	79.1	
Belgium	77.8	78.1	78.2	78.2	78.9	79.1	79.5
Finland	77.7	78.2	78.3	78.5	79.0	79.1	79.5

Country							
Denmark	76.9	77.0	77.1	77.4	77.8	78.3	78.4
United States	76.8	77.-	77.2	77.5	77.8	77.8	78.3
Portugal	76.7	77.0	77.2	77.4	78.3	78.1	78.9
Ireland	76.6	77.2	77.9	78.4	78.9	79.5	79.7
Korea	76.0	76.4	77.0	77.4	78.0	78.5	79.1
Czech Republic	75.1	75.4	75.4	75.3	75.9	76.1	76.7
Mexico	74.1	74.4	74.6	74.9	75.2	75.5	75.7
Poland	73.9	74.3	74.6	74.7	75.0	75.1	75.3
Slovak Republic	73.3	73.6	73.8	73.9	74.1	74.0	74.3
Hungary	71.7	72.3	72.6	72.6	72.8	72.8	73.2
Turkey	70.5	70.6	70.8	71.0	71.2	71.4	71.6

e, estimate.

Source: From OECD Health Data 2008. Retrieved October 12, 2009, from http://www.ecosante.org/index2.php?base=OCDE&langs=ENG&langh=ENG.

TABLE 2-12   Current Operations of US Healthcare System: Life Expectancy, Females at age 65

Countries	2000 Females at age 65 (years)	2001 Females at age 65 (years)	2002 Females at age 65 (years)	2003 Females at age 65 (years)	2004 Females at age 65 (years)	2005 Females at age 65 (years)
Japan	22.4	22.7	23.0	23.0	23.3	23.2
France	21.4	21.5	21.3	21.0	22.1	22.0
Switzerland	20.9	21.3	21.3	21.1	21.6	21.7
Spain	20.8	21.0	21.0	20.8	21.5	21.3
Italy	20.7	21.0	21.0	20.6	21.5	
Australia	20.4	20.7	20.8	21.0	21.1	21.4
Canada	20.4	20.6	20.6	20.8	21.0	21.1
Luxembourg	20.1	19.7	20.0	18.9	20.5	20.4
Sweden	20.0	20.1	20.0	20.3	20.6	20.6
Norway	19.9	19.9	19.8	20.3	20.7	20.9
New Zealand	19.8 e	20.0	20.0	20.1	20.4	20.5
Belgium	19.7	19.9	19.7	19.6	20.2	20.2
Iceland	19.7	20.3	20.4	20.3	20.5	20.7
Germany	19.6	19.8	19.6	19.5	20.1	20.1
Finland	19.5	19.8	19.8	20.0	20.7	21.0
Austria	19.4	19.8	19.7	19.9	20.3	20.3
Netherlands	19.2	19.3	19.3	19.5	19.8	20.0
United States	19.2	19.4	19.5	19.8	20.0	20.0
United Kingdom	19.0	19.2	19.2	19.1	19.4	19.5

Portugal	18.9	19.1	19.2	19.0	19.7	19.4
Denmark	18.3	18.3	18.2	18.5	19.0	19.1
Greece	18.3	18.7	18.8	18.9	19.2	19.4
Mexico	18.3	18.4	18.5	18.6	18.6	18.7
Korea	18.2	18.4	18.7	19.0	19.4	19.9
Ireland	18.0	18.5	18.9	19.2	19.7	20.0
Poland	17.5	17.6	17.9	17.9	18.4	18.6
Czech Republic	17.3	17.3	17.3	17.2	17.6	17.7
Hungary	16.5	16.7	17.0	16.9	16.9	16.9
Slovak Republic	16.5	16.8	16.9	16.9	16.9	16.9
Turkey	14.6	14.7	14.8	14.9	14.9	15.0

e, estimate.

Source: From OECD Health Data 2008. Retrieved October 13, 2009, from http://www.ecosante.org/index2.php?base=OCDE&langs=ENG&langh=ENG.

TABLE 2-13 — Current Operations of US Healthcare System: Life Expectancy, Males at age 65

Countries	2000 Males at age 65 (years)	2001 Males at age 65 (years)	2002 Males at age 65 (years)	2003 Males at age 65 (years)	2004 Males at age 65 (years)	2005 Males at age 65 (years)
Iceland	18.1	17.6	17.5	18.1	17.9	18.0
Japan	17.5	17.8	18.0	18.0	18.2	18.1
Switzerland	17.0	17.3	17.6	17.6	18.2	18.1
Australia	16.9	17.2	17.4	17.6	17.8	18.1
Canada	16.8	17.1	17.2	17.4	17.7	17.9
France	16.8	17.0	17.0	17.0	17.7	17.7
Mexico	16.8	16.9	17.0	17.1	17.1	17.1
Italy	16.7	16.9	17.0	16.8	17.5	
Spain	16.7	16.9	16.9	16.8	17.3	17.3
Sweden	16.7	16.9	16.9	17.0	17.4	17.4
New Zealand	16.5 e	16.7	16.9	17.1	17.5	17.8
United States	16.3	16.4	16.6	16.8	17.1	17.2
Greece	16.2	16.6	16.7	16.8	17.0	17.2
Norway	16.1	16.2	16.2	16.8	17.2	17.2
Austria	16.0	16.3	16.3	16.4	16.9	17.0
Germany	15.8	16.1	16.2	16.2	16.7	16.9
United Kingdom	15.8	16.1	16.2	16.3	16.8	17.0
Belgium	15.6	15.9	15.8	15.9	16.4	16.6
Finland	15.5	15.7	15.8	16.2	16.5	16.8
Luxembourg	15.5	16.0	15.9	15.3	16.5	16.7

Portugal	15.4	15.7	15.7	16.3	16.1
Netherlands	15.3	15.5	15.6	16.3	16.4
Denmark	15.2	15.2	15.4	15.9	16.1
Ireland	14.6	15.0	15.4	16.2	16.8
Korea	14.3	14.6	14.9	15.5	15.8
Czech Republic	13.8	14.0	13.9	14.2	14.4
Poland	13.6	13.9	14.0	14.2	14.4
Slovak Republic	12.9	13.0	13.3	13.3	13.2
Turkey	12.9	12.9	13.0	13.1	13.1
Hungary	12.7	13.0	13.1	13.1	13.1

e, estimate

Source: From OECD Health Data 2008. Retrieved October 12, 2009, from http://www.ecosante.org/index2.php?base=OCDE&langs=ENG&langh=ENG.

Iceland was the lead country for males' life expectancy at age 65 with 18.1 years, which did decrease to 18 years of age by 2006. The United States ranked 12th in this category. In 2000, the male expectancy after age 65 was 16.3 years, which increased to 17.2 years by 2006. The lowest ranked countries were Turkey and Hungary, which had 12.9 and 12.7 years, respectively. These statistics support the general international statistics of female life expectancy that are longer than males. These statistics further support the quality of care provided to the elderly.

2000–2005 Infant Mortality Rates per 1000 Births (Table 2-14, pages 57–58)

According to the OECD, the infant mortality rate is the number of deaths per 1000 live births occurring among the population of a designated area during the same calendar year. In 2000, Turkey and Mexico had infant mortality rates of 28.9 and 23.3 per 1000 live births. Fortunately, by 2005, these rates decreased to 23.6 and 18.8 per 1000 live births. The lowest infant mortality rates are in Iceland, Japan, and Sweden. Their rates in 2000 were 3.0, 3.2, and 3.4, respectively. By 2005, the rates dropped to 2.4, 2.8, and 2.3, which points to the quality of prenatal care in their healthcare system. The United States ranks sixth from the bottom out of the 30 countries. In 2000, the infant mortality rates were 6.9, which remained the same for 2005. One of the criticisms of the US delivery system is the poor prenatal care received by different ethnic groups.

2000–2005 Diabetes Deaths per 100,000 Population (Table 2-15, pages 59–60)

Diabetes mellitus is a disease in which the body does not produce or properly use insulin, a hormone that is needed to convert sugar and starches that are needed for energy (American Diabetes Association [ADA], 2009). It has become a common chronic disease that can cause serious health conditions worldwide. There are different types of diabetes but a common form of diabetes, type 2, is often the result of being overweight. Although these statistics do not differentiate the different forms of this disease, it can be fatal if not addressed. In 2000, Mexico was clearly the leader of deaths due to diabetes at 90.2, which increased to 109 by 2005. The second highest rate was Korea, which reported rates of 33.7 in 2000 which decreased to 30.2 by 2005. In 2000, the United States ranked fourth in this category at 20.6, which slightly decreased to 20.3 by 2005. These high rates are a result, in part, of the increase in overweight individuals in the United States.

The lowest 2000 rates occurred in Greece and Iceland at 5.5 and 5.3. In 2006, Greece's rate decreased slightly to 5.4 but Iceland's increased slightly to 5.9.

2000–2006 Overweight or Obese Percentage of Total Population (Table 2-16, pages 61–62)

An individual is considered overweight with a body mass index of 25–30 kg/m^2. An individual is considered obese with a body mass index >30 kh/m^2. The top three countries had 60% or greater of their total population either obese or overweight. In 2000, the United States had a 64.5% of either overweight or obese in their population. This has increased to 67.3%. This indicates a serious problem in the US population. The second highest was Mexico with 62.3% with an increase to 69.5% in 2006. Being overweight or obese can lead to other health problems such as hypertension, diabetes, and other major health issues. There have been recent studies indicating that overweight and obese individuals are becoming an international problem. A major reason is the change in lifestyles. People are more sedentary than in previous decades. There are also more options for unhealthy eating. Franchises such as McDonalds and Burger King have expanded worldwide and are very popular.

CONCLUSION

The US healthcare system is a complicated system that is comprised of both public and private resources. Health care is available to those who have health insurance or who are entitled to health care through a public program. One can think of the healthcare system as several concentric circles that surround the most important stakeholders in the center circle; the most important stakeholders are the healthcare consumers and providers. Immediately surrounding this relationship are the healthcare insurance companies and the government programs, the healthcare facilities, the pharmaceutical companies, and the laboratories that all provide services to the consumer to ensure they receive quality health care and support the provider to ensure they provide quality health care. The next circle consists of peripheral stakeholders that do not have immediate impact on the main relationship but are still important to the industry. These consist of the professional associations, the research organizations, and the medical and training facilities.

It is important to assess the system from an international perspective. Comparing different statistics from the OECD is valuable to assess the health of the United States.

TABLE 2-14	Current Operations of US Healthcare System: Infant Mortality Deaths per 1000 Live Births					
Countries	2000 Infant mortality, deaths per 1000 live births	2001 Infant mortality, deaths per 1000 live births	2002 Infant mortality, deaths per 1000 live births	2003 Infant mortality, deaths per 1000 live births	2004 Infant mortality, deaths per 1000 live births	2005 Infant mortality, deaths per 1000 live births
Turkey	28.9	27.8	26.7	28.7	24.6	23.6
Mexico	23.3	22.4	21.4	20.5	19.7	18.8
Hungary	9.2	8.1	7.2	7.3	6.6	6.2
Slovak Republic	8.6	6.2	7.6	7.9	6.8	7.2
Poland	8.1	7.7	7.5	7.0	6.8	6.4
United States	6.9	6.8	7.0	6.9	6.8	6.9
New Zealand	6.3	5.6	6.2	5.4	5.9	5.0
Ireland	6.2	5.7	5.0	5.3	4.6	4.0
United Kingdom	5.6	5.5	5.2	5.2	5.1	5.1
Portugal	5.5	5.0	5.0	4.1	3.8	3.5
Greece	5.4	5.1	5.1	4.0	4.1	3.8
Canada	5.3	5.2	5.4	5.3	5.3	5.4
Denmark	5.3	4.9	4.4	4.4	4.4	4.4
Australia	5.2	5.3	5.0	4.8	4.7	5.0
Luxembourg	5.1	5.9	5.1	4.9	3.9	2.6
Netherlands	5.1	5.4	5.0	4.8	4.4	4.9
Switzerland	4.9	5.0	5.0	4.3	4.2	4.2
Austria	4.8	4.8	4.1	4.5	4.5	4.2

continues

TABLE 2-14   Current Operations of US Healthcare System: Infant Mortality Deaths per 1000 Live Births *(Continued)*

Countries	2000 Infant mortality, deaths per 1000 live births	2001 Infant mortality, deaths per 1000 live births	2002 Infant mortality, deaths per 1000 live births	2003 Infant mortality, deaths per 1000 live births	2004 Infant mortality, deaths per 1000 live births	2005 Infant mortality, deaths per 1000 live births
Belgium	4.8	4.5	4.4	4.3	4.3	3.7
France	4.5	4.6	4.2	4.2	4.0	3.8
Italy	4.5	4.6	4.3	3.9	3.9	3.9
Germany	4.4	4.3	4.2	4.2	4.1	3.9
Spain	4.4	4.1	4.1	3.9	4.0	3.8
Czech Republic	4.1	4.0	4.1	3.9	3.7	3.4
Finland	3.8	3.2	3.0	3.1	3.3	3.0
Norway	3.8	3.9	3.5	3.4	3.2	3.1
Sweden	3.4	3.7	3.3	3.1	3.1	2.4
Japan	3.2	3.1	3.0	3.0	2.8	2.8
Iceland	3.0	2.7	2.3	2.4	2.8	2.3
Korea			5.3			

Source: From OECD Health Data 2008. Retrieved October 12, 2009, from http://www.ecosante.org/index2.php?base=OCDE&langs=ENG&langh=ENG.

TABLE 2-15 Current Operations of US Healthcare System: Diabetes Mellitus Deaths per 100,000 Population

Countries	2000 Diabetes mellitus, deaths per 100,000 population (standardized rates)	2001 Diabetes mellitus, deaths per 100,000 population (standardized rates)	2002 Diabetes mellitus, deaths per 100,000 population (standardized rates)	2003 Diabetes mellitus, deaths per 100,000 population (standardized rates)	2004 Diabetes mellitus, deaths per 100,000 population (standardized rates)	2005 Diabetes mellitus, deaths per 100,000 population (standardized rates)
Mexico	90.2	93.1	98.9	103.2	104.5	109.0
Korea	33.7	34.7	35.3	33.8	31.5	30.2
Portugal	20.9	25.6	28.0	27.8		
United States	20.6	20.8	20.9	20.9	20.2	20.3
Denmark	18.4	17.1				
New Zealand	18.3	17.6	17.5	18.2	17.5	
Canada	17.8	18.3	19.6	19.3	18.4	
Italy	17.7	17.2	16.4	17.9		
Hungary	16.9	13.2	16.9	18.4	16.5	24.8
Germany	15.5	15.6	16.6	16.7	16.2	16.4
Netherlands	15.4	19.5	18.1	16.5	16.3	15.8
Spain	13.9	14.0	13.8	13.8	13.2	13.3
Slovak Republic	13.7	13.6	12.8	13.5	12.7	12.0
Switzerland	13.1	13.1	12.9	14.4	12.0	10.8
Australia	13.0	12.7	13.1	13.2		
Poland	12.6	12.1	11.9	11.9	11.3	11.8
France	11.5	11.5	11.4	11.9	10.8	10.9

continues

TABLE 2-15 Current Operations of US Healthcare System: Diabetes Mellitus Deaths per 100,000 Population (*Continued*)

Countries	2000 Diabetes mellitus, deaths per 100,000 population (standardized rates)	2001 Diabetes mellitus, deaths per 100,000 population (standardized rates)	2002 Diabetes mellitus, deaths per 100,000 population (standardized rates)	2003 Diabetes mellitus, deaths per 100,000 population (standardized rates)	2004 Diabetes mellitus, deaths per 100,000 population (standardized rates)	2005 Diabetes mellitus, deaths per 100,000 population (standardized rates)
Austria	11.2	11.4	16.2	24.2	28.8	27.1
Czech Republic	11.1	9.4	9.7	10.9	10.0	10.3
Sweden	10.7	11.1	11.6	11.3	11.5	
Ireland	10.2	9.5	9.7	9.5	10.1	10.0
Norway	9.2	9.9	9.3	9.5	8.1	10.1
Luxembourg	8.5	9.6	9.3	8.9	7.1	7.4
Finland	7.9	7.1	7.2	6.9	7.0	6.6
Japan	6.1	5.8	5.9	5.8	5.5	5.7
Iceland	5.5	8.1	4.5	6.3	6.0	5.4
Greece	5.3	4.4	4.9	5.1	5.8	5.9
United Kingdom		7.6	7.5	7.6	7.1	6.7

Source: From OECD Health Data 2008. Retrieved October 12, 2009, from http://www.ecosante.org/index2.php?base=OCDE&langs=ENG&langh=ENG.

TABLE 2-16 Current Operations of US Healthcare System: Overweight or Obese Population Percentages

Countries	2000 Overweight or obese population, % of total population	2001 Overweight or obese population, % of total population	2002 Overweight or obese population, % of total population	2003 Overweight or obese population, % of total population	2004 Overweight or obese population, % of total population	2005 Overweight or obese population, % of total population	2006 Overweight or obese population, % of total population
United States	64.5 d		65.7 d		56.3 d		67.3 d
Mexico	62.3					69.2	69.5
United Kingdom	60.0 d	62.0 d	61.0 d	60.0 d	62.0 d	60.0 d	62.0 d
Hungary	51.4			52.8			
Luxembourg	50.1	51.8	51.6	52.8	52.8	53.3	
Netherlands	44.1	44.8	44.8	46.1	46.5	44.9	46.5
Finland	43.4	44.1	45.3	45.0	45.3	49.2	47.7
Sweden	42.7	42.7	44.4	42.8	42.6	44.0	
Denmark	41.7					44.6	
Italy	41.1	42.4	42.0	42.6		44.6	45.1
France	36.2		37.5		34.7		37.0
Japan	23.8 d	24.4 d	25.7 d	24.7 d	24.0 d	24.9 d	
Australia							
Austria							47.7 b
Belgium		44.4			44.1		
Canada		45.1 b		46.5		49.9	
Czech Republic			51.1			52.0 d	
Germany				49.2		49.6	

continues

TABLE 2-16 Current Operations of US Healthcare System: Overweight or Obese Population Percentages (*Continued*)

Countries	2000 Overweight or obese population, % of total population	2001 Overweight or obese population, % of total population	2002 Overweight or obese population, % of total population	2003 Overweight or obese population, % of total population	2004 Overweight or obese population, % of total population	2005 Overweight or obese population, % of total population	2006 Overweight or obese population, % of total population
Greece				57.1			
Iceland			48.3				
Ireland			47.0				
Korea		30.6				30.5	
New Zealand				60.5 d			d
Norway			42.7			43.0	
Poland					45.3		
Portugal							
Slovak Republic				47.6	50.1	51.6	
Spain		48.3		48.4			
Switzerland			37.1				51.1
Turkey				43.4			

b, break in series; d, differences in methodology.

Source: From OECD Health Data 2008. Retrieved October 12, 2009, from http://www.ecosante.org/index2.php?base=OCDE&langs=ENG&langh=ENG.

Despite the cost of the healthcare system, many of the US statistics ranked lower than other countries that spend less on their healthcare system. These statistics may point to the fact that other countries' healthcare systems are more effective than the US system or that their citizens have healthier lifestyles although obesity rates throughout the world are increasing in all of the countries evaluated.

PREVIEW OF CHAPTER THREE

The government's role in health care evolved as a regulatory mechanism to ensure that the elderly and the poor were able to receive health care. The passage of the 1935 Social Security Act and the implementation of Medicare and Medicaid increased the role of government in healthcare coverage. The chapter will focus on the different roles the federal, state, and local government play in the US healthcare system. It is important to note that these government agencies were established to enforce regulations that were implemented to protect individuals. The chapter will highlight different programs and regulations that may help you as a consumer so you will be able to understand how health care is provided and how it is regulated.

VOCABULARY

American Association of Homes and Services for the Aging (AAHSA)

American Health Care Association (AHCA)

American Hospital Association (AHA)

Bad debt and charitable care

Blue Cross and Blue Shield

Bureau of Labor Statistics (BLS)

Commonwealth Fund

Complementary and alternative medicine (CAM)

Diabetes mellitus

Duty to treat

Home health care

Infant mortality rates

Life expectancy rates

Medical and diagnostic laboratories

National Center for Health Statistics (NCHS)

Organisation for Economic Co-operation and Development (OECD)

Outpatient care centers

Pew Charitable Trust

Pharmaceutical companies

Professional associations

Residential care facilities

Robert Wood Johnson Foundation

Stakeholder

REFERENCES

American Association of Home and Services for the Aging. (2009). Retrieved November 9, 2009, from http://www.aahsa.org/about.aspx.

American Diabetes Association. (2009). Retrieved November 9, 2009, from http://www.diabetes.org/diabetes-basics/.

American Health Care Association. (2009). Retrieved November 9, 2009, from http://www.ahcancal.org/about_ahca/who_we_are/Pages/default.aspx.

American Hospital Association. (2009). Retrieved June 21, 2009, from http://www.aha.org.

Centers for Disease Control and Prevention. (2007). *Chartbook on trends in the health of Americans*. Retrieved April 30, 2009, from http://www.cdc.gov/nchs/data/hus/hus07.pdf.

HealthReform.gov. (2009). *Health disparities: A case for closing the gap*. Retrieved June 25, 2009, from http://www.healthreform.gov.

Jonas, S. (2003). *An introduction to the U.S. health care system* (pp. 17–45). New York: Springer Publishing.

National Center for Health Statistics. (2008). *The use of complementary and alternative medicine in the United States*. Retrieved November 9, 2009, from http://nccam.nih.gov/news/camstats/2007/.

Organisation for Economic Co-operation and Development. (2009). Retrieved April 30, 2009, from http://www.oecd.org/pages/0_3417_36761863_1_1_1_1_1,00.html.

Pharmaceutical Research and Manufacturers of America. (2009). Retrieved April 29, 2009, from http://www.phrma.org/about_phrma/.

Pointer, D., Williams, S., Isaacs, S., & Knickman, J. (2007). *Introduction to U.S. health care*. Hoboken, NJ: Wiley Publishing.

Smith, D. (2008). The uninsured in the U.S. health care system. *Journal of Health Care Management, 53*, 2, 79–81.

Sultz, H., & Young, K. (2006). *Health care USA: Understanding its organization and delivery* (5th ed.). Sudbury, MA: Jones and Bartlett.

US Bureau of Labor Statistics. (2010). Retrieved January 12, 2010, from http://data.bls.gov/cgi-bin/print.pl/oco/cg/cgs/035.htm.

US Census Bureau. (2009). Retrieved April 30, 2009, from http://www.census.gov.

NOTES

STUDENT ACTIVITY 2-1

CROSSWORD PUZZLE

Instructions: Please complete the puzzle using the vocabulary words found in the chapter. There may be multiple-word answers. The number in the parenthesis indicates the number of words in the answer.

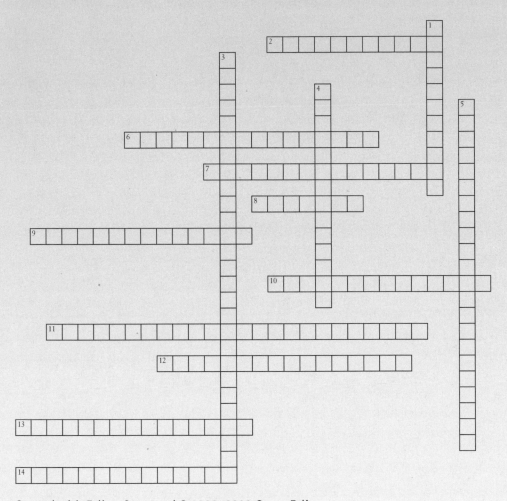

Created with EclipseCrossword © 1999–2009 Green Eclipse

STUDENT ACTIVITY 2-1

Across

2. The principle of the healthcare system that says all individuals have the right to basic health care. (3 words)

6. These types of variables include ethnicity, marital status, education, and occupational class. (1 word)

7. These facilities provide this type of care, which includes around-the-clock social and personal care to patients. (2 words)

8. The provider provides care even though they suspect that all efforts to secure payment will fail. (2 words)

9. This type of care is becoming more popular because consumers prefer this type of treatment and it is more cost effective. (3 words)

10. This industry is responsible for developing and producing medication for the healthcare industry. (1 word)

11. These associations represent physicians, hospitals, nurses, and other stakeholders and lobby for them at all government levels to ensure regulations are fair to them. (2 words)

12. This chronic condition is often the result of being overweight and can cause serious health conditions. (2 words)

13. This rate focuses on the number of deaths of a child under 12 months of age during a calendar year in a specific geographic location. (2 words)

14. The healthcare provider provides care even though they know the patient will not be able to pay. (2 words)

Down

1. An individual or organization that has an interest or participates in an industry. (1 word)

3. Examples of this type of medicine include yoga, vitamin therapy, and acupuncture. (3 words)

4. These types of centers include kidney dialysis, mental health, and substance abuse care. (2 words)

5. These types of facilities include medical, nursing, and public health schools, and allied health programs. (3 words)

STUDENT ACTIVITY 2-2

IN YOUR OWN WORDS

Based on Chapter 2, please provide a definition of the following vocabulary words in your own words. DO NOT RECITE the text definition.

Duty to treat: _____

_____

_____

Infant mortality rate: _____

_____

_____

Life expectancy rates: _____

_____

_____

Bad debt and charitable care: _____

_____

_____

Residential care facilities: _____

_____

_____

Complementary and alternative medicine: _____

_____

_____

Outpatient care centers: _____

_____

_____

Professional associations: _____

_____

_____

Residential care facilities: _____

_____

_____

STUDENT ACTIVITY 2-3

REAL LIFE APPLICATIONS: CASE STUDY

You have decided to become a health education teacher for a high school. One of your first class lessons will be on explaining the complexity of the US healthcare system to your students. You want to be creative so you decide to have a role play in which you select students to play the stakeholders in the healthcare system. You also want to them to understand how the United States compares to other countries. You develop two lesson plans that are outlined below. Your first lesson plan outlines the major stakeholders in the system and how they interact with each other. The second lesson plan focuses on selecting five health statistics that compare the United States to another country.

RESPONSES

_____

_____

_____

_____

_____

_____

_____

_____

_____

_____

_____

STUDENT ACTIVITY 2-4

INTERNET EXERCISES

Write your answers in the space provided.

- Visit each of the Web sites listed here.
- Name the organization.
- Locate their mission statement or statement of purpose on their Web site.
- Provide a brief overview of the activities of the organization.
- How do these organizations participate in the US healthcare system?

Web Sites

http://www.rwjf.org

Organization Name: _____

Mission Statement:

_____

_____

_____

Overview of Activities:

_____

_____

_____

Importance of organization to US health care:

_____

_____

_____

http://www.commonwealthfund.org

Organization Name: _____

Mission Statement:

_____

_____

_____

Overview of Activities:

_____

_____

_____

Importance of organization to US health care:

_____

_____

_____

http://www.phrma.org

Organization Name: _____

Mission Statement:

_____

_____

_____

Overview of Activities:

_____

_____

_____

Importance of organization to US health care:

_____

_____

_____

http://www.oecd.org

Organization Name: _____

Mission Statement:

_____

_____

_____

Overview of Activities:

_____

_____

_____

Importance of organization to US health care:

_____

_____

_____

STUDENT ACTIVITY 2-4

http://www.bls.gov

Organization Name: _____

Mission Statement:

_____

_____

_____

Overview of Activities:

_____

_____

_____

Importance of organization to US health care:

_____

_____

_____

http://www.ahcancal.org

Organization Name: _____

Mission Statement:

_____

_____

_____

Overview of Activities:

_____

_____

_____

Importance of organization to US health care:

_____

_____

_____

Chapter 3

The Role of Government in Health Care

LEARNING OBJECTIVES

The student will be able to:

- Describe five government organizations and their roles in health care.

- Explain the importance of the National Association of County and City Officials in health care.

- Analyze the integration of the collaboration of the Department of Homeland Security and the Federal Emergency Management Agency and its importance in health care.

- Describe the role of the National Institutes of Health in healthcare research.

- Discuss the US Food and Drug Administration's regulatory responsibility in health care.

- Evaluate the role of the Centers for Medicare and Medicaid Services in health care.

- Assess the importance of the Association of State and Territorial Health Officials on state health departments.

DID YOU KNOW THAT?

- There are 25 accrediting organizations that target certain sectors of health care.

- The US Surgeon General is the chief health educator in the United States.

- There are 3000 local health departments in the United States.

- Nearly 100% of local health departments have Internet access with 70% having a Web site.

- The Department of Homeland Security is responsible for ensuring that all government levels have an emergency preparedness plan for catastrophic events.

INTRODUCTION

As discussed in Chapter 1, during the Depression and World War II the United States had no funds to start a universal healthcare program—an issue that had been discussed for years. As a result, a private sector system was developed that did not provide healthcare services to all citizens. However, the government's role of providing healthcare coverage evolved as a regulatory body to ensure that the elderly and poor were able to receive health care. The passage of the Social Security Act of 1935 and the establishment of the Medicaid and Medicare programs in 1965 mandated government's increased role in providing healthcare coverage. Also, the State Children's Health Insurance Program (SCHIP), now the Children's Health Insurance Program, established in 1997 and reauthorized through 2010, continues to expand government's role in children's health care (Buchbinder & Shanks, 2007).

In both of these instances, the government increased accessibility to health care as well as provided financing for health care to certain targeted populations. This chapter will focus on the different roles the federal, state, and local governments play in the US healthcare system. This chapter will also highlight different government programs and regulations that focus on monitoring how health care is provided.

HISTORY OF THE ROLE OF GOVERNMENT IN HEALTH CARE

Social regulation focuses on organizations' actions, such as those in the healthcare industry, that impact individual's safety. Social regulations focus on protecting individuals as employees and consumers (Carroll & Buchholtz, 2006). These types of regulations are common in the US healthcare system. The healthcare industry claims it is the most regulated industry in the world. It is important to mention that government regulations aside, there are nongovernmental regulations of US health care by accrediting bodies such as The Joint Commission, which began over 80 years ago. There are currently 25 accrediting organizations that target certain sectors of health care (Walshe & Shortell, 2004). However, regulatory oversight is mainly handled at the federal, state, and local government levels.

US GOVERNMENT AGENCIES

Regulatory healthcare power is shared among federal and state governments. State government has a dominant role of regulating constituents in their jurisdiction. To assure success in this regulatory process, state governments also developed local government levels to provide direct services to constituents and regulate their geographic region. Their legal authority is derived from legislatures that establish the legal framework for their authority (Jonas, 2003).

Important Federal Government Agencies

Many federal agencies are responsible for a sector of healthcare. The **US Department of Health and Human Services** (HHS) is the most important federal agency. HHS collaborates with state and local governments because many HHS services are provided at those levels. There are 11 operating divisions: the **Centers for Disease Control and Prevention** (CDC), **National Institutes of Health** (NIH), **Agency for Toxic Substances and Disease Registry** (ATSDR),

Indian Health Service (IHS), the **Health Resources and Services Administration** (HRSA), the **Agency for Healthcare Research and Quality** (AHRQ), the **Substance Abuse and Mental Health Services Administration** (SAMHSA), and the **US Food and Drug Administration** (FDA). All of these agencies are part of the Public Health Service component of the HHS. The other three divisions that operate within the human services component are the **Administration for Children and Families** (ACF), **Administration on Aging** (AOA), and the **Centers for Medicare and Medicaid Services** (CMS). Each of these agencies will be discussed individually (HHS, 2009).

Centers for Disease Control and Prevention

Established in 1946 and headquartered in Atlanta, GA, the CDC's mission is to protect health and promote quality of life through the prevention and control of disease, injury, and disability. The CDC has created four health goals that focus on (1) healthy people in healthy places, (2) preparing people for emerging health threats, (3) positive international health, and (4) healthy people at all stages of their life. To achieve these goals, the CDC focuses on six areas: health impact, customer focus, public health research, leadership, globalization, and accountability (CDC, 2009b).

Agency for Toxic Substances and Disease Registry

Established in 1985, headquartered in Atlanta, GA, and authorized by the Comprehensive Environmental Response, Compensation, and Liability Act of 1980 (CERCLA; more commonly known as the Superfund law), ATSDR is responsible for finding and cleaning the most dangerous hazardous waste sites in the country. ATSDR's mission is to protect the public against harmful exposures and disease-related exposures to toxic substances. ATSDR is the lead federal public health agency responsible for determining human health effects associated with toxic exposures, preventing continued exposures, and mitigating associated human health risks. ATSDR is administered with the CDC (ATSDR, 2009).

National Institutes of Health

Established in 1930 and headquartered in Bethesda, MD, this agency is the primary federal agency for research toward preventing and curing disease. Its mission is the pursuit of knowledge about the nature and behavior of living systems and the application of that knowledge to extend healthy life and reduce the burdens of illness and disability. They have 27 institutes and centers that focus on different diseases and conditions including cancer, ophthalmology, heart and lung and blood, genes, aging, alcoholism and drug abuse, infectious diseases, chronic diseases, children's diseases, and mental health. Although they have sponsored external research, they also have a large internal research program (NIH, 2009; Turnock, 2007).

The Health Resources and Services Administration

Created in 1982 and headquartered in Rockville, MD, the HRSA is the primary federal agency for improving access to healthcare services for people in every state who are uninsured, isolated, or medically vulnerable. They have six bureaus: primary health care, health professions, health care systems, maternal and child, the HIV/AIDS bureau, and the Bureau of Clinician Recruitment and Service. HRSA provides funding to grantees that provide health care to those vulnerable populations. They train health professionals and improve systems of care in rural communities. They oversee 650 community and migrant health centers, plus 150 primary care programs for the homeless and residents of public housing. Service is provided to individuals with AIDS through the Ryan White Care Act programs (Turnock, 2007). They also oversee organ, bone marrow, and cord blood donation; support programs against bioterrorism; and maintain databases that protect against healthcare malpractice and healthcare waste, fraud, and abuse (HRSA, 2009).

The Agency for Healthcare Research and Quality

Created in 1989 and headquartered in Rockville, MD, the agency's mission is to improve the quality, safety, efficiency, and effectiveness of health care for all US citizens. AHRQ's cutting edge research helps people make more informed decisions and improve the quality of healthcare services. AHRQ focuses on the following areas of research: healthcare costs and utilization, information technology, disaster preparedness, medication safety, healthcare consumerism, prevention of illness, and special needs populations (AHRQ, 2009). There is a **Coalition for Health Services Research** (CHSR) an organization of volunteers who advocate group for the AHRQ. It is comprised of more than 250 nonprofit organizations that support the AHRQ (CHSR, 2009). They send letters to Congress encouraging more funds for research.

Indian Health Service

Established in 1921 and headquartered in Rockville, MD, the mission of IHS is to raise the physical, mental, social, and spiritual health of American Indians and Alaska Natives to the highest level. It is also their mission to assure that comprehensive, culturally acceptable personal and public health services are available and accessible to American Indian and Alaska Native people. They are also responsible to promote their communities and cultures and to honor and protect the inherent sovereign rights of these people (IHS, 2009).

The Substance Abuse and Mental Health Services Administration

Established in 1992, the SAMHSA is the main federal agency for improving access to quality substance abuse and mental health services in the United States by working with state, community, and private organizations. SAMHSA is the umbrella agency for mental health and substance abuse services, which includes the **Center for Mental Health Services** (CMHS), the **Center for Substance Abuse Prevention** (CSAP), and the **Center for Substance Abuse Treatment** (CSAT). The **Office of Applied Studies** (OAS) is the destination for data collection, analysis, and dissemination of critical health data to assist policymakers, providers, and the public for the use in making informed decisions regarding the prevention and treatment of mental and substance use disorders (SAMHSA, 2009; Turnock, 2007).

US Food and Drug Administration

Established in 1906 as a result of the **Federal Food, Drug, and Cosmetic Act**, the FDA is responsible for ensuring that the following products are safe: food, human and veterinary products, biologic products, medical devices, cosmetics, and electronic products. The FDA is also responsible for ensuring that product information is accurate (FDA, 2009b). The agency monitors approximately $1 trillion worth of goods on an annual basis (Turnock, 2007). The following is a summary of FDA responsibility for each category:

1. Food: The FDA ensures that labeling of food has accurate information. Also, they regulate the safety of all food except poultry and meat. They also oversee bottled water.

2. Veterinary products: The FDA has oversight of the production of livestock feed, pet food, and veterinary drugs and devices.

3. Human drugs: The FDA has regulatory oversight of both prescription and over-the-counter (OTC) drug development and labeling, which includes the manufacturing standards for these drug products.

4. Medical devices: The FDA has the authority for premarket approval for any new devices as well as developing standards for their manufacturing and performance. They also must track reports of any malfunction of these devices.

5. Cosmetics: The FDA oversees both the safety and labeling of cosmetic products.

6. Electronic products: The FDA must develop and regulate standards for microwaves, televisions receivers, and diagnostic equipment such as x-ray equipment, laser products, ultrasonic therapy equipment, and sunlamps. They also must accredit and inspect any mammography facilities.

The FDA is also responsible for advancing the public health by speeding up innovations to make medicine and food more effective, safer, and more affordable. They are also responsible for ensuring that the public receives accurate information to be able to make informed decisions about using medicine and food products (FDA, 2009b).

Administration on Aging

Established in 1965 as part of the **Older Americans Act** (OAA), the AOA is one of the largest providers of home- and community-based care for older persons. Their mission is to develop a cost effective and efficient system of long-term care that helps the elderly to maintain dignity in their homes and communities. The AOA is a partnership of federal, state, and local networks called the **National Network on Aging** (NNOA) that services 7 million elderly and their caregivers in the United States.

Services provided by the AOA include supportive community services such as transportation to medical appointments, nutritional services, preventive health services, and caregiver services. In 2000, the National Family Caregiver Support Program was funded and it assists caregivers with education and additional services to care for their elderly. The AOA also protects the rights of the elderly and provides services to Native Americans (AOA, 2009).

The Administration for Children and Families

The ACF, which has 10 regional offices, is responsible for federal programs that promote the economic and social well-being of families, children, individuals, and communities. Their mission is to empower people to increase their own economic well-being, support communities that have a positive impact on the quality of life of its residents, partner with other organizations to support Native American tribes, improve needed access to services, and work with those who are special needs populations (ACF, 2009).

Centers for Medicare and Medicaid Services

CMS was established when the Medicare and Medicaid programs were signed into law in 1965 by President Lyndon B. Johnson, as a result of the **Social Security Act**. At that time, only half of those 65 years or older had health insurance. Medicaid was established for low income children, elderly, the blind, and the disabled and was linked with the Supplemental Security Income program (SSI). In 1972, Medicare was extended to cover people under the age of 65 with permanent disabilities. CMS also has oversight of SCHIP, Title XXI of the Social Security Act, which is financed by both federal and state funding and is administered at the state level.

Headquartered in Baltimore, MD, the CMS has over 20 offices that oversee different aspects of their programs. Their primary responsibility is to provide policy, funding, and oversight to the elderly and poor healthcare programs. For years, their organizational oversight was a geographically based structure with 10 field offices. In 2007, CMS was reorganized to a consortia structure based on the priorities of Medicare health plans and financial management, Medicare fee for service, Medicaid and children's health, surveys and certification, and quality assurance and improvement. The consortia are responsible for oversight of the 10 regional offices for each priority (CMS, 2009). The restructuring of the organization was to improve performance of the strategic plan.

Occupational Safety and Health Administration

Established on December 29, 1970, the **Occupational Safety and Health Administration** (OSHA) was established to govern workplace environments to ensure that employees have a safe and healthy environment (OSHA, 2009). The **Hazard Communication Standard** (HCS) ensures that all hazardous chemicals are properly labeled and that companies are informed of these risks. The **Medical Waste Tracking Act** requires companies to have medical waste disposal procedures so that there is no risk to employees and the environment. The **Occupational Exposure to Bloodborne Pathogen Standard** developed behavior standards for employees who deal with blood products such as wearing gloves and other equipment, disposal of blood collection materials, etc. (Pointer, Williams, Isaacs, & Knickman, 2007).

Surgeon General/US Public Health Service

The **Surgeon General** is the US chief health educator who provides information on how to improve the health of the US population. The Surgeon General, who is appointed by the President of the United States, and the Office of the Surgeon General oversee the operations of the commissioned **US Public Health Service Corps** who provide support to the Surgeon General. The US Public Health Service Commissioned Corps consists of 6000 public health professionals that are stationed within federal agencies and programs. These commissioned employees include many professionals such as dentists, nurses, physicians, mental health specialists, environmental health specialists, veterinarians, and therapists.

The Surgeon General serves a 4-year term and reports to the Secretary of Health and Human Services. The Surgeon General focuses on certain health priorities for the United States and publishes reports on these issues. Currently, the priorities for the Surgeon General are disease prevention, eliminating health disparities, disaster preparedness, and improving health literacy (Office of the Surgeon General, 2009).

Department of Homeland Security

The **Department of Homeland Security** (DHS) was established in 2002 as a result of the 2001 terrorist attack on the United States. The **Federal Emergency Management Agency** (FEMA), which is responsible for managing catastrophic events, was integrated into DHS in 2003. Together, they are responsible for coordinating efforts at all government levels to ensure emergency preparedness for any catastrophic events such as bioterrorism, chemical and radiation emergencies, mass casualties as a result of explosions, natural disasters and severe weather, and disease outbreaks. They coordinate with the CDC to ensure there are plans in place to quickly resolve these events (CDC, 2009a; DHS, 2009). DHS has also developed a **National Incident Management System** (NIMS) that provides a systematic, proactive approach to all levels of government and private sector agencies to collaborate to ensure there is a seamless plan to manage any major incidents. NIMS also works with the **National Response Framework** (NRF) that provides the structure for national policy for emergency management (DHS, 2009). Both programs are housed in the DHS's National Incident Management System Resource Center. For more information about both of these programs, see Chapter 4.

Council of State and Territorial Epidemiologists

Established in 1992 and headquartered in Atlanta, GA, the **Council of State and Territorial Epidemiologists** (CSTE) is a professional organization of over 1000 public health epidemiologists that work in state and local health department who provide technical assistance to the **Association of State and Territorial Health Officials** (ASTHO) and to the CDC for research and policy issues. They provide expertise in the areas of maternal child health, infectious diseases, environmental health, injury epidemiology, occupational health, and public health informatics (CSTE, 2009).

State Health Departments' Role in Health Care

The US constitution gives state governments the primary role in providing health care for their citizens. Most states have several different agencies that are responsible for specific public health services. There is usually a lead state agency with approximately 20 agencies that target health issues like aging, living and working environments, and alcoholism and substance abuse. Many state agencies are responsible for implementing several different federal acts such as the Clean Water Act; Clean Air Act; Food, Drug, and Cosmetic Act; and Safe Drinking Water Act (Turnock, 2007). **State health departments** have the authority to collect health data, manage vital statistics, declare health emergencies, and conduct health planning and formulate health policy. They also manage disease and tumor registries and provide health education and laboratory services. Vital statistics collected include deaths, births, marriages, and health and disease statuses of the population. These statistics are important to collect because they serve as a basis for funding. CSTE decides which diseases should be considered reportable to the CDC and produced in a weekly report *Morbidity and Mortality Weekly Report* (*MMWR*). The *MMWR* is an estimate of the prevalence of disease throughout the country (CDC, 2009b). Also, as result of the September 11, 2001 terrorist attacks, all states must have a crisis management plan in place for any type of health crisis that may occur.

State health departments also license health professionals such as physicians, dentists, chiropractors, nurses, pharmacists, optometrists, and veterinarians who practice within the state. They also inspect and license healthcare facilities such as hospitals and nursing homes. Most state agencies provide technical assistance to their local health departments in the following areas: (1) quality improvement, (2) data management, (3) public health law, (4) human resource management, and (5) policy development. It is important to emphasize that the state health department provides oversight to their local health departments who are directly responsible for providing public health activities for their community (Mays, 2008).

States also provide prevention services in the following areas: (1) tobacco use, (2) obesity, (3) injury, (4) HIV/AIDS, (5) diabetes, and (6) sexually transmitted infections. State agencies are funded primarily by federal sources (45%), state resources (24%), and Medicaid/Medicare (15%), with the remaining sources supplied by fines and fees (4%), indirect federal funding (3%), and other minor sources (9%) (ASTHO, 2009).

The Association of State and Territorial Health Officials

ASTHO is a not-for-profit organization that provides support for state and territorial health agencies. They provide research, expertise, and guidance for health policy issues. The federal government looks to ASTHO for their expertise in developing health policy. They frequently testify in front of Congress regarding major health issues. They advocate for increased public health funding and campaign against any funding reductions. ASTHO provides training opportunities for state public health leaders. All states and US territories and the District of Columbia belong to ASTHO (ASTHO, 2009).

Local Health Departments' Role in Health Care

Local health departments are the government organizations that provide the most direct services to the population. There are approximately 3000 local health departments across the United States (Pointer et al., 2007). Although their organizational structures may differ across the United States, their basic role is to provide direct public health services to their designated areas. It is difficult to generalize what types of services are offered by local health departments because they do vary according to geographic location, but most are involved in communicable disease control. According to a recent **National Association for County and City Health Officials** (NACCHO) survey, the following are highlights of what types of services are offered by local health departments:

- Nearly 75% of local health departments have a local board of health that support policy making.
- Over 90% offer child immunizations and adult immunizations either directly or indirectly through collaboration with local healthcare providers.
- Over two thirds provide sexually transmitted infection testing and treatment for those diseases.
- Nearly 75% offer treatment for tuberculosis.
- Approximately 60% provide family planning services.
- Approximately 70% offer tobacco prevention services.
- Nearly 70% provide women, infants, and children (WIC) services.
- Almost 90% of local health departments provide surveillance and assessment activities and environmental health protection.
- Approximately 75% provide food safety education (NACCHO, 2005).

Although funding for emergency preparedness has increased, local health departments, which fall under public health funding, are traditionally underfunded. Local health departments receive funding from their state government, the federal government, direct funding such as from the CDC, reimbursement for services from Medicaid and Medicare, private health insurance, and fees for services. Because of population size and coverage, local health department funding varies from state to state. Local sources are the greatest contributor to funding local health departments (29%), followed by state allocations (23%) and federal funding (13%). As a result of this continued lack of funding, more local health departments are collaborating with schools, community organizations, other local government organizations such as social services, and healthcare providers to provide services (NACCHO, 2009).

Regionalization of Local Health Departments

Over the last 10 years, there has been a trend to regionalize local health departments in order to maximize the service provided to their populations. Counties that normally provide health services separately have formed regional health departments, which means that smaller local health departments unite as one operation to provide services within a geographic area. This type of organizational restructure reduced redundancy in services. Usually, one larger county health department will serve as the leader of the region (Mays, 2008). For example, when bioterrorism grants were distributed, those regional areas received more funds than counties that were not regionalized. The **regionalization** in many states has been voluntary. Individual counties still have autonomy for funding and regulatory issues but have become more efficient in providing services regionally. Kansas and Massachusetts have developed regionalization projects to assess the effectiveness of this type of reorganization (Functional Regionalization, 2009).

Emergency Preparedness in Local Health Departments

Centers for Disease Control and Prevention Funding for Emergency Preparedness

As a result of the threat of bioterrorism to the United States, all local health departments' roles have changed since September 11, 2001. The CDC awarded funding to state health agencies who, in turn, allocated funding to the local health departments to develop plans for bioterrorism attacks. Although bioterrorism is a new public health threat, emergency preparedness also includes responses to natural disasters or disease outbreaks. The CDC has developed a checklist to guide local health departments when a disaster occurs. These activities should be included in their emergency preparedness plan:

- Assess the situation: The local health department has to assess the capability of the community and itself to respond quickly to a threat. It is also important to assess the impact of the threat.
- Epidemiologic capability and laboratory analyses: Local health departments should have a surveillance component in place to track susceptible populations and ensure access to laboratory services as needed.

- Communication: Communication protocols need to be in place for key health and medical agencies. The protocols should be practiced to ensure that when a public health threat occurs, the protocols will be implemented smoothly.
- Community reassurance: Address requests for assistance and information.
- Clinical interventions: Depending on the type of disaster, interventions must be readily available to the population.
- Coordination of healthcare systems: Coordinate with onsite federal and state assistance.
- Workforce training: It is vital that all workers involved in the disaster plan be trained. Volunteers also need to be trained so they understand the hierarchy of implementing a disaster plan.
- Special populations: Address the needs of the elderly, disabled, and young children.
- Legal issues: Stay apprised of any legal issues (CDC, 2009a).

National Association for County and City Health Officials

NACCHO is the advocacy organization for local health departments. Established in 1993 and located in Washington, DC, NACCHO provides support to nearly 3000 local health department members that include city, county, district, metro, and tribal agencies. They are staffed by nearly 100 physicians and public health experts and a 32-member board of directors that lobbies Congress for their public health agenda, promotes public health, and provides support for their members (NACCHO, 2009). Table 3-1 provides an outline of the local health departments' responsibilities according to NACCHO.

NACCHO also developed standards for local health department's activities. Activities include (1) food safety, (2) sanitation services, (3) waste disposal, (4) pest control, (5) drinking water purification, (6) restaurant inspection and licensing, (7) communicable disease surveillance, (8) control of sexually transmitted infections, and (9) public health education (Pointer et al., 2007). Other frequent local contributors to public health activities include social service agencies, elementary and secondary public schools, housing departments, fire and police departments, parks and recreation, libraries, waste management, and water and sewer authorities (Mays, Miller, & Halverson, 1999).

TABLE 3-1	Operational Definition of a Functional Local Health Department

- Monitor health status and understand community health issues.

- Protect people from health problems and health hazards.

- Provide information so individuals may make healthy choices.

- Engage the community to identify and solve health issues.

- Develop public health policies and plans.

- Enforce public health laws and regulations.

- Help people receive health services.

- Maintain a competent public health workforce.

- Evaluate and improve programs and interventions.

- Contribute to and apply the evidence base of public health.

Source: Operational Definition of a Functional Local Health Department. Washington, DC National Association of County and
City Health Officials, 2005.

NACCHO has recently focused on providing guidance to local health departments on ways to market public health activities and their role in public health. In collaboration with World Ways Social Marketing, NACCHO has developed a logo with the tagline of "Prevent, Promote, Protect," which can be used nationally by local health departments to help the public understand their role. NACCHO has also developed a communications toolkit with fact sheets regarding public health departments (NACCHO, 2009).

In May 2007, the **Public Health Accreditation Board** (PHAB) was established as a nonprofit organization to administer the voluntary, national accreditation program for state and local health departments based on the recommendations of the steering committee of the Exploring Accreditation project. Development of the program's components began in June 2007. The development process will allow sufficient time for the creation of a successful program, which will include:

- Development of standards and metrics for state and local health departments

- Creation of an assessment process for applicants

- Establishment of a process to determine recognition/approval of existing state-based accreditation programs

- Implementation of a pilot testing phase for state and local public health departments

Voluntary standards have been developed and are in the process of receiving public comments. It is anticipated that the first applications for accreditation will be accepted no later than winter 2011 (PHAB, 2009).

CONCLUSION

The government plays an important role in the quality of the US healthcare system. The federal government provides funding for state and local government programs. Federal healthcare regulations are implemented and enforced at the state and local levels. Funding is primarily distributed from the federal government to the state government, which consequently allocates funding to their local health departments. Local health departments provide the majority of services for their constituents. More local health departments are working with local organizations such as schools and physicians to increase their ability to provide services such as immunizations, education, and prevention services.

NACCHO and ASTHO are important support organizations for both state and local governments by providing policy expertise, technical advice, and lobbying at the federal level for appropriate funding and regulations. DHS and FEMA now play an integral role in the management and oversight of any catastrophic events such as natural disasters, earthquakes, floods, pandemic diseases, and bioterrorism. DHS and FEMA collaborate closely with the CDC to ensure that both the state and local health departments have a crisis management plan in place for these events. These attacks are often horrific and frightening with a tremendous loss of life, and as a result, the state and local health departments need to be more prepared to deal with catastrophic events. They are required to develop plans and be trained to deal effectively with many of these catastrophic issues.

PREVIEW OF CHAPTER FOUR

According to the Institute of Medicine (IOM), the concept of public health is an organized community effort that addresses health issues in the community by applying specific knowledge to promote health (IOM, 2008). Chapter 4 will discuss the concept of public health and its vital role in the US healthcare system. This chapter will discuss the history of public health and core public health activities including the collaboration of public health in natural disasters and terrorist activities. The chapter will also address the collaboration of public health and traditional medicine. As a consumer, public health is very important to you because public health activities focus on the collective health of your community. Public health officials are focused on ensuring there are programs in place for primary prevention activities such as education and screening for disease.

VOCABULARY

Administration for Children and Families (ACF)

Administration on Aging (AOA)

Agency for Healthcare Research and Quality (AHRQ)

Agency for Toxic Substances and Disease Registry (ATSDR)

Association of State and Territorial Health Officials (ASTHO)

Center for Mental Health Services (CMHS)

Center for Substance Abuse Prevention (CSAP)

Center for Substance Abuse Treatment (CSAT)

Centers for Disease Control and Prevention (CDC)

Centers for Medicare and Medicaid Services (CMS)

Coalition for Health Services Research (CHSR)

Council of State and Territorial Epidemiologists (CSTE)

Department of Homeland Security (DHS)

Federal Emergency Management Agency (FEMA)

Federal Food, Drug, and Cosmetic Act (FDCA)

Hazard Communication Standard (HCS)

Health Resources and Services Administration (HRSA)

Indian Health Service (IHS)

Local health departments

Medical Waste Tracking Act

Morbidity and Mortality Weekly Report (MMWR)

National Association for County and City Health Officials (NACCHO)

National Incident Management System (NIMS)

National Institutes of Health (NIH)

National Network on Aging (NNOA)

National Response Framework (NRF)

Occupational Exposure to Bloodborne Pathogen Standard

Occupational Safety and Health Administration (OSHA)

Office of Applied Studies (OAS)

Older Americans Act (OAA)

Over-the-counter (OTC) drugs

Public Health Accreditation Board (PHAB)

Regionalization

Social regulation

Social Security Act

State health departments

Substance Abuse and Mental Health Services Administration (SAMHSA)

Surgeon General

US Department of Health and Human Services (HHS)

US Food and Drug Administration (FDA)

US Public Health Service Corps

REFERENCES

Administration for Children and Families. (2009). Retrieved November 9, 2009, from http://www.acf.hhs.gov/acf_about.html#mission.

Administration on Aging. (2009). Retrieved November 9, 2009, from http://www.aoa.gov/AoARoot/About/index.aspx.

Agency for Healthcare Research and Quality. (2009). Retrieved November 9, 2009, from http://www.ahrq.gov/about/profile.htm.

Agency for Toxic Substances and Disease Registry. (2009). Retrieved November 9, 2009, from http://www.atsdr.cdc.gov/about/mission_vision_goals.html.

Association of State and Territorial Health Officials. (2009). Retrieved November 9, 2009, from http://www.astho.org/about/.

Buchbinder, S., & Shanks, S. (2007). *Introduction to health care management*. Sudbury, MA: Jones and Bartlett.

Carroll, A., & Buchholtz, A. (2006). *Business and society: Ethics and stakeholder management*. Mason, OH: Southwestern Learning.

Centers for Disease Control and Prevention. (2009a). *Public health emergency response guide for state, local, and tribal public health directors*. Retrieved July 15, 2009, from http://www.bt.cdc.gov/planning/responseguide.asp.

Centers for Disease Control and Prevention. (2009b). Retrieved March 12, 2009, from http://www.cdc.gov.

Centers for Medicare and Medicaid Services. (2009). Retrieved November 9, 2009, from http://www.cms.hhs.gov/home/aboutcms.asp.

Coalition for Health Services Research. (2009). Retrieved November 9, 2009, from http://www.chsr.org/about.htm.

Council of State and Territorial Epidemiologists. (2009). Retrieved November 9, 2009, from http://www.cste.org/dnn/AboutCSTE/AboutCSTE/tabid/56/Default.aspx.

Department of Homeland Security. (2009). Retrieved November 9, 2009, from http://www.dhs.gov/xabout/index.shtm.

Functional Regionalization Project. (2009). Retrieved November 9, 2009, from http://www.kalhd.org/en/cms/?1109.

Health and Human Services. (2009). Retrieved November 9, 2009, from http://www.hhs.gov/about/.

Health Resources and Services Administration. (2009). Retrieved November 9, 2009, from http://www.hrsa.gov/about/budgetjustification09/performance/StrategicPlan.htm.

Indian Health Service. (2009). Retrieved November 9, 2009, from http://www.ihs.gov/PublicInfo/PublicAffairs/Welcome_Info/IHSintro.asp.

Institute of Medicine of the National Academies. (2008). Retrieved November 9, 2009, from http://www.iom.edu/en/About-IOM.aspx.

Jonas, S. (2003). *An introduction to the U.S. health care system* (pp. 17–45). New York: Springer Publishing.

Mays, G. (2008). Organization of the public health delivery system. In L. Novick & C. Morrow (Eds.). *Public health administration: Principles for population-based management* (pp. 69–126). Sudbury, MA: Jones and Bartlett.

Mays, G., Miller, C., & Halverson, P. (1999). *Local public health practice: Trends and models*. Washington, DC: American Public Health Association.

National Association of County and City Health Officials. (2005). *Operational definition of a functional local health department*. Retrieved March 31, 2009, from http://www.naccho.org/topics/infrastructure/accreditation/upload/OperationalDefinitionBrochure-2.pdf.

National Association for County and City Health Officials. (2009). Retrieved November 9, 2009, from http://www.naccho.org/topics/infrastructure/profile/index.cfm.

National Institutes of Health. (2009). Retrieved November 9, 2009, from http://www.nih.gov/about/NIHoverview.

Occupational Safety and Health Administration. (2009). Retrieved November 9, 2009, from http://www.osha.gov/about.html.

Office of the Surgeon General. (2009). Retrieved November 9, 2009, from http://www.surgeongeneral.gov/about/index.html.

Pointer, D., Williams, S., Isaacs, S., & Knickman, J. (2007). *Introduction to U.S. health care*. Hoboken, NJ: Wiley Publishing.

Public Health Accreditation Board. (2009). Retrieved November 9, 2009, from http://www.phaboard.org/about/.

Substance Abuse and Mental Health Services Administration. (2009). Retrieved November 9, 2009, from http://www.oas.samhsa.gov/.

Turnock, B. (2007). *Essentials of public health*. Sudbury, MA: Jones and Bartlett.

US Food and Drug Administration. (2009a). Retrieved November 9, 2009, from http://www.fda.gov/RegulatoryInformation/Legislation/FederalFoodDrugandCosmeticActFDCAct/default.htm.

US Food and Drug Administration. (2009b). Retrieved November 9, 2009, from http://www.fda.gov/AboutFDA/WhatWeDo/WhatFDARegulates/default.htm.

Walshe, K., & Shortell, S. (2004). Social regulation of health care organizations in the United States: Developing a framework for evaluation. *Health Services Management, 17*, 79–99.

CROSSWORD PUZZLE

Instructions: Please complete the puzzle using the vocabulary words found in the chapter. There may be multiple-word answers. The number in the parenthesis indicates the number of words in the answer.

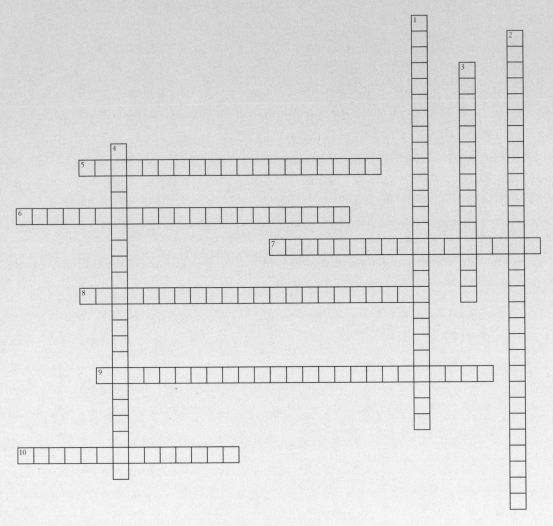

Created with EclipseCrossword © 1999–2009 Green Eclipse

STUDENT ACTIVITY 3-1

Across

5. Their mission is to raise the physical, mental, social, and spiritual health of American Indians and Alaskan Natives to their highest level. (3 words)

6. State and local health departments are required to have this type of plan in place for catastrophic events such as bioterrorism. (2 words)

7. This 1935 Act increased the government's role in providing healthcare coverage. (3 words)

8. This federal government agency has 11 operating divisions. (4 words)

9. This federal agency was established as a result of the 1906 Food, Drug, and Cosmetic Act. (4 words)

10. This person is the chief health educator in the United States. (2 words)

Down

1. This federal agency has 27 institutes that focus on diseases and conditions. (4 words)

2. Established as a nonprofit organization to administer the voluntary national accreditation program for state and local health departments. (4 words)

3. This process combined several small local health departments into one larger health department to serve as the leader. (1 word)

4. This federal agency is one of the largest providers of home- and community-based care for older persons. (3 words)

STUDENT ACTIVITY 3-2

IN YOUR OWN WORDS

Based on Chapter 3, please provide a description of the following concepts in your own words. DO NOT RECITE the text description.

Over-the-counter (OTC) drugs:

_____

_____

_____

Hazard Communication Standard:

_____

_____

_____

Regionalization of public health departments:

_____

_____

_____

Administration on Aging:

_____

_____

_____

National Network on Aging:

_____

_____

_____

US Public Health Service Corps:

_____

_____

_____

Morbidity and Mortality Weekly Report:

_____

_____

_____

National Incident Management System:

_____

_____

_____

STUDENT ACTIVITY 3-2

Association of State and Territorial Health Officials:

_____

_____

_____

US Surgeon General:

_____

_____

_____

STUDENT ACTIVITY 3-3

REAL LIFE APPLICATIONS: CASE STUDY

You will be graduating from college soon with a degree in healthcare management. You are considering different career choices and would like to work for the government. You are thinking of applying to both state and local health departments but are unsure of what types of activities you may be involved with as a healthcare manager.

ACTIVITY

(1) Discuss the role that state and local health departments have in health care, (2) identify the services that are provided by both levels, (3) using the Internet, look up the state and local health departments in your state and provide an overview of their activities, and (4) decide on where you are going to apply and explain your decision.

RESPONSES

_____

_____

_____

_____

_____

_____

_____

_____

_____

_____

_____

_____

_____

_____

_____

STUDENT ACTIVITY 3-4

INTERNET EXERCISES

Write your answers in the space provided.

- Visit each of the Web sites listed here.
- Name the organization.
- Locate their mission statement on their Web site.
- Provide a brief overview of the activities of the organization.
- How do these organizations participate in the US healthcare system?

Web Sites

http://www.atsdr.cdc.gov

Organization Name: _____

Mission Statement:

_____

_____

_____

Overview of Activities:

_____

_____

_____

Importance of organization to US health care:

_____

_____

_____

http://www.hrsa.gov

Organization Name: _____

Mission Statement:

_____

_____

_____

Overview of Activities:

_____

_____

_____

STUDENT ACTIVITY 3-4

Importance of organization to US health care:

_____

_____

_____

http://www.fda.gov

Organization Name: _____

Mission Statement:

_____

_____

_____

Overview of Activities:

_____

_____

_____

Importance of organization to US health care:

_____

_____

_____

www.ihs.gov

Organization Name: _____

Mission Statement:

_____

_____

_____

Overview of Activities:

_____

_____

_____

Importance of organization to US health care:

_____

_____

_____

STUDENT ACTIVITY 3-4

http://www.aoa.gov

Organization Name: _____

Mission Statement:

_____

_____

_____

Overview of Activities:

_____

_____

_____

Importance of organization to US health care:

_____

_____

_____

http://www.acf.hhs.gov

Organization Name: _____

Mission Statement:

_____

_____

_____

Overview of Activities:

_____

_____

_____

Importance of organization to US health care:

_____

_____

_____

Chapter 4

Public Health's Role in Health Care

LEARNING OBJECTIVES

The student will be able to:

- Define and discuss the determinants of health.

- Describe the core public health functions of assessment, policy, and assurance and their role in public health organizations.

- Define and discuss the epidemiology triangle and its importance to public health.

- Analyze five major public health issues.

- Evaluate the roles of John Snow, Lemuel Shattuck, and Edwin Chadwick in the development of public health.

- Analyze the importance of data and surveillance systems in public health policy.

DID YOU KNOW THAT?

- In 1842, Edwin Chadwick reported that the poor had higher rates of disease—a fact that still exists today.

- Established in 1905, the civic organization Rotary International has played a huge role in eradicating polio through international vaccine programs.

- In 1916, the Johns Hopkins University, located in Baltimore, Maryland, established the first school of public health.

- In 1992, a national exercise program for Medicare patients, Silver Sneakers, was created to provide free access to organized exercise at national fitness chains.

- Established in 2001, the Department of Homeland Security, the federal agency responsible for national security, has become an integral component of public health policy because of the continual threat of terrorist activities on US soil.

- In 2002, the federal government provided grants to hospitals and public health organizations to prepare for bioterrorism attacks on the United States.

INTRODUCTION

There are two important definitions of public health. In 1920, **public health** was defined by Charles Winslow as the science and art of preventing disease, prolonging life, and promoting physical health and efficiency through organized community efforts for the sanitation of the environment, control of community infections, and education of individuals regarding hygiene to ensure a standard of living for health maintenance (Winslow, 1920). Sixty years later, the **Institute of Medicine** (IOM), in its 1988 *Future of Public Health* report, defined public health as an organized community effort to address public health by applying scientific and technical knowledge to promote health (IOM, 1988). Both definitions point to broad community efforts to promote health activities to protect the population's health status.

The development of public health is important to note as part of the basics of the US healthcare system because its development was separate from the development of private medicine practices. Public health specialists view health from a collectivist and preventative care viewpoint: to protect as many citizens as possible from health issues and to provide strategies to prevent health issues from occurring. The definitions cited in the previous paragraph emphasize this viewpoint. Public health concepts were in stark contrast to traditional medicine, which focused on the sole relationship between a provider and patient. Private practitioners held an individualistic viewpoint—citizens more often would be paying for their services from their health insurance or from their own pockets. Physicians would be providing their patients guidance on how to cure their diseases, not preventing disease.

This chapter will discuss the concept of health and healthcare delivery and the role of public health in delivering health care. The concepts of primary, secondary, and tertiary prevention and the role of public health in those delivery activities will be highlighted. Discussion will also focus on the origins of public health, the major role epidemiology plays in public health, the role of public health in disasters, core public health activities, the collaboration of public health and private medicine, and the importance of public health consumers.

WHAT IS HEALTH?

The World Health Organization (WHO) defines **health** as the state of complete physical, mental, and social well-being and not merely the absence of disease or infirmity (WHO, 2008). IOM defines health as a state of well-being and the capability to function in the face of changing circumstances. It is a positive concept emphasizing social and personal resources as well as physical capabilities (IOM, 1997). According to the Society for Academic Emergency Medicine (SAEM), health is a state of physical and mental well-being that facilitates the achievement of individual and societal goals (SAEM, 1992). All of these definitions focus on the impact an individual's health status has on their quality of life.

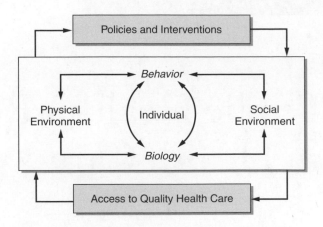

Figure 4-1 (From US Department of Health and Human Services. Available at http://www.healthypeople.gov.)

As indicated in Figure 4-1, health has several **determinants** or influences that impact the status of an individual's health. Within the immediate environment of an individual, there is the social and physical environment—external influences on health. The **physical environment** would include pollutants, hazardous exposure at work, water contamination, etc. The **social environment** would include socioeconomic status, which relates directly to quality of health. Individuals with a higher income level are less exposed to environmental risks and have increased access to quality health care. The individual's health status is also impacted by their personal behavior and their biology or genetic makeup. An individual's **lifestyle** or **behavior** includes diet, exercise, sexual activity, and stressful job, which all have an impact on health. Also, **genetic factors** or a **person's biology** predispose individuals to certain diseases. The **determinants of health** depicted here tie into the role of public health in the healthcare delivery system because public health focuses on the impact of these determinants on an individual's health. Public health provides health education and other preventive activities to a consumer so they will understand the negative impact these determinants may have on their health status. These activities are often categorized as primary, secondary, and occasionally tertiary prevention.

PRIMARY, SECONDARY, AND TERTIARY PREVENTION

Primary prevention activities focus on reducing disease development. Smoking cessation programs, immunization programs, educational programs for pregnancy, and employee safety education are all examples of primary prevention programs. **Secondary prevention** activities refer to early detection and treatment of diseases. The goal of secondary prevention is to stop the progression of disease. Blood pressure screenings, colonoscopies, and mammograms are examples of secondary prevention. **Tertiary prevention** activities focus on activities to rehabilitate and monitor individuals during disease progression. Activities may also include patient behavior education to limit disease impact and reduce progression (Shi & Singh, 2008). Although public health professionals may participate in each area of prevention activities, they focus primarily on primary and secondary prevention.

ORIGINS OF PUBLIC HEALTH

During the 18th and 19th centuries, the concept of public health was born. Edwin Chadwick, Dr. John Snow, and Lemuel Shattuck demonstrated a relationship between the environment and disease that established the foundation of public health.

In 1842, **Edwin Chadwick** published the *General Report on the Sanitary Condition of the Labouring Population of Great Britain*. His report highlighted the relationship between unsanitary conditions and disease (Rosen, 1958). As Chief Commissioner of the Poor Law Commission, Chadwick was responsible for relief to the poor in England and Wales. He became the champion of reform for working conditions. His report illustrated that the poor had higher rates of disease than the upper class, a fact that still exists today. His activities became the basis for US public health activities (Rosen, 1958). He was also responsible for the implementation of the 1848 Public Health Act, which created England's first national board of health. Unfortunately, in 1854, the Parliament did not renew the Act which consequently dissolved the board of health. Although dissolved, the concept of public health was born because this act, using data, identified several public health issues that were assigned to national and local boards (Ashton & Sram, 1998). Public health issues such as water, sewerage, environment, safety, and food were a focus of the act. By identifying these community issues, they were focused on improving the community's health status (Ashton & Sram, 1998).

Dr. John Snow, a famed British anesthesiologist, is more famous for investigating the cholera epidemics in London in the 1800s. He made the connection between contaminated water and the spread of cholera. Dr. Snow surveyed local London residents

and discovered that those who were ill had retrieved water from a specific neighborhood pump on Broad Street. When the pump handle was removed, the disease ceased. This famous Broad Street pump incident became a classic example of an epidemiologic investigation that studies the causes between disease and external sources (Ellis, 2008).

During the same time, in the United States, **Lemuel Shattuck** in his *Census of Boston* report discussed high mortality rates among lower income populations and unsanitary living conditions. In 1850, he published a plan for health promotion to combat unsanitary conditions. He was considered the American advocate for environmental health (Rosen, 1958).

As a result of their work, public health law was enacted and, by the 1900s, public health departments were focused on the environment and its relationship to disease outbreaks. Disease control and health education also became integral components of public health departments.

WHAT IS PUBLIC HEALTH?

A Discussion of Core and Essential Public Health Functions

In 1945, in conjunction with Haven Emerson and CEA Winslow, the American Public Health Association (APHA) issued a set of guidelines for the basic functions of the local health department, including:

- Vital statistics: data management of the essential facts births, deaths, and reportable diseases
- Communicable disease control: management of tuberculosis, venereal disease, and malaria
- Sanitation: management of the environment including milk, water, and dining
- Laboratory services
- Maternal and child health: management of school aged children's health
- Health education of the general public (Emerson, 1945)

These functions remained the cornerstone of public health until the 1960s when the APHA, reacting to cultural and political changes, revised the definition of the core public health functions. The APHA issued the following guidelines for the core public health functions:

- Health surveillance, planning, and program development

- Health promotion of local health activities
- Development and enforcement of sanitation standards
- Health services provisions (APHA, 2008)

The IOM, as a result of an in-depth study of public health, stated that the three **core public health functions** of public health are:

- Assessment, which includes surveillance, identifying problems, data collection, and analysis
- Policy development, which includes developing policies to address public problems
- Assurance, which includes evaluation of policies meeting program goals (IOM, 1988)

These core public health functions became accepted by public health departments; however, there was some confusion about the terminology. In 1994, the Public Health Steering Committee, as part of the US Public Health Service, issued a list of essential public health services that provided specific information on the implementation of the core public health functions and how they should be implemented.

These services include:

- Monitoring community health status
- Diagnosing and investigating community health problems
- Educating people about potential health problems
- Developing community partnerships to resolve health problems
- Developing policies that support individual and community health problems
- Enforcing laws and regulations that protect community and individual health
- Sustaining a competent healthcare workforce
- Evaluating the effectiveness, access, and long-term sustainability of community health services
- Linking people to needed health services
- Researching and developing health problem solutions (APHA, 2008)

THE EPIDEMIOLOGY TRIANGLE

Epidemiology is the study of disease distribution and patterns among populations. Epidemiologists search for the relationship of those patterns of disease to the causes of the disease. They scientifically collect data to

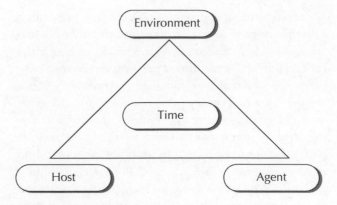

Figure 4-2 (From Centers for Disease Control and Prevention. Available at http://www.bam.gov.)

determine what has caused the spread of the disease. Epidemiology is the foundation for public health because its focus is to prevent disease from reoccurring (Centers for Disease Control and Prevention [CDC], 2008b). Epidemiologists identify three major risk factor categories for disease. These three factors are called the **epidemiology triangle** (Figure 4-2) that consists of the host, which is the population that has the disease; the agent or organism, which is causing the disease; and the environment, or where the disease is occurring (CDC, 2009a). Public health workers attempt to assess each factor's role in why a disease occurs. Based on this research, public health workers develop prevention strategies to alter the interaction between the host, disease, and the environment so the disease occurrences will be less severe or will not occur again.

For example, a person (host) can be vaccinated against a disease to prevent the host from carrying the disease (agent). Procedures can be implemented such as sanitary regulations to protect the community condition (environment) from contamination.

EPIDEMIOLOGIC SURVEILLANCE

An important component of epidemiology is **surveillance**, which is the monitoring of patterns of disease and investigating disease outbreaks to develop public health intervention strategies to combat disease. A new form of surveillance involves **biosurveillance**, which focuses on early detection of unusual disease patterns that may be due to human intervention. Historically, surveillance activities have been passive and been initiated by public health workers through routine disease reports. However, public health has become more proactive by initiating contact with providers to assess any unusual disease pattern. New surveillance techniques can include pattern recognition software and geographic information systems to determine disease patterns (Turnock, 2007). Depending on the severity of the disease outbreaks, these activities will be investigated by the CDC, a federal public health agency, although public health mostly remains a state responsibility.

ENVIRONMENTAL HEALTH

Since John Snow linked disease with environmental factors, the field of **environmental health** is an integral component of public health. Environmental health workers often are responsible for investigating environmental hazards in the community and monitoring and enforcing environmental regulations. A subset of environmental health workers is occupational health workers who focus on ensuring employees' environments have safe working conditions. Both state and local health departments have environmental health departments who are responsible for investigating and enforcing local regulations.

EMERGENCY PREPAREDNESS

Federal Response

Public health emergency preparedness is a term used for planning protocols that are in place to manage a large scale event such as a natural disaster like a hurricane or massive flooding, or a manmade disaster such as a terrorist attack like September 11, 2001. During a public health emergency, such as Hurricane Katrina in Louisiana and food contamination outbreaks in 2008 with salmonella cases nationwide, risk communication protocols are implemented to inform the public regarding the health issue and what the public should do during a severe situation. Dissemination of information is handled through multimedia efforts such as the radio, television, and print media. Depending on the level of disease threat, the federal government may intervene in a disease outbreak. If not, state and local public health departments are responsible for monitoring the disease threat. Unfortunately, severe public health crises such as these noted can create secondary disease threats. These crises also can have an extreme psychological impact on the public. The public needs to be informed. Since the terrorist attacks in 2001, simulations of public health emergencies have been staged across vulnerable areas of the United States like large urban areas such as New York City and Las Vegas to plan for these possible events. Public health funding

for state activities such as these are largely from CDC grants and budget allocations (Turnock, 2007).

September 11, 2001, Terrorist Attack Impact on Public Health

As result of the terrorist attacks on the United States in 2001, the Department of Homeland Security (DHS) was created from 23 federal agencies, programs, and offices to coordinate an approach to emergencies and disasters. Several public health functions were transferred to the DHS in 2003 (Turnock, 2007). Within the DHS, the Emergency Preparedness and Response Directorate coordinates emergency medical response in the event of a public health emergency. Some states have created their own Homeland Security offices that coordinate with the federal DHS.

The **National Response Framework** (NRF), created by DHS, presents the guiding principles that enable all response partners to prepare for and provide a unified national response to disasters and emergencies. It establishes a comprehensive, national, all-hazards approach to domestic incident response. The National Response Plan was replaced by the NRF effective March 22, 2008 (Federal Emergency Management Agency [FEMA], 2008).

The NRF defines the principles, roles, and structures that organize how we respond as a nation. The NRF describes how communities, states, the federal government, the private sector, and nongovernment partners collaborate to coordinate national response and describes "best practices" for managing incidents and builds on the **National Incident Management System** (NIMS), which provides a framework for managing incidents. Information on the NRF including documents, annexes, references, and briefings/trainings can be accessed from the NRF Resource Center (FEMA, 2008).

STATE AND LOCAL RESPONSE TO DISASTERS

Incident Command System and Public Health

Incident Command System (ICS) is used by police, fire, and emergency management agencies. ICS eliminates many communication problems, spans of control, organizational structures, and differences in terminology when multiple agencies respond to emergency events (FEMA, 2008). The ICS is a coordinator for an emergency event. They are in control of a situation and make decisions about how to manage an emergency. They coordinate all responders to the event, which increases management effectiveness. Local public health agencies work with first responders such as fire and rescue, emergency medical service, law enforcement, physicians, and hospitals in managing health-related emergencies. Most local public health agencies provide epidemiology and surveillance, food safety, communicable disease control, and health inspections. Many state public health agencies provide laboratory services.

Public health has traditionally been underfunded from federal sources. As a consequence of medicine's focus on technology, the medical establishment has relegated public health to a level of minor importance (Shi & Singh, 2008). Because public health is now considered an integral component to battling terrorism and, consequently, a matter of national security, federal funding has dramatically increased. Since 2002, the federal budget for public health activities at all government levels increased by $2 billion with continued funding through the next 5 years (Turnock, 2007).

BIOTERRORISM: A NEW PUBLIC HEALTH THREAT

According to the CDC, **bioterrorism** is an attack on a population by deliberately releasing viruses, bacteria, or other germs or agents that will contribute to illness or death in people (CDC, 2008a). These can be spread throughout the environment through the air, water, or in food. These agents can be difficult to detect and may take a period of time to spread. DHS, American Red Cross (ARC), the American Medical Association (AMA), and the Environmental Protection Agency (EPA) have developed educational campaigns regarding the US response to bioterrorism. Since the September 11, 2001, terrorist attack on the United States, bioterrorism has become a reality.

More than 20 federal departments and agencies have roles in preparing for a bioterrorist attack. In 2002, the **Public Health Security and Bioterrorism Preparedness and Response Act** provided grants to hospitals and public health organizations to prepare for bioterrorism as a result of September 11, 2001. Funding will support increased public health infrastructures and programs, increase laboratory testing, and develop programs to detect bioterrorist threats. The **US Food and Drug Administration** (FDA) also has additional responsibilities in the detection of food as a threat to community health (FDA, 2009).

Bioterrorism preparedness involves federal, state, and local health departments as well as input from other organizations. When a disaster occurs such as a bioterrorist attack, responses from both the federal and state level may take 24 hours; therefore, it is vital that local health departments, because they are at the front line of public health interventions, need to have a plan in place for immediate intervention. In terms of emergency responders, local health departments are the frontline organizations to assess an emergency situation (Turnock, 2007).

PUBLIC HEALTH FUNCTIONS AND ADMINISTRATION

Accreditation of Public Health Departments

The 2003 IOM report discussed previously recommends a national accreditation system for public health agencies because there is no national accrediting body to institute standards. In 2004, the CDC and the Robert Wood Johnson Foundation (RWJF) funded a study, the **Exploring Accreditation Project** (EAP), to assess accreditation of public health agencies.

Mobilizing for Action through Planning and Partnership

The cooperative agreement of Mobilizing for Action through Planning and Partnership (MAPP), between the CDC and the **National Association of County and City Health Officials** (NACCHO), is a strategic plan for community health. A strategic or long-range plan for community health is developed based on a community health assessment, which is an evaluation of the health program needs for the local community. Based on the needs assessment of the community, a long-range plan is developed that establishes goals and a set of actions to accomplish these goals. This tool is an interactive tool for public health departments that can enhance their performance. Communities such as Chicago and San Antonio are examples of MAPP utilization (NACCHO, 2009).

The Influence of the Institute of Medicine Reports on Public Health Functions

Published in 1988, the IOM published a report, *The Future of Public Health*, which indicated that although the health of the American people has been accomplished through public health measures such as consumer food regulations, water safety standards, and epidemic control of disease, the public has come to take public health measures for granted. The report indicated that there was an attrition of public health activities in protecting the community because of this attitude (IOM, 1988). The report established recommendations for reorganizing public health that emphasized population-based strategies rather than personal healthcare delivery. There was poor collaboration between public health and private medicine, no strong mission statement, weak leadership, and politicized decision making. Three core public health functions were identified: **assessment**, **policy development**, and **assurance**. Assessment was recommended because it focused on systematic continuous data collection of health issues, which would ensure that public health agencies were vigilant in protecting the public. Policy development was also mentioned but the recommendation was to ensure that any policies were based on valid data to avoid any political decision making. Policy development was recommended to include planning at all health levels, not just at the federal level. Federal agencies should support local health planning. Assurance focused on evaluating any processes that had been put in place to assure that the programs were being implemented appropriately (IOM, 1988). These core functions will ensure that public health remains focused on the community, has programs in place that are effective, and has an evaluation process in place to ensure that the programs do work.

In 2002, the IOM published a second more in-depth report, *The Future of the Public's Health in the 21st Century*, based on the 1988 report that analyzed public health as a system and discussed several deficiencies first noted in their 1988 report. Deficiencies included:

- Fragmented government public health infrastructures
- Passive community participation in public health activities
- Lack of healthcare delivery coordination
- Lack of participation of businesses in influencing health activities
- Lack of coordination of media with the health arena
- Lack of academic institutions in community-based health activities

Recommendations to rectify these deficiencies included:

- Development of a national commission to establish a framework for state public health law reform
- Development of active partnerships between public health agencies and communities
- Insurance plans should offer preventive services as part of their plans
- Businesses should collaborate with communities to develop health promotion programs
- Media outlets should increase their public service announcements to include health promotion marketing
- Increase funding for researchers who are interested in public health practice research (IOM, 2002)

HEALTHY PEOPLE REPORTS

The **Healthy People** series is a federal public health planning tool that assesses the most significant health threats and sets objectives to challenge these threats (Novick & Morrow, 2008). The first major report, published in 1979, *Healthy People: The Surgeon General's Report on Health Promotion and Disease Prevention*, discussed five goals of public health: reduce mortality rates among children, adolescents, young adults, and adults and increase independence among older adults. Objectives were set for 1990 to accomplish these goals (US Department of Health and Human Services [HHS], 1979).

The **Healthy People 2000** report released in 1990, the *National Health Promotion and Disease Prevention Objectives*, was created to implement a new national prevention strategy with three major goals: increase life expectancy, reduce health disparities, and increase access to preventive services. Three categories (health promotion, health prevention, and preventive services) and surveillance activities were emphasized. Healthy People 2000 provided a vision to reduce preventable disabilities and death. Year 2000 target objectives were set throughout the years to measure progress. An evaluation report in 2002 found that only 21% of the objectives were met with an additional 41% indicating progress. Unfortunately, in the critical areas of mental health, there were significant reversals in any progress. There was also minor progress in the areas chronic diseases and diabetes (CDC, 2009b).

The **Healthy People 2010** report, *Understanding and Improving Health*, based on the previous Healthy People reports and their progress, was released in 2000 (HHS, 2000). The report contained a health promotion and disease prevention focus to identify preventable threats to public health and to set goals to reduce the threats. They had two major goals: to increase the quality and years of healthy life and to eliminate health disparities. Nearly 500 objectives were developed according to 28 focus areas. Focus areas ranged from access to care, food safety, education, and environmental health to tobacco and substance abuse. An important component of the Healthy People 2010 was the development of an infrastructure to ensure public health services are provided in a systematic approach. Infrastructure includes skilled labor, information technology, organizations, and research (CDC, 2008b). Like Healthy People 2000, its major goals were to increase quality and life expectancy and to reduce health disparities. The goals for these reports are consistent with both Winslow's and the IOM's definitions of public health.

PUBLIC HEALTH INFRASTRUCTURE

US public health activities are delivered by many organizations, including government agencies at the federal, state, and local levels and nongovernment organizations including healthcare providers, community organizations, educational institutions, charitable organizations, philanthropic organizations, and businesses (Mays, 2008).

GOVERNMENT CONTRIBUTIONS TO PUBLIC HEALTH

Federal

The federal government has the ability to formulate and implement a national policy agenda for public health (Lee, 1994). It also has the power to allocate funding to both government and nongovernment organizations for public health programs at the state government level. If there is a major health threat in a community, direct federal activity may occur such as investigating a disease outbreak or providing assistance during a major disaster. The majority of their activities focus on policy and regulatory development and funding allocation to public health programs. The major federal agency responsible for public health

activities is HHS. They are responsible for the following activities:

- Data gathering and analysis, and surveillance and control
- Conducting and funding research
- Providing assistance to state and local government programs
- Formulating health policy
- Ensuring food and drug safety
- Ensuring access to health services for the poor and elderly
- Providing direct services to special populations (Pointer, Williams, Isaacs, & Knickman, 2007)

State

State public health agencies follow two basic models: a freestanding agency structure that reports directly to the state's governor or an organizational unit with a larger agency structure that includes other healthcare activities. The key feature of state agencies is their relationship with their local public health agencies that are responsible for implementing state policy and regulations. Most states have public health activities distributed across many agencies which include environmental protection, human services, labor, insurance, transportation, housing, and agriculture (Mays, 2008).

Additional activities include:

- Licensure of healthcare professionals
- Inspection and licensure of healthcare facilities
- Collection of vital statistics
- Epidemiologic studies
- Crisis management of disease outbreaks
- Disease registry
- Laboratory services
- Implementation and analysis of health policy
- Community health education (Pointer et al., 2007)

Local

Local government agencies are directly responsible for performing the majority of community public health services. On November 1, 2005, NACCHO, which is the national advocacy organization for local health departments, released the operational definition of a local health department, which is defined as the "public health government entity at a local level including a locally governed health department, state-created district, department serving a multi-county area or any other arrangement with governmental authority and responsibilities for public health at the local level" (NACCHO, 2009).

The 2003 IOM report *The Future of Public Health in the 21st Century* recommended a voluntary national accreditation program for public health agencies that would create national standards for their agencies. In 2004, RWJF and CDC funded the EAP to assess the feasibility of their recommendation. The Steering Committee of the EAP made the following recommendations: (1) have an objective administrator to administer the program, (2) there are 11 areas for standard development, (3) have financing options to support the accreditation process, (4) include performance incentives to maintain accreditation, and (5) include a program evaluation component (Bender et al., 2007).

NATIONAL ACCREDITATION OF PUBLIC HEALTH AGENCIES

The 1988 IOM report made recommendations to improve the public health system. Based on the report, the RWJF funded the **Turning Point**, which provided funding to 21 states for 6 years to assess the public health system. Interviews were conducted of public health administrators in 17 states who indicated repeatedly that they needed guidance on how to maximize their funding through comprehensive planning and developing strategic partnerships (RWJF, 2008). The Turning Point initiative has facilitated the development of valuable partnerships, gave public health partners experience and training in planning and collaboration, and helped communities and public health agencies understand the need for effective public health infrastructures. In spring 2002, the CDC asked public health departments to write emergency preparedness plans for their states. Many Turning Point states found they were at an advantage because of their Turning Point work, which had laid the groundwork for effective collaboration and comprehensive planning that enabled them to move into the planning and application process effectively (Bekemeier, Riley, Padgett, & Berkowitz, 2007).

NONGOVERNMENT PUBLIC HEALTH ACTIVITIES

Community hospitals have been important to public health. The Hill-Burton Act of 1943, which financed hospital construction projects, required them to provide charitable services, which established a tradition of charitable services among community hospitals.

Hospitals may operate primary care clinics and sponsor health education programs and health screening fairs. The Joint Commission on Accreditation of Healthcare Organizations (now The Joint Commission [TJC]) requires hospitals to participate in community health assessment activities (TJC, 2009).

Ambulatory or outpatient care providers such as physician practices also contribute to community public health. Physicians may serve on local public health organizations or provide services to the uninsured for reduced fees. Hospitals, clinics, and nursing homes may also contribute to public health. Health insurers and managed care providers also make important public health contributions. All types of healthcare providers cooperate with state and local health departments by providing immunizations, offering patient education, screening for communicable diseases, and reporting disease information to health departments (Pointer et al., 2007). Health insurers and managed care providers have a large network of clients to encourage health promotion and health education activities. For example, a physical activity program for senior citizens, **Silver Sneakers**, was developed in 1992 and encouraged the elderly to participate in organized exercise at national fitness chains. Data is being collected to assess if those seniors visited their providers less because their health status increased. It is a free program to Medicare or Medicare supplement participants (Healthways Silver Sneakers Fitness Program, 2008).

Nonprofit agencies such as the **American Cancer Society**, **American Heath Association**, and **American Lung Association** have active health promotion and health screening programs at the national, state, and local levels. The **United Way** is a civic organization that is active in identifying health risks and implementing community public health programs to target these risks. Established in 1905, the civic organization **Rotary International** is responsible for efforts to eradicate polio through vaccine programs throughout the world (Rotary International, 2008). Philanthropic organizations such as RWJF have provided funding for public health activities such as community education and intervention programs. The RWJF's goal is to improve the health of all Americans and have provided substantial funds for research activities to combat public health issues such as obesity and smoking (RWJF, 2008).

Public health, nursing, and medical schools are also major contributors to public health activities. Faculty from these schools often provide technical assistance to local public health organizations and often partner with organizations to establish health programs. The schools may also provide specific educational programs that are tailored to community needs. Educational accreditation organizations are also encouraging educational programs to participate in community health activities. The Harvard University's School of Public Health has established several centers to advance research in public health such as health communication, injury control, AIDS, health promotion, and population and development studies (Harvard School of Public Health, 2008)

PUBLIC HEALTH EDUCATION AND HEALTH PROMOTION

Public health educational strategies are a crucial component to public health interventions. **Health education** focuses on changing health behavior through educational interventions such as multimedia education and classes. **Health promotion** is a broader intervention term in public health that encompasses not only educational objectives and activities but also organizational, environmental, and economic interventions to support activities conducive to healthy behavior (Pointer et al., 2007).

Public Health Education Campaign

Educational strategies inform the community about positive health behavior, targeting those at risk to change or maintain positive health behavior. Many public health campaigns are performed by the local public health department and in collaboration with community organizations. There are several steps to planning and developing a successful public health educational campaign.

- The first step in implementing a public health education campaign is to perform a community assessment to determine at-risk populations. Developing an effective educational campaign to target high-risk populations requires community participation.

- The next step is collaborating with the community for their input on health issues and prioritizing target health issues.
- The third step is performing surveillance activities for specific data related to mortality and morbidity rates.
- The fourth step is to develop a pilot study to assess the effectiveness of the proposed campaign.
- The fifth step is to revise the campaign based on the pilot study.
- The sixth step is to implement the chosen campaign for a period of time.
- The seventh step is to perform an evaluation of the impact of the campaign and revise, if needed (Minnesota Department of Health, 2009).

Public Health Education Evaluation

Educational activities can be difficult to measure because of their abstract nature. It is important that specific outcome measures are developed prior to the campaign. Each measure should address the following parameters: (1) specific target group, (2) change in and type of behavior, (3) time frame for change, and (4) defined geographic area of change (Novick & Morrow, 2008).

Health Promotion Activities

Most health promotion campaigns have more community health objectives than health educational campaigns that focus on specific target populations. **Health promotion** focuses on a comprehensive coordinated approach to long-term health behavior changes by influencing the community through educational activities (Minnesota Department of Health, 2009). When a focus is at the community level, it is necessary to address lifestyle behavior which includes cultural, economic, psychologic, and environmental factors. Examples of health promotion include nutritional, genetic, or family counseling which would include health education activities. Health promotion may also include other community development activities such as occupational and environmental control and immunization programs (Turnock, 2007).

Public Health Marketing

According to the CDC, **health marketing** is an innovative approach to public health practice. Public health marketing draws from the business discipline of marketing theory and adds science-based health strategies of promotion and prevention. It involves creating, communicating, and delivering health information and interventions using customer-oriented and science-based strategies to protect and promote health in diverse populations (CDC, 2009c). Marketing research is used to deliver messages to educate the public on priority health issues.

MAJOR PUBLIC HEALTH ISSUES

It is important to mention the impact the terrorist attack on the United States on September 11, 2001, the anthrax attacks, the outbreak of global diseases such as AIDS, and the natural disaster of Hurricane Katrina had on the scope of public health responsibilities. As a result of these major events, public health has expanded their area of responsibility. The term bioterrorism and disaster preparedness have more frequently appeared in public health literature and have become part of strategic planning. The Public Health Security and Bioterrorism Preparedness and Response Act of 2002 provided grants to hospitals and public health organizations to prepare for bioterrorism as a result of September 11, 2001 (CDC, 2008c).

COLLABORATION OF PUBLIC HEALTH AND PRIVATE MEDICINE

Public health and private medicine have traditionally focused on different aspects of US health. Public health focuses on primary prevention, which focuses on the prevention of disease. Public health practitioners' approach is to develop strategies to promote community health. Private medicine has traditionally focused on tertiary care or providing a cure to individuals or patients. These approaches have traditionally been in conflict. In the 1920s, when public health clinics were treating the poor, private medicine felt threatened because these clinics were viewed as competitors (Reiser, 1996).

Prior to these activities, there were some collaborative activities in the early 1800s and early 1900s—many physicians were involved in public health. They realized the importance of public health in the role of infectious diseases. However, public health efforts were later resisted by physicians. They resented mandatory tuberculosis reporting, as well as immunization programs (Council on Scientific Affairs, 1990). When antibiotics were developed to combat diseases and the

financial benefit of reimbursement of tertiary care by health insurance companies was realized, physicians' interest in public health dissipated (Lasker, 1997). They became more hostile because public health was viewed as a direct competitor.

Over the last decade, there has been an increase in the collaboration between public health and private medicine. In 1994, there was a long-term commitment established between the AMA and the APHA that established the following initiatives to formalize a partnership: creation of joint research and local and national networks, development of a strategic plan, and development of a shared vision of health care. There has been an increase in collaborative efforts between the AMA and the CDC to develop healthcare programs to combat disease (AMA, 2009). With the increased prevalence of obesity, diabetes, and other chronic health conditions, this collaboration is crucial to develop strategies to reduce the rates of these diseases in the United States.

CONCLUSION

Public health is challenged by its very success because consumers now take public health measures for granted. There are several successful vaccines that have targeted all childhood diseases, tobacco use has decreased significantly, accident prevention has increased, there are safer workplaces because of Occupational Safety and Health Administration (OSHA), the fluoridation of water is established, and a decrease in mortality from heart attacks (Novick & Morrow, 2008). When some major event occurs like anthrax or severe acute respiratory syndrome (SARS), people immediately think that public health will automatically control these problems. The public may not realize how much effort and dedication and research takes place to protect the public.

As a healthcare consumer, it is important to recognize the role that public health plays in our health care. If you are sick, you go to your physician for medical advice which may mean providing you with a prescription. However, there are oftentimes that you may not go see your physician because you do not have health insurance or you do not feel that sick or you would like to change one of your lifestyle behaviors. Public health surrounds consumers with educational opportunities to change a health condition or behavior. You can visit the CDC's Web site that is discussed in several chapters, which provides information about different diseases and health conditions. You can also visit your local health department.

The concept of public health has been more publicized over the last 7 years because of the terrorist attacks of 2001, the anthrax attacks in post offices, the natural disaster of Hurricane Katrina, and the flooding in the Midwest. Funding has increased for public health activities because of these events. The concept of bioterrorism is now a topic of conversation. Because public health is now considered an integral component to battling terrorism and consequently a matter of national security, federal funding has dramatically increased. Since 2002, the federal budget for public health activities at all government levels has increased by billions with continued funding expected over the next several years (Turnock, 2007). However, in order to continue to receive increased funding levels, it is important that public health markets itself to both the policy makers and the public so they understand the increased importance of public health's role in national security.

PREVIEW OF CHAPTER FIVE

Historically, the US healthcare system involved inpatient services provided by hospitals and outpatient services provided by physicians. Over the past two centuries, hospitals have evolved from serving the poor and homeless to offering the latest technology to serve the ill. As a result of cost containment issues that have focused on hospital inpatient services and consumer preferences for being treated on an outpatient basis, more ambulatory and outpatient services are being offered by hospitals and more standalone outpatient services such as surgery and home health care have been successfully developed. This chapter will discuss the evolution of outpatient and inpatients health services in the United States.

VOCABULARY

American Cancer Society

American Lung Association

Assessment

Assurance

Biosurveillance

Bioterrorism

Core public health functions

Determinants of health

Edwin Chadwick

Environmental health

Epidemiology

Epidemiology triangle

Exploring Accreditation Project (EAP)

Federal Emergency Management Agency (FEMA)

Genetic factors

Health

Health education

Health marketing

Health promotion

Healthy People 2000 Report

Healthy People 2010 Report

Incident Command System

Institute of Medicine

John Snow

Lemuel Shattuck

Lifestyle behaviors

Mobilizing for Action through Planning and Partnership (MAPP)

National Association of County and City Officials (NACCHO)

National Incident Management System (NIMS)

National Response Framework (NRF)

Physical environment

Policy development

Primary, secondary, and tertiary prevention

Public health

Public health education

Public health emergency preparedness

Public Health Security and Bioterrorism Preparedness and Response Act

Rotary International

REFERENCES

American Medical Association. (2009). Retrieved November 9, 2009, from http://www.ama-assn.org/ama/pub/advocacy/current-topics-advocacy.shtml.

American Public Health Association. (2008). 10 essential public health services. Retrieved August 23, 2009, from http://www.apha.org/programs/standards/performancestandardsprogram/resexxentialservices.htm.

Ashton, J., & Sram, I. (1998). Millennium report to Sir Edwin Chadwick. *British Medical Journal*, *317*, 592–596.

Bender, K., Benjamin, G., Fallon, M., Gorenflo, G., Hardy, G., Jarris, P., et al. (2007). Final recommendations for a voluntary national accreditation program for state and local health departments: Steering committee report. *Journal of Public Health Management Practice*, *13*, 4, 342–348.

Bekemeier, B., Riley, C., Padgett, S., & Berkowitz, B. (2007). Making the case: Leveraging resources toward public health system improvement in turning point states. *Journal of Public Health Management Practice*, *13*, 6, 649–654.

Centers for Disease Control and Prevention. (2008a). *Bioterrorism*. Retrieved July 15, 2009, from http://emergency.cdc.gov/bioterrorism/.

Centers for Disease Control and Prevention. (2008b). *Epidemiology in the classroom*. Retrieved July 5, 2008, from http://www.cdc.gov/excite/classroom.

Centers for Disease Control and Prevention. (2008c). *Public health emergency response guide for state, local, and tribal public health directors*. Retrieved September 6, 2008, from http://www.bt.cdc.gov/planning/responseguide.asp.

Centers for Disease Control and Prevention. (2009a). *Understanding the epidemiologic triangle through infectious disease*. Retrieved October 26, 2009, from http://www.bam.gov/teachers/activities/epi_1_triangle.pdf.

Centers for Disease Control and Prevention. (2009b). *National Health Promotion and Disease Prevention Objectives*. Retrieved November 8, 2009, from http://www.cdc.gov/mmwr/preview/mmwrhtml/00001788.htm.

Centers for Disease Control and Prevention. (2009c). *What is Health Marketing?* Retrieved November 8, 2009, from http://www.cdc.gov/healthmarketing/whatishm.htm.

Council on Scientific Affairs. (1990). The IOM report and public health. *Journal of American Medical Association*, *264*, 4, 508–509.

Ellis, H. (2008). John Snow: Early anaesthetist and pioneer of public health. *British Journal of Hospital Medicine*, *69*, 2, 113.

Emerson, H. (1945). *Local health units for the nation* (p. viii). New York: The Commonwealth Fund.

Federal Emergency Management Agency. (2008). NRF Resource Center. Retrieved August 1, 2008, from http://www.fema.gov/nrf.

Harvard School of Public Health. (2008). Research centers. Retrieved July 7, 2008, from www.hsph.harvard.edu/research/.

Healthways Silver Sneakers Fitness Program. (2008). Retrieved July 7, 2008, from http://www.silversneakers.com.

Institute of Medicine. (1988). *The future of public health*. Washington, DC: National Academies Press.

Institute of Medicine. (1997). *Improving health in the community*. Washington, DC: National Academies Press.

Institute of Medicine. (2002). *The future of the public's health in the 21st century*. Washington, DC: National Academies Press.

The Joint Commission. (2009). Retrieved November 9, 2009, from http://www.jointcommission.org/Accreditation Programs/Hospitals/.

Lasker, R. (1997). *Medicine & public health: The power of collaboration*. New York: Academy of Medicine.

Lee, B. (1994). *Health policy and the politics of health care: Nation's health* (4th ed.). Sudbury, MA: Jones and Bartlett.

Mays, G. (2008). Organization of the public health delivery system. In L. Novick & C. Morrow (Eds.). *Public health administration: Principles for population-based management* (pp. 69–126). Sudbury, MA: Jones and Bartlett.

Minnesota Department of Health. (2009). *Community health promotion*. Retrieved October 26, 2009, from http://www.health.state.mn.us/divs/hpcd/chp/hpkit/index.htm.

National Association of County and City Health Officials. (2009). Mobilizing for action through planning and partnerships. Retrieved October 26, 2009, from http://naccho.org/topics/infrastructure/mapp/index.cfm?&render.

Novick, L., & Morrow, C. (2008). A framework for public health administration and practice. In L. Novick & C. Morrow (Eds.). *Public health administration: Principles for population-based management* (pp. 35–68). Sudbury, MA: Jones and Bartlett.

Pointer, D., Williams, S., Isaacs, S., & Knickman, J. (2007). *Introduction to U.S. health care*. Hoboken, NJ: Wiley Publishing.

Reiser, S. (1996). Medicine and public health. *Journal of American Medical Association*, *276*, 17, 1429–1430.

Robert Wood Johnson Foundation. (2008). Retrieved November 9, 2009, from http://www.rwjf.org/about/.

Rosen, G. (1958). *A history of public health*. New York: MD Publications.

Rotary International. (2008). Retrieved July 7, 2008, from http://www.rotary.org.

Shi, L., & Singh, D. (2008). *Essentials of the U.S. health care system*. Sudbury, MA: Jones and Bartlett.

Society for Academic Emergency Medicine, Ethics Committee. (1992). An ethical foundation for health care: An emergency medicine perspective. *Annals of Emergency Medicine*, *21*, 11, 1381–1387.

Turnock, B. (2007). *Essentials of public health*. Sudbury, MA: Jones and Bartlett.

US Department of Health and Human Services. (1979). *Healthy people: The Surgeon General report on health promotion and disease prevention*. Publication no. 79-55071. Washington, DC: Public Health Service.

US Department of Health and Human Services. (2000). *Healthy people 2010*. Retrieved October 26, 2009, from http://www.healthypeople.gov/document/html/uih/uih_bw/uih_2.htm#determanats.

US Food and Drug Administration. (2009). *Counterterrorisim legislation*. Retrieved November 8, 2009, from http://www.fda.gov/EmergencyPreparedness/Counterterrorism/BioterrorismAct/default.htm.

World Health Organization. (2008). *Health promotion*. Retrieved July 20, 2008, from http://www.who.int/healthpromotion/en/.

Winslow, C. (1920). The untitled fields of public health. *Science*, *51*, 23.

NOTES

STUDENT ACTIVITY 4-1

CROSSWORD PUZZLE

Instructions: Please complete the puzzle using the vocabulary words found in the chapter. There may be multiple-word answers. The numbers in the parenthesis indicate the number of words in the answers.

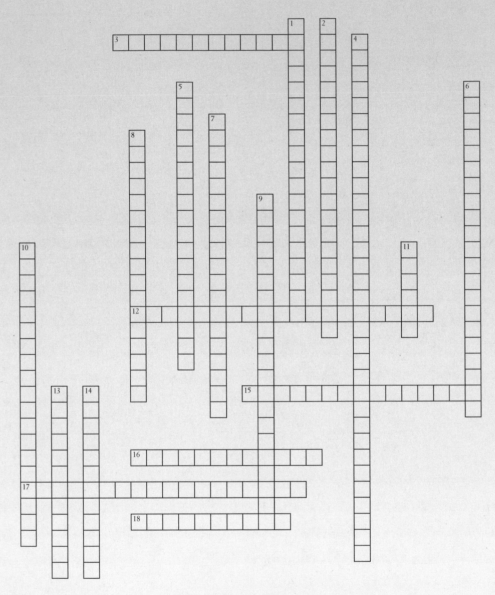

Created with EclipseCrossword © 1999–2009 Green Eclipse

STUDENT ACTIVITY 4-1

Across

3. Science and art of preventing disease, prolonging life, and promoting physical health through organized community efforts. (2 words)

12. The investigation of environmental hazards in the community and the monitoring and enforcing of environmental regulations. (2 words)

15. Educational, organizational, environmental, and economic interventions to support healthy behavior. (2 words)

16. Examples of these are diet, exercise, genetics, and income level. (1 word)

17. Rehabilitation. (2 words)

18. Pubic health action of systematic continuous data collection of health issues. (1 word)

Down

1. Pollutants, hazardous work exposure, water contamination. (2 words)

2. The relationship between the population, the disease, and the environment. (2 words)

4. Planning protocols that are implemented to manage a large-scale disaster. (4 words)

5. Elderly, disabled people, and children. (2 words)

6. Innovative approach to delivering health interventions by drawing from the business discipline. (3 words)

7. These types of providers see patients on an outpatient basis. (2 words)

8. Smoking cessation programs. (2 words)

9. Changing health behavior through educational interventions such as classes. (3 words)

10. Blood pressure screenings. (2 words)

11. The state of complete physical, mental, and social well-being. (1 word)

13. An attack on a population by deliberately releasing viruses, bacteria, or other germs. (1 word)

14. Study of disease distribution and patterns among populations. (1 word)

STUDENT ACTIVITY 4-2

IN YOUR OWN WORDS

Based on Chapter 4, please provide a description of the following concepts in your own words. DO NOT RECITE the text description.

Exploring Accreditation Project: _____

_____

_____

Determinants of health: _____

_____

_____

Mobilizing for Action through Planning and Partnership (MAPP):

_____

_____

_____

Turning Point: _____

_____

_____

Incident Command System: _____

_____

_____

Institute of Medicine: _____

_____

_____

Health promotion: _____

_____

_____

National Response Framework: _____

_____

_____

Public health marketing: _____

_____

_____

STUDENT ACTIVITY 4-3

REAL LIFE APPLICATIONS: CASE STUDY

Because of all of the media attention on terrorism, your grandparents, who are elderly, are very concerned about terrorist attacks on the United States. They hear the concept of "bioterrorism" and are worried they will be poisoned. They do not understand the role public health departments play in protecting the public from terrorism. As the director of the local health department, you explain that you have a disaster plan prepared in case there is a natural or manmade disaster in the community.

ACTIVITY

(1) Define bioterrorism and how it can impact a community; (2) describe the coordination of the federal, state, and local health departments in a catastrophic event such as bioterrorism; and (3) explain the role that the public health department has in protecting special groups such as the disabled and elderly.

RESPONSES

_____

_____

_____

_____

_____

_____

_____

_____

_____

_____

_____

_____

_____

_____

STUDENT ACTIVITY 4-4

INTERNET EXERCISES

Write your answers in the space provided.

- Visit each of the Web sites listed here.
- Name the organization.
- Locate their mission statement on their Web site.
- Provide a brief overview of the activities of the organization.
- How do these organizations participate in the US healthcare system?

Web Sites

http://www.fema.gov/nrf

Organization Name:_____

Mission Statement:

_____

_____

_____

Overview of Activities:

_____

_____

_____

Importance of organization to US health care:

_____

_____

_____

http://www.saem.org

Organization Name:_____

Mission Statement:

_____

_____

_____

Overview of Activities:

_____

_____

_____

STUDENT ACTIVITY 4-4

Importance of organization to US health care:

_____
_____
_____

http://www.apha.org

Organization Name: _____

Mission Statement:

_____
_____
_____

Overview of Activities:

_____
_____
_____

Importance of organization to US health care:

_____
_____
_____

http://www.hsph.harvard.edu/research

Organization Name: _____

Mission Statement:

_____
_____
_____

Overview of Activities:

_____
_____
_____

Importance of organization to US health care:

_____
_____
_____

STUDENT ACTIVITY 4-4

http://www.silversneakers.com

Organization Name:_____

Mission Statement:

_____

_____

_____

Overview of Activities:

_____

_____

_____

Importance of organization to US health care:

_____

_____

_____

http://www.naccho.org

Organization Name:_____

Mission Statement:

_____

_____

_____

Overview of Activities:

_____

_____

_____

Importance of organization to US health care:

_____

_____

_____

Inpatient and Outpatient Services

LEARNING OBJECTIVES

The student will be able to:

- Identify and discuss three milestones of the history of the hospital.

- Define and discuss the different hospitals by ownership classification.

- Describe the difference between hospitals by service.

- Identify the different types of outpatient care settings.

- Analyze the utilization trends of both inpatient and outpatient services.

- Evaluate the difference between inpatient and outpatient services.

- Assess the impact of outpatient services on healthcare delivery.

DID YOU KNOW THAT?

- Other terms related to "hospital" include hospitality, host, hotel, and hospice.

- Voluntary hospitals are called voluntary because their funding comes from the community voluntarily.

- Over 50% of urgent care centers are owned by physicians.

- Nearly 1 in 20 individuals in the United States relies on community health centers for primary care.

- Women seek healthcare services more frequently than men.

INTRODUCTION

Inpatient services are services that involve an overnight stay of a patient. Historically, the US healthcare industry was based on the provision of inpatient services provided by hospitals and outpatient services provided by physicians. As our healthcare system evolved, hospitals became the mainstay of the healthcare system offering primarily inpatient with limited outpatient services. Over the past 2 centuries, hospitals have evolved from serving the poor and homeless to providing the latest medical technology to serve the seriously ill and injured (Shi & Singh, 2008). Although their primary revenue is derived from inpatient services, as a result of cost containment and consumer preferences, more outpatient services are being offered by hospitals.

Hospitals have evolved into medical centers that provide the most advanced service. Hospitals can be classified by who owns them, length of stay, and the type of services they provide. Inpatient services typically focus on acute care, which includes secondary and tertiary care levels that most likely require inpatient care. Inpatient care is very expensive and, throughout the years, has been targeted for cost containment measures. Hospitals began offering more outpatient services that do not require an overnight stay and were less financially taxing on the healthcare system. As the US healthcare expenditures have increased as part of the gross domestic product, more cost containment measures have evolved. Outpatient services have become more popular because they are less expensive and they are preferred by consumers. This chapter will discuss the evolution of outpatient and inpatient healthcare services in the United States.

HISTORY OF HOSPITALS

The word hospital comes from the Latin word *hospes*, which means a visitor or host who receives a visitor. From this root word, the Latin *hospitalia* evolved, which means an apartment for strangers or guests. The word hospital was a word in the Old French language. As it evolved, in the 15th century, England shifted the meaning to a home for the infirmed, poor, or elderly. The modern definition of "an institution where sick or injured are given medical or surgical care" was developed in the 16th century. The name Hotel-Dieu was commonly given to hospitals in France during the Middle Ages and means the hotel of God (MedicineNet, Inc., 2009).

Over 5000 years ago, Greek temples were the first type of hospital with similar institutions in Egyptian, Hindu, and Roman cultures (Longest & Darr, 2008). They were the precursor of the **almshouses** or **poorhouses** that were developed in the 1820s to primarily serve the poor. Hospitals provided food and shelter to the poor and consequently treated the ill. **Pesthouses**, operated by local governments, were used to quarantine people who had contagious diseases such as cholera. The framework of these institutions set up the concept of the hospital. Initially, wealthy people did not want to go to hospitals because the conditions were deplorable and the providers were not skilled, so hospitals, which were first built in urban areas, were used by the poor. In 1789, the Public Hospital of Baltimore was established for the indigent and, in 1889, it became Johns Hopkins Hospital, which exists today as one of the best hospitals in the world (Sultz & Young, 2006). In the 1850s, a hospital system was finally developed, but the conditions were deplorable because of the staff of unskilled providers. Hospitals were owned primarily by

the physicians who practiced in them (Relman, 2007). The hospitals became more cohesive among providers because the physicians had to rely on each other for referrals and access to hospitals, which gave them more professional power (Rosen, 1983).

In the early 20th century, with the establishment of more standardized medical education, hospitals became more accepted across socioeconomic classes and became the symbol of medicine. With the establishment of the American Medical Association (AMA) who protected the interests of providers, the reputation of providers became more prestigious. In the 1920s, because of the development of medical technological advances, increases in the quality of medical training and specialization, and the economic development of the United States, the establishment of hospitals became the symbol of the institutionalization of health care and the acknowledgment of the medical profession as a powerful presence (Torrens, 1993). During the 1930s and 1940s, the ownership of the hospitals changed from physician-owned to church-related and government operated (American Hospital Association [AHA], 2009a; Starr, 1982). Religious orders viewed hospitals as an opportunity to perform their spiritual good works so religion played a major role in the development of hospitals. Several religious orders established hospitals that still exist today.

In 1973, the first Patient Bill of Rights was introduced to represent the healthcare consumer in hospital care (AHA, 2009a). In 1972, the AHA had all hospitals display a "Patient Bill of Rights" in their institutions (Sultz & Young, 2006). In 1974, the National Health Planning and Resources Development Act required states to have certificate of need (CON) laws to ensure the state approved any capital expenditures associated with hospital/medical facilities' construction and expansion (AHA, 2009a). The Act was repealed in 1987, but 36 states still have some type of CON mechanism (National Conference of State Legislatures, 2009). The concept of CON was important because it encouraged state planning to ensure their medical system was based on need.

Hospitals are the foundation of our healthcare system. As our health insurance system evolved, the first type of insurance was hospital insurance. As society's health needs increased, expansion of different medical facilities increased. There was more of a focus on ambulatory or outpatient services because US healthcare consumers prefer outpatient services and, secondly, it is more cost-effective. In 1980, the AHA estimated that 87% of hospitals offered outpatient surgery (Duke University Libraries, 2008). Although hospitals are still an integral part of our healthcare delivery system, the method of their delivery has changed. "Hospitalists," created in 1996, are providers that focus specifically on the care of a patient when they are hospitalized (Longest & Darr, 2008; Shi & Singh, 2008; Sultz & Young, 2006). This new type of provider recognized the need of providing quality hospital care. More hospitals have recognized the trend of outpatient services and have integrated those types of services in their delivery. In 2000, as a result of the Balanced Budget Act cuts of 1997, the federal government authorized an outpatient Medicare reimbursement system (Centers for Disease Control and Prevention [CDC], 2009a), which has supported hospital outpatient services efforts. In 2007, hospitals employed over 5 million individuals, were the second largest source of private sector jobs, provided outpatient care to over 600 million patients, and performed 27 million surgeries (AHA, 2009b).

HOSPITAL TYPES BY OWNERSHIP

There are three major types of hospitals by ownership: (1) public, (2) voluntary, and (3) proprietary hospitals. **Public hospitals** are the oldest type of hospital and are owned by the federal, state, or local government. **Federal hospitals** generally do not serve the general public but operate for federal beneficiaries such as military personnel, veterans, and Native Americans. The Veterans Affairs (VA) hospitals are the largest group of federal hospitals. They have high utilization rates by veterans. Taxes support part of their operations. In 2007, there were 213 federal hospitals (Pointer, Williams, Isaacs, & Knickman, 2007). County and city hospitals are open to the general hospital and are supported by taxes. Many of these hospitals are located in urban areas to serve the poor and the elderly. Larger public hospitals may be affiliated with medical schools and are involved in training medical students and other healthcare professionals (Shi & Singh, 2008). Their services are primarily reimbursed by Medicare and Medicaid services and have high utilization rates. In 2007, there were 1111 state and local hospitals (AHA, 2009b).

Voluntary hospitals are not government owned, private, and not for profit. They are considered voluntary because their financial support is the result of community organizational efforts. Their focus is their community. Private, not-for-profit hospitals are the largest group of hospitals. In 2007, there were nearly 3000 not-for-profit hospitals. **Proprietary hospitals** or investor-owned hospitals are for-profit institutions and are owned by corporations, individuals, or partnerships. Their primary goal is to generate a profit. They have the lowest utilization rates. In 2007, there were 873 proprietary hospitals (AHA, 2009b).

HOSPITAL TYPES BY SPECIALTY

Hospitals may be classified by what type of services they provide and their target population. A general hospital provides many different types of services to meet the general needs of their population. Most hospitals are general hospitals. Specialty hospitals are hospitals that provide services for a specific disease or target population. Some examples are psychiatric, children's, women's, cardiac, cancer, rehabilitation, and orthopedic hospitals.

OTHER HOSPITAL CLASSIFICATIONS

Hospitals can be classified by single- or multiunit operations. Two or more hospitals may be owned by a central corporation. Multiunit hospitals are the result of the merging or acquiring of other hospitals that have financial problems. These chains can be operated as for profit, not for profit, or government owned. These hospitals often formed systems because it was more cost-efficient. In 2007, there were over 2700 hospital systems. Hospitals can also be classified by length of stay. A short stay or **acute care hospital** focuses on patients who stay on an average of less than 30 days. Community hospitals are short term. A **long-term care hospital** focuses on patients who stay on an average of more than 30 days. Rehabilitation and chronic disease hospitals are examples of long-term care hospitals. More than 90% of hospitals are acute or short-term. (AHA, 2009a; Longest & Darr, 2008)

Hospitals can be classified by geographic location—rural or urban. Urban hospitals are located in a county with designated urban or city geographic areas. Rural hospitals are located in a county that has no urban areas. Urban hospitals tend to pay higher salaries and consequently offer more complex care because of the highly trained providers and staff. In 2007, there were nearly 3000 urban hospitals. Rural hospitals tend to see more poor and elderly and, consequently, have financial issues. In 2007, there were nearly 2000 rural hospitals (AHA, 2009b). As a result of this issue, the **Medicare Rural Hospital Flexibility Program** (MRHFP) was created as part of the Balanced Budget Act of 1997. The MRHFP allows some rural hospitals to be classified as critical access hospitals if they have no more than 25 acute care beds and provide emergency care. This classification enables them to receive additional Medicare reimbursement called cost plus. **Cost plus reimbursement** allows for capital costs, which enables these facilities to expand (Centers for Medicare and Medicaid Services [CMS], 2009).

Teaching hospitals are hospitals that have one or more graduate resident programs approved by AMA. **Academic medical centers** are hospitals organized around a medical school. There are approximately 400 teaching hospitals including 64 VA medical centers that are members of the **Council of Teaching Hospitals and Health Systems** in the United States and Canada. These institutions offer substantial programs and are considered elite teaching and research institutions affiliated with large medical schools (Shi & Singh, 2008).

As discussed previously, **church-related hospitals** are developed as a way to perform spiritual work. The first church-affiliated hospitals were established by Catholic nuns. These hospitals are community general hospitals. They could be affiliated with a medical school. **Osteopathic hospitals** focus on a holistic approach to care. They emphasize diet and environmental factors that influence health as well as the manipulation of the body. Their focus is preventive care. There are approximately 200 osteopathic hospitals in the United States. Historically, osteopathic hospitals were developed as a result of the antagonism between the different approaches to medicine—traditional or allopathic medicine versus holistic. Current trends indicate that both branches of medicine now serve in each others' hospitals and respect the focus of each others' treatment (Shi & Singh, 2008).

HOSPITAL GOVERNANCE

Hospitals are governed by a **chief executive officer** (CEO), a board of trustees or board of directors, and the chief of medical staff. The CEO or president is ultimately responsible for the day-to-day operations of the hospital and is a board of trustees member. CEOs provide leadership to achieve their mission and vision. The **board of trustees** is legally responsible for hospital operations. It approves strategic plans and budgets and has authority for appointing, evaluating, and terminating the CEO. Boards often form different committees such as quality assurance, finance, and planning. There

are two standing committees: the executive committee that monitors the hospital activities and makes policy recommendations and the medical staff committee that is charged with medical staff relations. The **chief of medical staff** or **medical director** is in charge of the medical staff/physicians that provide clinical services to the hospital. The physicians may be in private practice and have admitting privileges to the hospital and are accountable to the board of trustees. The medical staff is divided according to specialty or department such as obstetrics, cardiology, radiology, etc. There may be a **chief of service** that leads each of these specialties. There is also the **operational staff** that is a parallel line of staff with the medical staff. They are responsible for managing nonmedical staff and performing nonclinical, administrative, and service work (Longest & Darr, 2008; Pointer et al., 2007). It is in the best interest of the institution that both the operational staff and medical staff collaborate to ensure smooth management of the facility.

The medical staff also have committees such as a **credentials committee** that reviews and grants admitting privileges to physicians, a **medical records committee** that oversees patient records, a **utilization review committee** that ensures inpatient stays are clinically appropriate, an **infection control committee** that focuses on minimizing infections in the hospital, and a **quality improvement committee** that is responsible for quality improvement programs (Shi & Singh, 2008).

HOSPITAL LICENSURE, CERTIFICATION, AND ACCREDITATION

State governments oversee the licensure of healthcare facilities including hospitals. States set their own standards. It is important to note that all facilities must be licensed but do not have to be accredited. **State licensure** focuses on building codes, sanitation, equipment, and personnel. Hospitals must be licensed to operate with a certain number of beds.

Certification of hospitals enables them to obtain Medicare and Medicaid reimbursement. This type of certification is mandated by the Department of Health and Human Services (HHS). All hospitals that receive Medicare and Medicaid reimbursement must adhere to **conditions of participation** that emphasize patient health and safety. **Accreditation** is a private standard developed by accepted organizations as a way to meet certain standards. For example, accreditation of a hospital by The Joint Commission (TJC) means that hospitals have met

Medicare and Medicaid standards and do not have to be certified. Medicare and Medicaid have also authorized the American Osteopathic Organization to jointly accredit their types of hospitals with TJC (TJC, 2009).

It is important to mention that TJC has had tremendous impact on how healthcare organizations are accredited. Since its formation in 1951, TJC has expanded its accreditation beyond hospitals. They accredit ambulatory care, assisted living, behavioral health care, home care, hospitals, laboratory services, long-term care, and office-based surgery centers. Accreditation of managed care organizations such as preferred providers and managed behavioral organizations ended in 2006 (Longest & Darr, 2008).

International Organization for Standardization

Established in 1947 in Geneva, Switzerland, the **International Organization for Standardization** (ISO) is a worldwide organization that promotes standards from different countries. Although this is not an accrediting organization, those organizations that register with the ISO are promoted as having higher standards. ISO 9000 (quality management focus) and ISO 14000 (environmental management focus) are management standards that are applicable to any organization, including healthcare organizations, and many healthcare organizations are registered with the ISO (ISO, 2009)

PATIENT RIGHTS

The **Patient Self-Determination Act of 1990** requires hospitals and other facilities that participate in the Medicare and Medicaid programs to provide patients, on admission, with information on their rights and is referred to as the Patient Bill of Rights. If you enter any hospital, you will see the Bill of Rights posted on their walls. This law requires that the hospital maintains confidentiality of their personal and medical information. The patient also has the right to be provided accurate and easy-to-understand information about their medical condition so they may give **informed consent** for any of their medical care.

CURRENT STATUS OF HOSPITALS

Many hospitals have become the dinosaurs of the healthcare industry. Nearly two thirds of hospitals have financial problems. As a result of the increased competition of outpatient services (which are often more cost-effective, efficient, and consumer friendly) and reduced reimbursement from Medicare and Medicaid, many hospitals are developing strategies to increase their financial stability. In the 1990s, many hospitals merged with other hospitals, were acquired by other hospitals, or became part of a hospital chain. These strategies were an attempt to become more cost-efficient in the management of these organizations (Sultz & Young, 2006).

Interestingly, outpatient services have become the major competitors of hospitals. Advanced technology has enabled more ambulatory surgeries and testing, which has resulted in the development of many specialty centers for radiology and imaging, chemotherapy treatment, kidney dialysis, etc. These services were often performed in a hospital. What is even more interesting is that many physicians or physician groups own these centers. They are receiving revenue that used to be hospital revenue (Buchbinder & Shanks, 2007; Shi & Singh, 2008). Although hospitals have operated outpatient clinics since the 19th century, these clinics were used to care for the indigent population. As revenues continued to fall, these clinics gradually generated revenue by offering more hospital services. In 2003, outpatient services accounted for nearly 40% of the total hospital revenue (Sultz & Young, 2006). Hospitals have to continue to focus on revenue generation by operating more outpatient service opportunities.

Unfortunately, as a result of the economic recession, there are less insured citizens and therefore less inpatient care and fewer patients who can pay for their care. A 2008 AHA survey of 736 hospitals from 30 states indicated that 40% of the respondents reported a drop in overall admissions. Uncompensated care in 2008 was up 8% from July to September compared to 2007 data, and there was a moderate to significant decline in elective procedures (AHA, 2009b).

OUTPATIENT SERVICES

As discussed previously, **outpatient services** are services that are provided that do not require an overnight stay. Often, the term **ambulatory care** is used interchangeably with outpatient services. Ambulatory literally means a person is able to walk to receive a service, which may not always be necessarily true. The term outpatient is a more general term for services other than inpatient services (Jonas, 2003). Hospitals also offer outpatients services in their emergency departments and their outpatient clinics.

Physician Offices

The basic form of an outpatient service is a patient seeing their physician in the physician's office. Both general practitioners and specialists offer ambulatory care. They offer ambulatory care as either a solitary practitioner or in group practice. Traditionally, physicians established solitary practices but the cost of running a practice became too expensive so more physicians are establishing group practices. Approximately two thirds of physicians now operate as a group practice. Approximately 70% of group practices are single specialty groups while the remaining 30% are multispecialty group practices (Jonas, 2003; Pointer et al., 2007).

Hospital Emergency and Outpatient Services

Hospitals traditionally provide inpatient services although nearly all community hospitals provide emergency services that are considered outpatient services. Although emergency departments have the technology to treat emergency situations, many emergency rooms are used for nonemergency issues. In 2006, there were 119 million visits to hospital emergency rooms. The rate per 100 persons was 36.1 for white persons, 79.9 for black persons, and 35.3 for Hispanic persons. Individuals who are 75 years or older use an emergency room 66% more frequently than the general population (CDC, 2009b).

Hospital and Nonhospital-Based Outpatient Clinics

Many outpatient clinics are found in teaching hospitals. They use outpatient clinics as an opportunity to teach and perform research. The clinics are categorized as surgical, medical, and other. Larger teaching hospitals may have 100 specialty and subspecialty clinics (Jonas, 2003). They may operate as part of the hospital or as a hospital-owned entity.

Nonhospital-based freestanding ambulatory or outpatient facilities may be owned or operated by hospitals, hospital systems, or hospital chains; physicians; or for-profit or not-for-profit organizations. These facilities may provide several different types of services that used to be offered as inpatient services. As a result of advanced technology, surgery can be performed as an outpatient service. Also, any type of rehabilitation service, elective surgery such as cosmetic procedures, kidney dialysis, substance abuse treatment, sports medicine, and other specialty services are offered as ambulatory services (Longest & Darr, 2008).

Urgent/Emergent Care Centers

Urgent/emergent care centers were first established in the 1970s. **Urgent/emergent care centers** are used for consumers who need medical care but their situation is not life-threatening. This would take the place of the hospital emergency room visit. The medical issue usually occurs outside traditional physician office hours so they see patients in the evenings, weekends, and on holidays. Many of these centers are both walk-in and appointment facilities. They do not take the place of a patient's primary care provider. These centers are conveniently located and may be in strip malls or medical buildings so they are accessible for consumers. It is important to note that many managed care organizations will reimburse member visits because they are less expensive than an emergency room visit (Sultz & Young, 2006). The urgent care centers relieve the emergency departments from seeing patients who do not have life-threatening situations. It is anticipated that there will be an increase in urgent care centers because of this need.

The Urgent Care Association of America (UCAOA) estimates there are 8000 urgent care centers in 2008 (Pointer et al., 2007). According to an UCAOA survey, approximately 54% of urgent centers are owned by physicians, 25% are hospital owned, and 18% are corporately owned. Approximately 85% of the centers have a physician onsite at all times, and 75% of the physicians are board certified in a primary specialty (UCAOA, 2009).

Ambulatory Surgery Centers

Ambulatory surgery centers (ASCs) are for surgeries that do not require an overnight stay. Advances in technology and newer anesthesia drugs that enable patients to recover more quickly from grogginess have enabled more surgeries to be performed on an outpatient basis. ASCs may focus on general surgical procedures that involve the abdomen. Specialized surgical centers focus on orthopedic surgery, plastic surgery, and gynecologic surgery. Some centers offer a combination of both general and specialized surgeries (Pointer et al., 2007). Outpatient surgery is a major contributor to growth in ambulatory care. Approximately 8 million surgeries are performed in 4000 ASCs annually. The most common procedures include ophthalmology; gastroenterology; orthopedic; ear, nose, and throat; gynecology; and plastic surgery. ASCs contribute to healthcare cost containment. Procedures at ASCs cost nearly 50% less than inpatient surgeries (Ambulatory Surgery Center Association, 2009).

Community Health Centers

Community health centers (CHCs), which originated in the 1960s as part of the war on poverty, are organizations that provide healthcare services to the uninsured or indigent population such as minorities, infants, patients with HIV, substance abusers, and the homeless (Sultz & Young, 2006). Their focus is primary care. In order for the individual to receive CHC services, a patient should be a resident of the state, be uninsured, and be considered poor in accordance with the federal poverty guidelines. They also cannot be eligible for any state or federal indigent insurance programs.

CHCs often are located in urban and rural areas where there is a designated need. They enter a contract with the state or local health department to provide services to these populations. They also provide links with social workers, Medicaid, and Children's Health Insurance program (CHIP) (Pointer et al., 2007). CHCs receive funding under section 330 of the Public Health Service Act with grants from HHS of approximately $1 billion. CHCs may be organized as part of the local health department or another health service organization or organized as a not-for-profit organization (Sultz & Young, 2006).

It is estimated that 1 of every 19 individuals in the United States rely on CHCs for primary care. Nearly 16 million were treated at CHCs in 2008. On March 2, 2009, President Barack Obama released $155 million in grant money to support 126 additional CHCs nationwide, which will provide services to an additional 750,000 Americans and create nearly 6000 jobs. It is anticipated that within a 2-year period, an additional $2 billion will be invested in CHCs to support investments in health care (HHS, 2009c).

Home Health Agencies

Home health agencies and **visiting nurse agencies** provide medical services in a patient's home. The earliest form of home healthcare was developed by Lillian Wald who created the Visiting Nurse Service of New York in 1893 to service the poor. In 1909, she persuaded the Metropolitan Life Insurance Company to include nursing home care in their policies (Longest & Darr, 2008). This care is often provided to the elderly, disabled, or a patient who is too weak to come to the hospital or

physician's office or has just been released from the hospital. Contemporary home health services include both medical and social services. Services include skilled nursing care and home health aide care such as dispensing medications, assisting with activities of daily living, and meal planning. Physical, speech, and occupational therapy can also be provided at home. Medical equipment such as oxygen tanks, hospital beds, etc., may also be provided. Annually, approximately 7 million people receive home health services that are provided by approximately 20,000 agencies. These agencies can be private not for profit, government, or private for profit (Longest & Darr, 2008; Pointer et al., 2008).

Although the home healthcare industry is very popular with patients, there have been continued problems with the quality of home health care being offered. Although most states offer licensing for home health agencies, it is important that home health agencies are Medicare certified because they are required to comply with CMS regulations. They can also receive accreditation from the Community Health Accreditation Program (CHAP). Approximately 40% of home healthcare agencies are certified by Medicare. Nearly 70% of individuals who received home health care are older than 65 years of age (CMS, 2009; Longest & Darr, 2008).

Occupational Health Programs

Occupational health programs are often located at employer sites. Their purpose is to maintain the safety of the employee. Larger companies may provide physical exams, drug screenings, and basic health care. Employee assistance programs (EAPs) are a type of occupational health program. Established in the 1970s as an intervention for employee drug and alcohol abuse, the program has expanded to offer other services such as tobacco cessation programs and mental health counseling and referrals. EAP services have expanded to meet the needs of employees (Occupational Safety and Health Association, 2009).

OTHER HEALTH SERVICES
Respite Care

Often, family and friends of chronically ill patients become the major caregivers of their friends and family. This continuous care often becomes stressful for those caregivers. These caregivers may still be working full-time and have other family members that need their attention. As a result of this issue, **respite care** or **temporary** care programs were formally established in the 1970s to provide relief to those caregivers. These programs provide systematic relief to those caregivers who need a mental break. It also forestalls the ill patient from being placed in a facility. There are a variety of programs that are considered respite programs such as adult day care, furloughs to facilities for the patient, and in-home aides.

Hospice

Hospice care provides care for patients who have a life-threatening illness and the patient's family. Medicare, private health insurance, and Medicaid (in 43 states) cover hospice care for qualified patients. Some hospice programs offer healthcare services on a sliding fee scale basis for patients with limited resources. A typical hospice care team includes the following:

- Doctor
- Nurses
- Home health aides
- Clergy or other spiritual counselors (e.g., minister, priest, rabbi)
- Social workers
- Volunteers
- Occupational, physical, and/or speech therapists (HHS, 2009a)

The family of the terminally ill patient is also involved in the caregiving. More than 90% of hospice services are utilized by those who are older than 65 years of age. Hospice services can be offered both as inpatient and outpatient services. Hospitals may have designated hospice units. Home health agencies may also offer a hospice program (Longest & Darr, 2008).

Adult Day Care

Adult day care centers are day programs that provide a medical model of care with medical and therapeutic services; a social model that provides meals, recreation, and some basic medical health; or a medical–social model that provides social interaction and intensive medical-related activities, all depending on the needs of the patients. These centers were developed in the 1960s based on research that indicated adult day care centers were an opportunity to provide a break for their informal caregivers as well as providing an opportunity to prolong the patient's life at home. The average age of the adult day care center recipient is 72 years old and two thirds are female (National Adult Day Services Association [NADSA], 2009; Sultz & Young, 2006).

In 1979, the NADSA was formed to promote these types of community services. They established national standard criteria for the operation of adult day care centers. Many adult day care centers are regulated by state licensing and may be certified by a particular community agency. According to surveys (1) there are currently 3500 adult day care centers in the United States that provide care for 150,000 recipients on a daily basis; (2) nearly 80% of these centers are not for profit or public; (3) they are often affiliated with larger formal home healthcare or skilled nursing care facilities, medical centers, or senior organizations; and (4) the average daily rate is $60 per day (8–10 hours per day) (NADSA, 2009).

Senior Centers

Established by the Older American Act of 1965, senior centers provide a broad array of services for the older population. According to 2004 statistics, there are 5,000 senior centers in the United States. Approximately 70% of users are women; users spend 3 hours per day, 1–3 times per week at the centers; and the average age of attendees is 75 years of age (National Council on Aging [NCOA], 2009). Funding is received from state and local governments, grants, and private donations. They serve as community focal points for seniors. Services provided include meal and nutrition programs, education, recreational programs, volunteer opportunities, counseling, and other services.

Located in Washington, DC, NCOA is a not-for-profit advocacy agency for the senior population. As part of the NCOA, the National Institute of Senior Centers (NISC) is a network of senior center professionals that promote senior centers. They are the only national program dedicated to the welfare of senior centers. They sponsor a national voluntary accreditation program for senior centers (NCOA, 2009). With the expected increase in life expectancy, senior centers will continue to expand and offer more services to deal with seniors who have chronic disease that can be managed on an outpatient basis.

Women's Health Centers

Women seek healthcare services more frequently than men (Shi & Singh, 2008). They have unique health needs that can be provided by a medical facility that focuses on their needs. Recognizing this need, in 1991, HHS established an Office on Women's Health (OWH). Their mission is to promote women's and girl's health by gender-specific health activities. The OWH has developed five innovative national programs for coordinated women's healthcare that are summarized on their Web site (HHS, 2009b).

The National Centers of Excellence in Women's Health

The National Centers of Excellence in Women's Health (CoE) are located in academic medical centers throughout the country. This program combines healthcare services addressing women's health needs, public and professional education and training, the promotion of community links, and the provision of leadership positions for women in academic medicine.

The National Community Centers of Excellence in Women's Health

The National Community Centers of Excellence in Women's Health (CCOE) program provides recognition and resources to community-based programs to develop and integrate six components: (1) health services delivery, (2) particularly preventive services, (3) training for healthcare professionals including allied health professionals and others, (4) community based research, (5) public education and outreach, (6) leadership development for women, and (7) technical assistance to other communities to replicate the CCOE model.

The CoE and CCOE Ambassador for Change Program

The purpose of the Ambassadors for Change (AFC) program is to continue the "one-stop shopping" or "centers without walls" models of women's health care that have been developed by these organizations at a new, more progressive, and focused leadership level, and the provision of advice and guidance to other organizations interested in developing or implementing these unique models of care. There are 18 programs across the country that focus on the following objectives:

- Develop and/or strengthen a framework to bring together a comprehensive array of services for women
- Train a cadre of diverse healthcare providers that include allied health professionals and community health workers
- Promote leadership/career development for diverse women in the health professions,

including allied health professions and community health workers

- Enhance public education and outreach activities in women's health with an emphasis on gender-specific and age-appropriate prevention and/or reduction of illness or injuries
- Participate in any national evaluation of the CoE and/or CCOE program
- Conduct basic, clinical, and/or community-based research in women's health
- Provide advice and guidance to other organizations interested in learning more about the OWH CoE and CCOE programs

The CoE Region VIII Demonstration Program

There are three demonstration programs located at the University of Utah, University of North Dakota, and the University of South Dakota. The University of Utah Health Sciences Center in Salt Lake City was awarded a Region VIII CoE Demonstration Project contract in September 2005. The CoE program implements a national model for comprehensive, integrated, and multi- and interdisciplinary approaches to women's health care.

The University of North Dakota School of Medicine and Health Sciences in partnership with Altru Health System was selected for a CoE in Women's Health Region VIII Demonstration Project contract in September 2004. The project, the North Dakota Women's Health **CORE** (clinical, outreach, research, education) strives for an integrated model of health care, bringing together four key areas into a single setting. The ideal clinical concept is a one-stop shop for women's health care integrated with the other components. The CORE focuses on the needs of women of all ages, with particular emphasis toward women in rural areas as well as the needs of diverse populations.

The Sanford School of Medicine of The University of South Dakota in partnership with Sioux Valley Hospital and Clinics and University Physicians Clinics was awarded a contract to be a CoE in Women's Health Region VIII Demonstration Project in September 2004. The project is entitled HERS (health, education, resources, and support) for South Dakota Women. The goal of the project is to improve the health of South Dakota women by teaching health professionals about evidence-based women's health topics while improving the health literacy of women.

The Rural Frontier Women's Health Coordinating Centers

The OWH has funded eight new second-generation National Rural/Frontier Women's Health Coordinating Centers (RFCCs) on September 30, 2005. These centers are located in Arizona, Colorado, Nevada, Utah, Kentucky, Wisconsin, New Hampshire, Tennessee, and New Mexico. HHS Secretary Tommy G. Thompson began an Initiative on Rural Communities in 2001 to improve and enhance health care and human services for the 65 million people who live in rural America. It is estimated that approximately one fourth of the total US population lives in rural areas.

Rural residents have higher poverty rates, tend to be in poorer health, have fewer physicians, and fewer other health resources. Rural women are more likely to suffer from heart disease, hypertension, and cancer than urban women residents. The OWH has concluded that a comprehensive RFCC may be an effective strategy to address their health status.

Each of the centers must achieve the following objectives:

- Develop a comprehensive healthcare referral and tracking document
- Create a strategy for increasing the use of a gender-based approach to service delivery
- Develop innovative multidisciplinary health-care approaches to women
- Network in the community to form alliances that link existing resources efficiently
- Foster the leadership and advocacy skills of women to navigate access to health care
- Maximize access to healthcare services using existing transportation resources
- Facilitate research in women's health
- Include culturally and linguistically appropriate training and education in women's health for the public and healthcare professionals
- Develop community coalition
- Evaluate project outcomes and effectiveness (HHS, 2009b)

Meals on Wheels Association of America

The first **Meals on Wheels Association of America** (MOWAA) program started in Philadelphia, PA, in 1954 and is the largest and oldest organization in the United States that provides meal services those seniors in need. In 1954, the Philadelphia Health & Welfare Council funded a grant to pioneer a program to provide food to homebound seniors in the area. Most of the volunteers were high school students and they were dubbed Platter Angels. A fee of 40 to 80 cents per day was charged. Columbus, OH, was the second program in the country to start this type of program, followed by Rochester, NY, in 1958. Eventually, cities across the country established similar programs, which are continued today and represent an important component of senior citizen home health services (MOWAA, 2009). In 2008, the MOWAA released a study that indicated 1 in 9 seniors (5 million citizens) are at risk of food insecurity, which means they may have financial constraints, disabilities, or diseases that preclude them from having ready access to food. The study estimates that by 2025, there will be 10 million seniors that will experience food insecurity (Ziliak, Gunderson, & Haist, 2008).

In March 2009, Wal-Mart Foundation awarded $750,000 to Meals on Wheels programs in 40 states; the donations will help to continue those programs. Because of gasoline prices and the recession and an increase in request for services, it has been difficult to maintain many of these programs. These funds will sustain these programs for a period of time (Wal-Mart Stores, Inc., 2009).

Other Outpatient Health Services

There are many organizations that provide outpatient health services. These organizations can be for profit or not for profit. They can focus on specific populations such as migrant farm workers or the rural populations. There are too many to mention in this chapter but four organizations, Planned Parenthood of America (PPFA), the American Red Cross (ARC), Doctors Without Borders, and Remote Medical Access (RAM) will be discussed briefly. The common characteristic of all of these organizations are that they provide services in the United States and internationally.

Planned Parenthood Federation of America

PPFA is a 90-year-old organization that provides family services to local communities regarding sexual health, family planning, and more for men, women, and teens both online and at sites across the United States. They also provide health education. They accept Medicaid but also provide services based on a sliding fee scale. Their outreach provides over 1 million individuals with important health education (PPFA, 2009). They are also a founding member of the International Planned Parenthood Federation.

American Red Cross

Founded in 1881 and headquartered in Washington, DC, **ARC** provides emergency response to victims of war and natural and manmade disasters. They also provide services to the indigent and the military, analyze and distribute blood products, provide education, and organize international relief programs. Approximately 91 cents of every dollar spent is invested in humanitarian program. There are over 700 local chapters with 35,000 employees supported by 500,000 volunteers (ARC, 2009).

PPFA and ARC are examples of the types of outpatient services offered in different communities across the United States. Organizations have recognized that outpatient services are preferred by healthcare consumers and are cost-effective. Many physicians have established outpatient services as a way to satisfy consumer preference.

Doctors Without Borders

Established in 1971 by physicians and journalists, **Doctors Without Borders** is an international medical organization provides quality medical care to those individuals who are threatened by violence, catastrophe, lack of health care, natural disasters, epidemics, or wars. Nearly 90% of their funding is from private sources. Staff is derived from the communities where the crises are occurring as well as US aid workers. The organization won the Nobel Peace Prize in 1999. A US component of this organization was established in 1990. It recently raised $152.1 million in funding (Doctors Without Borders, 2009).

Remote Area Medical

RAM was founded in 1985 to develop a mobile efficient workforce to provide free health care to areas of need worldwide. Volunteer physicians, nurses, and other healthcare professionals provide general medical, surgical, eye, dental, and veterinary care to thousands of individuals worldwide. However, 60% of their services are provided to the United States (RAM, 2009). RAM determines where the centers are needed the most and set up a mobile healthcare unit for weekend services only. As a result of the economic downturn in the United States, there continues to be a huge need for their services.

Telehealth

Information technology will be discussed in depth in Chapter 9. **Telehealth** uses technology for providing healthcare services and is an efficient method of providing outpatient care. Telemedicine is a new model for delivering health care—it moves information electronically to consumers quickly and efficiently without a patient physically seeing a healthcare provider. Using technology is an efficient and cost-effective way to target underserved populations. SwiftMD, a telemedicine organization, was recently founded by a group of board-certified emergency physicians who have developed a membership-based model for providing health care. The membership is very inexpensive. The consultation costs approximately $75. The consumer member calls a toll-free number or asks for a consultation through their Web site at http://www.mySwiftMD.com. An emergency trained physician returns the call or contacts the patient within 30 minutes to determine if it is an emergency or not. The service is available 24 hours a day, 7 days a week. In order for this service to be effective, the organization requests that the patient uploads an electronic health record, which must be kept current in order to receive the best advice from the physicians. They can treat patients from 3 to 69 years of age. They do not treat pregnancy-related problems or mental health disorders. They treat conditions for which a patient would normally visit their physician's office (SwiftMD, 2009).

CONCLUSION

Although hospitals admit 35 million individuals annually, the healthcare industry has recognized that outpatient services are a cost-effective method of providing quality health care and has therefore evolved into providing quality outpatient care. This type of service is the preferred method of receiving health care by the consumer. In 2006, there were over 900 million visits to doctor's offices, which is the traditional method of ambulatory care (CDC, 2009). However, as medicine has evolved and more procedures can be performed on an outpatient basis such as surgeries, different types of outpatient care have evolved. As discussed previously, there are more outpatient surgical centers, imaging centers, urgent/emergent care centers, and other services that used to be offered on an inpatient basis. There will continue to be an increase in outpatient services being offered. As a consumer, technology will only increase the quality and efficiency of your health care. The implementation of the patient's electronic health record nationwide will be the impetus for the development of more electronic healthcare services.

PREVIEW OF CHAPTER SIX

The healthcare industry is one of the largest employers in the United States, employing more than 3% of the US workforce. There are approximately 200 health occupations and professions in a workforce of 13 million healthcare workers. Considering the aging of the US population, it is expected that the healthcare industry will continue to grow (Pointer et al., 2007; Sultz & Young, 2006). The healthcare industry is comprised of many different health services professionals. The healthcare industry includes dentists, optometrists, psychologists, chiropractors, podiatrists, nonphysician practitioners (NPPs), administrators, and allied health professionals. It is important to identify allied health professionals because they provide a range of essential healthcare services that complement the services provided by physicians and nurses. This category of health professionals is an integral component of providing quality health care and constitutes 60% of the US healthcare workforce (Shi & Singh, 2008). Chapter 6 will provide a description of the different types of healthcare professionals and their role in providing primary, secondary, and tertiary care in the healthcare system.

VOCABULARY

Academic medical centers

Accreditation

Acute care hospitals

Adult day care centers

Ambulatory surgery centers

American Red Cross

Board of trustees

Certification

Chief executive officer

Chief of medical staff

Chief of service

Church-related hospitals

Community health centers

Conditions of participation

CORE

Cost plus reimbursement

Council of Teaching Hospitals and Health Systems

Credentials committee

Doctors Without Borders

Federal hospitals

Home health agencies

Hospice care

Infection control committee

Informed consent

Inpatient services

International Organization for Standardization (ISO)

Long-term care hospitals

Meals on Wheels Association

Medical records committee

Medicare Rural Hospital Flexibility Program

National Adult Day Services Association

Occupational health programs

Osteopathic hospitals

Outpatient services

Patient Self-Determination Act of 1990

Planned Parenthood Federation of America

Proprietary hospitals

Psychiatric hospitals

Public hospitals

Quality improvement committee

Rehabilitation hospitals

Remote Area Medical

Respite care

Senior centers

State licensure

Teaching hospitals

Urgent/emergent care centers

Utilization review committee

Voluntary hospitals

REFERENCES

Ambulatory Surgery Center Association. (2009). Retrieved November 10, 2009, from http://ascassociation.org/faqs/faqaboutascs/#1.

American Hospital Association. (2009a). A patient bill of rights. Retrieved November 10, 2009, from http://www.patienttalk.info/AHA-Patient_Bill_of_Rights.htm.

American Hospital Association. (2009b). *2009 Health and hospital trends*. Retrieved July 1, 2009, from http://www.aha.org/aha/research-and-trends/health-and-hospital-trends/2009.html.

American Red Cross. (2009). Retrieved November 10, 2009, from http://www.redcross.org/portal/site/en/menuitem.d8aaecf214c576bf971e4cfe43181aa0/?vgnextoid=477859f392ce8110VgnVCM10000030f3870aRCRD&vgnextfmt=default.

Buchbinder, S., & Shanks, N. (2007). *Introduction to health care management*. Sudbury, MA: Jones and Bartlett.

Centers for Disease Control and Prevention. (2009a). *Ambulatory care use and physician visits*. Retrieved July 3, 2009, from http://www.cdc.gov/nchs/fastats/docvisit.htm.

Centers for Disease Control and Prevention. (2009b). *National hospital medical care ambulatory survey*. Retrieved November 9, 2009, from http://www.cdc.gov/nchs/data/nhsr/nhsr007.pdf.

Centers for Medicare and Medicaid Services. (2009). Retrieved November 10, 2009, from http://www.cms.hhs.gov/center/hha.asp.

Department of Health and Human Services. (2009a). *Elder care locator*. Retrieved September 5, 2009, from http://www.eldercare.gov/Eldercare.NET/Public/Resources/Fact_Sheets/hospice_care.aspx.

Department of Health and Human Services. (2009b). *The Office of Women's Health*. Retrieved April 6, 2009, from http://www.4woman.gov/owh/about/.

Department of Health and Human Services. (2009c). *Recovery act: Community health centers*. Retrieved November 10, 2009, from http://www.hhs.gov/recovery/hrsa/healthcentergrants.html.

Doctors Without Borders. (2009). Retrieved November 10, 2009, from http://www.doctorswithoutborders.com/aboutus/?ref=main-menu.

Duke University Libraries. (2008). Timeline of medicine. Retrieved June 2, 2008, from http://library.duke.edu/digitalcollections/mma/timeline.html.

International Organization for Standardization. (2009). Retrieved June 13, 2009, from http://www.iso.org.

The Joint Commission. (2009). Retrieved November 10, 2009, from http://www.jointcommissioninternational.org/Quality-and-Safety-Risk-Areas/Accreditation-and-Certification/.

Jonas, S. (2003). *An introduction to the U.S. health care system*. New York: Springer Publishing.

Longest, B., & Darr, K. (2008). *Managing health services organizations and systems*. Baltimore: Health Professions Press.

Meals on Wheels Association of America. (2009). Retrieved November 10, 2009, from http://www.mealsonwheels.org/about/index.html.

MedicineNet, Inc. (2009). *Medical dictionary*. Retrieved June 13, 2009, from http://www.medterms.com/script/main/art.asp?articlekey=8390.

National Adult Day Services Association. (2009). *Adult day services: Overview and facts*. Retrieved April 7, 2009, from http://www.nadsa.org/adsfacts/default.asp.

National Conference of State Legislatures. (2009). Retrieved November 10, 2009, from http://www.ncsl.org/default.aspx?tabid=14373.

National Council on Aging. (2009). Retrieved November 10, 2009, from http://www.ncoa.org/content.cfm? sectionID=46.

Occupational Safety and Health Association. (2009). Retrieved November 10, 2009, from http://www.osha.gov/as/opa/worker/employer-responsibility.html.

Planned Parenthood Federation of America. (2009). Retrieved November 10, 2009, from http://www.plannedparenthood.org/about-us/index.htm.

Pointer, D., Williams, S., Isaacs, S., & Knickman, J. (2007). *Introduction to U.S. health care*. Hoboken, NJ: Wiley Publishing.

Relman, A. (2007). *A second opinion: Rescuing America's health care* (pp. 15–67). New York: PublicAffairs.

Remote Area Medical Volunteer Corps. (2009). Retrieved November 10, 2009, from http://www.ramusa.org/about/history.htm.

Rosen, G. (1983). *The structure of American medical practice 1875–1941*. Philadelphia: University of Pennsylvania Press.

Shi, L., & Singh, D. (2008). *Delivering health care in America*. Sudbury, MA: Jones and Bartlett.

Starr, P. (1982). *The social transformation of American medicine*. Cambridge, MA: Basic Books.

Substance Abuse and Mental Health Services Administration. (2009). Retrieved April 6, 2009, from http://www.samsha.gov.

Sultz, H., & Young, K. (2006). *Health care USA: Understanding its organization and delivery* (5th ed.). Sudbury, MA: Jones and Bartlett.

SwiftMD. (2009). Retrieved December 30, 2009, from http://www.swiftmd.com/how-much-does-it-cost.

Torrens, P. R. (1993). Historical evolution and overview of health services in the United States. In S. J. Williams & P. R. Torrens (Eds.). *Introduction to health services* (4th ed.). Clifton Park, NY: Delmar Publishers.

Urgent Care Association of America. (2009). Retrieved November 10, 2009, from http://www.ucaoa.org/home_abouturgentcare.php.

Wal-Mart Stores, Inc. (2009). Retrieved November 10, 2009, from http://walmartstores.com/CommunityGiving/9054.aspx.

Ziliak, J., Gunderson, C., & Haist, M. (2008). *The causes, consequences and future of senior hunger in America*. Lexington, KY: University of Kentucky Center for Poverty Research.

NOTES

STUDENT ACTIVITY 5-1

CROSSWORD PUZZLE

Instructions: Please complete the puzzle using the vocabulary words found in the chapter. There may be multiple-word answers. The numbers in the parenthesis are the number of words in the answer.

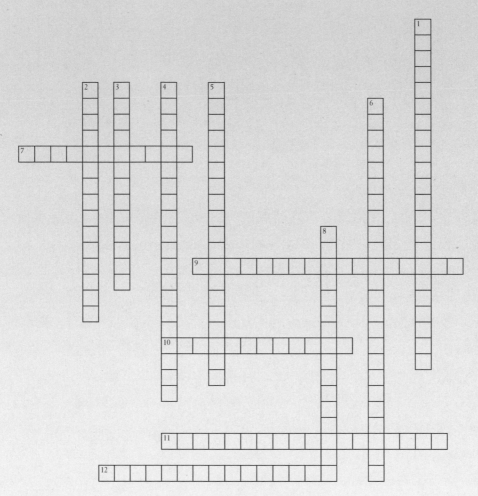

Created with EclipseCrossword © 1999–2009 Green Eclipse

STUDENT ACTIVITY 5-1

Across

7. Temporary care given to caregivers who are providing constant care to those who are ill. (2 words)

9. Founded in 1985, they provide medical services to those in need. This international organization provides 60% of their services to the United States. (3 words)

10. A new medical model that moves information electronically to the consumer efficiently and effectively. (1 word)

11. Nongovernment owned, private, and not for profit, these institutions rely on community financial giving. (2 words)

12. This hospital entity is legally responsible for hospital operations. (3 words)

Down

1. Originated in the 1960s as a result of the war on poverty, these organizations provide healthcare services to the indigent population and often enter a contract with the local health department to provide services. (3 words)

2. These are the oldest types of hospitals. (2 words)

3. This type of standard is private and developed by accepted organizations as a way to meet certain standards. (1 word)

4. Investor-owned for-profit institutions that can be owned by corporations, individuals, or partnerships. (2 words)

5. Day programs that provide a medical model and a social model depending on the needs of the patients. (4 words)

6. This is the oldest and largest organization in the United States that provides meal services to those seniors in need. (4 words)

8. This organization was founded in 1881 and provides emergency response to victims of natural disasters. Also processes blood products. (3 words)

STUDENT ACTIVITY 5-2

IN YOUR OWN WORDS

Based on Chapter 5, please provide an explanation of the following concepts in your own words. DO NOT RECITE the text.

Cost plus reimbursement: _____
_____
_____

Respite care: _____
_____
_____

Occupational health programs: _____
_____
_____

Public hospitals: _____
_____
_____

Voluntary hospitals: _____
_____
_____

Proprietary hospitals: _____
_____
_____

Certification: _____
_____
_____

Accreditation: _____
_____
_____

Acute care: _____
_____
_____

CORE: _____
_____
_____

REAL LIFE APPLICATIONS: CASE STUDY

You just received your Master of Health Administration degree and decided you would like to pursue a career in hospital management. You cannot decide what type of hospital you would like to apply to and decide to investigate the different types of hospitals that are available.

ACTIVITY

(1) Identify and list the different types of hospitals that are available for your employment, (2) compare and contrast the different types of hospitals, and (3) based on your research, select a hospital type and state why you chose this type of hospital.

RESPONSES

_____

_____

_____

_____

_____

_____

_____

_____

_____

_____

_____

_____

_____

_____

STUDENT ACTIVITY 5-4

INTERNET EXERCISES

Write your answers in the space provided.

- Visit each of the Web sites listed here.
- Name the organization.
- Locate their mission statement on their Web site.
- Provide a brief overview of the activities of the organization.
- How do these organizations participate in the US healthcare system?

Web Sites

http://www.doctorswithoutborders.org

Organization Name: _____

Mission Statement:

_____

_____

_____

Overview of Activities:

_____

_____

_____

Importance of organization to US health care:

_____

_____

_____

http://www.4woman.gov

Organization Name: _____

Mission Statement:

_____

_____

_____

Overview of Activities:

_____

_____

_____

STUDENT ACTIVITY 5-4

Importance of organization to US health care:

_____

_____

_____

http://www.ramusa.org

Organization Name: _____

Mission Statement:

_____

_____

_____

Overview of Activities:

_____

_____

_____

Importance of organization to US health care:

_____

_____

_____

http://www.swiftmd.com

Organization Name: _____

Mission Statement:

_____

_____

_____

Overview of Activities:

_____

_____

_____

Importance of organization to US health care:

_____

_____

_____

STUDENT ACTIVITY 5-4

http://ncoa.org

Organization Name: _____

Mission Statement:

_____

_____

_____

Overview of Activities:

_____

_____

_____

Importance of organization to US health care:

_____

_____

_____

http://www.ascassociation.org

Organization Name: _____

Mission Statement:

_____

_____

_____

Overview of Activities:

_____

_____

_____

Importance of organization to US health care:

_____

_____

_____

Chapter 6

Healthcare Professionals

LEARNING OBJECTIVES

The student will be able to:

- Describe five types of physicians and their roles in health care.

- Describe six types of nurse professionals and their roles in health care.

- Describe six types of other health professionals and their roles in health care.

- Discuss the issue of geographic maldistribution of physicians and its impact on access to care.

- Describe the difference between primary, secondary, and tertiary care.

- Define allied health professionals and their role in the healthcare industry.

- Discuss five allied health-certified educational programs and their impact on health care.

DID YOU KNOW THAT?

- The healthcare industry is one of the largest employers in the United States.

- Approximately 59% of US physicians are specialists such as surgeons, cardiologists, and psychiatrists.

- The principle funding for graduate medical education is Medicare.

- Since the 1990s, physicians who specialize in the care of hospitalized patients are called "hospitalists."

- Nurses are the largest group of healthcare professionals in the United States.

INTRODUCTION

The healthcare industry is one of the largest employers in the United States, employing more than 3% of the US workforce. There are approximately 200 health occupations and professions in a workforce of 13 million healthcare workers. Considering the aging of the US population, it is expected that the healthcare industry will continue to grow (Pointer, Williams, Isaacs, & Knickman, 2007; Sultz & Young, 2006). Between 2005 and 2030, the section of the population that is 65 years and older will increase from 6% to 10% of the total population, which will place pressure on the healthcare system (National Center for Health Statistics, 2008). When we think of healthcare providers, we automatically think of physicians and nurses. However, the healthcare industry is comprised of many different health services professionals. The healthcare industry includes dentists, optometrists, psychologists, chiropractors, podiatrists, nonphysician practitioners (NPPs), administrators, and allied health professionals. It is important to identify allied health professionals because they provide a range of essential healthcare services that complement the services provided by physicians and nurses. This category of health professionals is an integral component of providing quality health care and constitutes 60% of the US healthcare workforce (Shi & Singh, 2008).

Health care can occur in varied settings. Many physicians have their own practices but they may also work in hospitals, mental health facilities, managed care organizations, or community health centers. They may also hold government positions or teach at a university. They could be employed by an insurance company. Health professionals, in general, may work at many different organizations, both for profit and nonprofit. However, hospitals employ nearly 43% of the healthcare industry (Pointer et al., 2007). Although the healthcare industry is one of the largest employers in the United States, there continues to be shortages of physicians in geographic areas of the country. Rural areas continue to suffer physician shortages, which limits consumer access to health care. There have been different incentive programs to encourage physicians to relocate to rural areas, but shortages still exist. In most states, only physicians, dentists, and only a few other practitioners may serve patients directly without the authorization of another licensed independent health professional. Those categories authorized include chiropractic, optometry, psychotherapy, and podiatry. Some states authorize midwifery and physical therapy (Jonas, 2003). There also continues to be a shortage of nurses nationwide. It is projected that nursing shortages will continue to lag 36% behind nursing staffing needs (Bradley, 2008). This chapter will provide a description of the different types of healthcare professionals and their role in providing primary, secondary, and tertiary care.

PRIMARY, SECONDARY, AND TERTIARY CARE

There are three important concepts of care that need to be emphasized: primary, secondary, and tertiary care. **Primary care** is the essential component of the US healthcare system because it is the point of entry into the system—where the patient makes first contact with the system. Primary care focuses on continuous and routine care of an individual. It may be delivered by a physician, nurse practitioner, midwife, or physician's assistant. Categories of primary care practitioners usually include family practitioners, pediatricians, internal medicine providers, obstetricians and gynecologists,

psychiatrists, and emergency medicine physicians (Jonas, 2003). The focus of a primary care provider is to ensure patient access to the system by coordinating the delivery of healthcare services. Primary care is often referred to as essential health care. Primary care services could include health education and counseling and other preventive services. **Secondary care** focuses on short-term interventions that may require a specialist's intervention. Examples of secondary care would include hospitalizations, routine surgery, specialty consultation, and rehabilitation (Shi & Singh, 2008). **Tertiary care** is the most complex level of medical care for uncommon conditions. This type of care is usually based on a referral from a primary care provider. It is highly specialized and usually is delivered in specialty or research hospitals. Examples of tertiary care are organ transplants, bone marrow transplants, and heart surgery. These procedures would also be performed by specialist physicians (Pointer et al., 2007).

PHYSICIAN EDUCATION

Physicians play a major role in providing healthcare services. They have been trained to diagnose and treat patient illnesses. Depending on their training, physicians have participated in primary, secondary, and tertiary care; however, some physicians are now providing primary prevention. All states require a license to practice medicine. Physicians must receive their medical education from an accredited school that awards either a **Doctor of Medicine** (MD) or a **Doctor of Osteopathic Medicine** (DO). Prior to entering medical school, many students prepare for medical school by majoring in a premedical undergraduate program, which often consists of science and mathematics. Undergraduate students are also required to take the MCAT—the Medical College Admission Test. There are 126 accredited medical schools that award the Doctor of Medicine (Sultz & Young, 2006). In order to provide direct patient care, the physician must take a licensing examination in the desired state of practice once they complete a residency. State licensing requirements may vary. This residency or training may take 3 to 8 years. The residency is important because it allows physicians to learn about a certain specialty of interest while providing them with on-the-job training. The length of the residency program can be as short as 3 years for a family practice and as long as 10 years for different surgery specialties. There are currently 8000 residency programs offered by hospitals. Most states require physicians to take continuing medical education (CMEs) activities to maintain state licensure (Buchbinder & Shanks, 2007; Pointer et al., 2007; Sultz & Young, 2006; Shi & Singh, 2008).

There are only 20 accredited medical schools that confer the DO degree. Their enrollment has doubled over the last 20 years. They represent approximately 5% of all US physicians (Sultz & Young, 2006). The major difference between an MD and a DO is their approach to treatment. DOs tend to stress preventive treatments and use a **holistic approach** to treating a patient, which means they do not focus only on the disease but on the entire person. Most DOs are generalists. MDs use an **allopathic approach**, which means MDs actively intervene in attacking and eradicating disease and focus their efforts on the disease (Pointer et al., 2007; Shi & Singh, 2008).

GENERALISTS AND SPECIALISTS

Generalists are also called primary care physicians. Family care practitioners are also called generalists as are general internal medicine physicians and general pediatricians. Their focus is preventive services such as immunizations, health examinations, etc. They treat less severe medical problems. They often serve as a gatekeeper for a patient, which means they coordinate patient care if the patient needs to see a specialist for more complex medical problems. **Specialists** are required to be certified in their area of specialization. This may require additional years of training, as discussed in the previous paragraph, and require a **board certifying** or **credentialing examination**. The most common specialties are dermatology, cardiology, pediatrics, pathology, psychiatry, obstetrics, anesthesiology, specialized internal medicine, gynecology, ophthalmology, radiology, and surgery (Shi & Singh, 2008). The board certification is often associated with the quality of the healthcare provider's services because board certification requires more training. A consumer is eligible to view a physician's credentials in the **National Practitioner Data Bank** (NPDB). The database was created to provide a nationwide system to prohibit any incompetent healthcare practitioners from moving state-to-state without disclosing any previous issues (Buchbinder & Shanks, 2007).

DIFFERENCES BETWEEN PRIMARY AND SPECIALTY CARE

Primary care is the initial contact between the healthcare provider and the patient. If needed, specialty care will be a result of a primary care evaluation. The primary care physician will ultimately coordinate the health care of the patient if additional specialty care is required. If a patient has a chronic condition, the primary care provider will coordinate the overall care of the individual. In a managed care environment, which focuses on cost containment, the primary care physician becomes the gatekeeper of the patient's care. The primary care physician refers a patient to a specialist for additional care. Primary care students spend most of their focus in ambulatory settings learning about different diseases, whereas the specialty care students spend time in an inpatient setting focusing on special patient conditions (Shi & Singh, 2008).

PATTERNS OF PHYSICIAN SUPPLY

The estimated number of physicians required to service the US population is 145 to 185 per 100,000 population. Currently, the ratio is approximately 300 per 100,000. Despite these numbers, there are still shortages of physicians in certain parts of the country (Shi & Singh, 2008). This concept of **geographic maldistribution** has occurred because physicians prefer to practice in urban and suburban areas where there is a higher probability of increased income. Recruiting physicians to rural areas is difficult because of the working conditions, reduced income, and reduced access to technology, which is more available in urban and suburban areas. Another issue in physician supply is the increasing number of specialists to generalists, which is called **specialty maldistribution**. The supply of specialists has increased more than 100% over the last 20 years, while the supply of generalists has increased only 18%. Nearly 60% of active physicians are specialists. Specialty maldistribution has occurred for the following four reasons: (1) medical technology advances, (2) specialty-oriented medical education, (3) higher income for specialty physicians, and (4) consumer preference for technological driven medicine (Sultz & Young, 2006). There have been major technological advances in medicine that both physicians and consumer prefer. Consumer preferences indicate that they feel they are receiving better care when technology is introduced into their care. These preferences, coupled with the fact that medical schools focus on specialty care rather than primary care, encourage specialty maldistribution and increase the number of specialists. Despite federal and state incentives for encouraging both specialty and geographic maldistribution, these two major problems continue to exist (Health Resources and Services Administration [HRSA], 2008).

TYPES OF HEALTHCARE PROVIDERS

Hospitalists

A **hospitalist** is a physician that provides care to hospitalized patients. They replace a patient's primary care physician while the patient is hospitalized. A hospitalist monitors the patient from admittance to discharge. They normally do not have a relationship with the patient prior to admittance. This new type of physician, which evolved in the 1990s, is usually a general practitioner and is becoming more popular—because they spend so much time in the hospital setting, they can provide more efficient care. From a hospital's viewpoint, the focus is maximization of profit, which means shorter lengths of stay, decreased complications, and increased patient satisfaction (Sultz & Young, 2006). There are approximately 12,000 hospitalists in the United States, a number that is expected to triple by 2010. Although they are not board certified as a specialty, they have their own medical journal, annual meetings, and association. This concept has proven to be very effective and is expected to play a larger role in health care (Shi & Singh, 2008).

Nonphysician Practitioners

It is important to mention the general term **NPP**, which includes nonphysician clinicians (NPCs) and midlevel practitioners (MLPs). The specific professionals of this category will be discussed in depth in this chapter but it is important to mention their importance generally in providing health care. They are sometimes called **physician extenders** because they often are used as a substitute for physicians. They are not involved in total care of a patient so they collaborate closely with physicians. Categories of NPPs include physician assistants (PAs), nurse practitioners (NPs), and certified nurse practitioners (CNPs) (Shi & Singh, 2008). NPPs have been favorably received by patients because they tend to spend more time with patients. They play an important role in areas that are underserved by physician shortages in urban areas, in community health centers, and the managed care environment. NPPs can perform repetitive technical tasks such as screenings for diseases. They may also take care of non–life-threatening cases in emergency departments and perform physicals, drug testing, and other routine activities. Their salaries are nearly 50% less than physician salaries so they are a cost-effective caregiver for patients. As NPPs become more involved in patient care, reimbursement for their services should be addressed. At this time,
reimbursement is usually directed toward their collaborating physician, which often results in payment delays. It is important to emphasize that as NPPs' roles increase in patient care because of cost-cutting measures by healthcare organizations, continued regulations and guidelines are needed to ensure high quality patient care by NPPs (Shi & Singh, 2008).

Physician Assistants

PAs, a category of NPPs, provide a range of diagnostic and therapeutic services to patients. They take medical histories, conduct patient examinations, analyze tests, make diagnoses, and perform basic medical procedures. They are able to prescribe medicines in all but three states. They must be associated and supervised by a physician but the supervision does not need to be direct. In many areas where there is a shortage of physician, PAs act as primary care providers. They collaborate with physicians by telephone and onsite visits. There are 129 accredited programs in the United States. Students take classes and participate in clinical settings. They are required to pass a national certification exam. They may take additional education in surgery, pediatrics, emergency medicine, primary care, and occupational medicine. Their average salary is $65,000 (Bureau of Labor and Statistics [BLS], 2009c).

TYPES OF NURSES

Nurses constitute the largest group of healthcare professionals. Nurses provide the majority of care to patients, accounting for 20% of the workforce (Pointer et al., 2007). They are the patient advocate. There are several different types of nurses that provide patient care. There are several different levels of nursing care based on education and training. The following is a summary of each type of nurse.

Licensed Practical Nurse or Licensed Vocation Nurse (California and Texas)

- There are approximately 700,000 licensed practical nurses (LPNs) in the United States. They are the largest group of nurses.
- Education is offered by community colleges or technical schools. Training takes approximately 12–14 months and includes both education and supervised clinical practice. There are 1100 programs in the United States. LPNs have a high school diploma and a licensing exam. Their salary is approximately $29,000.

- Their job responsibilities include patient observation, taking vital signs, keeping records, assisting patients with personal hygiene, and feeding and dressing patients, which are considered **activities of daily living** (ADLs).

- In some states, LPNs administer some medications.

- They work primarily in hospitals, home health agencies, and nursing homes.

- Many LPNs work full time and earn their Bachelor of Science in Nursing (BSN) degree to increase their career choices (BLS, 2009b).

Registered Nurse

- There are approximately 2.5 million **registered nurses** (RNs) in the United States and they represent the largest healthcare occupation. An RN is a graduate trained nurse who has been licensed by a state board after passing the national nursing examination. They can be registered in more than one state.

- There are different levels of registered nursing based on education.

- **Associate Degree in Nursing** (ADN): Two-year program offered by community colleges.

- Diploma programs: Three-year programs offered by hospitals. There is no degree offered but undergraduate credit may be earned. They are very expensive and are being offered less often. There are approximately 70 diploma programs left in the United States.

- **Bachelor of Science in Nursing** (BSN): The most rigorous of the nursing programs. Programs offered by colleges and universities normally take 4 to 5 years. They perform both classroom activity and clinical practice activity.

- Their job responsibilities include recording symptoms of any disease, implementing care plans, assisting physicians in examinations and the treatment of patients, administering medications and performing medical procedures, supervising other personnel such as LPNs, and educating patients and families about follow-up care.

- The majority of RNs work in hospitals. Depending on the level of education, the average annual income is $45,000.

- **Advanced practical nurse** (APN) or midlevel practitioners are nurses who have experience and education beyond the requirements of an RN. They operate between the RN and MD, which is why they are called **midlevel practitioners**. They normally obtain a Master of Science in Nursing (MSN) with a specialty in the field of practice. There are four areas of specialization: clinical nurse specialist (CNS), certified registered nurse anesthetist (CRNA), nurse practitioners (NP), and certified nurse–midwives (CNM).

- Many of these certifications allow for a nurse to provide direct care including writing prescriptions (BLS, 2009e).

Nurse Practitioners and Certified Nurse Midwives

As stated earlier, NPPs are an integral component of providing quality health care in the United States. **NPs** are the largest categories of advanced practice nurses (APNs). The first group of NPs was trained in 1965 at the University of Colorado. In 1974, the American Nursing Association developed the Council of Primary Care Nurse Practitioners, which helped substantiate the role of NPs in patient care. Over the last two decades, several specialty NP boards have been established such as pediatrics and reproductive health for certification of NPs. In 1985, the American Association of Nurse Practitioners (AANP) was established as a professional organization for NPs. As of 2007, there were approximately 120,000 practicing NPs with an average of 6000 NPs receiving training at over 325 education institutions (AANP, 2008). They are required to obtain an RN and a master's degree. They may receive a certificate program and complete direct patient care clinical training. NPs emphasize health education and promotion as well as disease treatment—referred to as care and cure. NPs spend more time with patients and, as a result, patient surveys indicate satisfaction with NPs care. NPs may specialize in pediatrics, family, geriatric, or psychiatric care. Most states allow NPs to prescribe medications. Recent statistics indicated that there were 600 million visits made to NPs annually (AANP, 2008).

Certified nurse–midwives (CNM) are RNs who have graduated from a nurse midwifery education program that has been accredited by the American College of Nurse–Midwives' Division of Accreditation. Nurse–midwives have been practicing in the United States for nearly 90 years. They must pass the national certification exam to receive the designation of CNM. Nurse–midwives are primary care providers for women who are pregnant. They must be recertified every 8 years. The **certified midwives** (CMs) are individuals who do not have a nursing degree but have a related health background. They must take the midwifery education program, which is accredited by the same organization. They must also pass the same national certification exam to be given the designation of CM (BLS, 2009e).

Certified Nursing Assistants or Aides

Certified nursing assistants (CNAs) are unlicensed patient attendants who work under the supervision of physicians and nurses. They answer patient call bells that need their service; assist patients with personal hygiene, changing beds, ordering their meals; and assist patients with their ADLs. Most CNAs are employed by nursing care facilities. There are approximately 1.5 million CNAs in the healthcare industry. They are required to receive 75 hours of training and are required to pass a competency examination. Their average pay is extremely low. They are often overlooked for pay and advancement and therefore there is a high turnover in their field despite the fact that they provide needed services to the patient (Pointer et al., 2007; Shi & Singh, 2008).

NURSING SHORTAGES

Although nursing supply and demand is cyclical, during recent years there continues to be a nursing shortage. The current shortage began a decade ago, making it the longest shortage in 50 years. According to the BLS, employment of RNs will increase by 23% by 2016. Without recruitment for nursing programs, the Health and Human Services Administration projects the supply of US nurses will lag behind 36% of nursing staffing needs (Bradley, 2008). Although community colleges have developed quality nursing programs nationally, there is increased pressure for students to obtain additional nursing education. A reason there is a shortage of nursing personnel is the lack of qualified nursing faculty available. Unlike faculty in other disciplines who are doctorally prepared, that is not the case for nursing faculty. Approximately 50% of faculty in BSN and advanced degree programs do not hold a doctorate. Many nursing faculty leave for higher pay in clinical and private sector settings. An average nursing faculty salary is $62,000. Nurse practitioners who own their own practice earned an average of $94,000 (Yordy, 2006).

OTHER INDEPENDENT HEALTHCARE PROFESSIONALS

Dentists

Dentists prevent, diagnose, and treat teeth, gum, and mouth diseases. They are required to complete 4 years of dental school from an accredited dental school once a bachelor's degree is completed. They are awarded a Doctor of Dental Surgery (DDS) or Doctor of Dental Medicine (DDM). Some states may require a specialty license. The first 2 years of dental school are focused on dental sciences. The last 2 years are spent in a clinical environment. Dentists may take an additional 2 to 4 years of postgraduate education in orthodontics (teeth straightening), oral surgery, public health dentistry, etc. There are nearly 170,000 dentists in the United States—over 90% are private practice and are primarily general practitioners. Their average annual income is $130,000 (Pointer et al., 2007). Dental practices are not in managed care environments. Dentists only serve those who have dental insurance and who can pay out of pocket. There are sections of underserved populations that will continue to be underserved because there is no industry priority to target those populations (Sultz & Young, 2006).

Dentists are often helped by **dental hygienists** and **dental assistants**. Dental hygienists clean patients' teeth and educate patients on proper dental care. They are required to be licensed to practice, which requires graduation from an accredited dental hygienist school and passing both a national and state licensing exam. Dental assistants work directly with dentists in the preparation and treatment of patients. They do not have to be licensed but there are certification programs available (BLS, 2009a).

Pharmacists

Pharmacists are responsible for dispensing medication that has been prescribed by physicians. They also advise both patients and healthcare providers on potential side effects of medications. Pharmacists must earn a Doctor of Pharmacy (PharmD) degree from an accredited college or school of pharmacy, which has replaced the Bachelor of Pharmacy degree, which is no longer being awarded. To be admitted to a PharmD program, an applicant must have completed at least 2 years of postsecondary study, although most applicants have completed 3 or more years, which include courses in mathematics and natural sciences. In 2007,

92 colleges and schools of pharmacy were accredited to confer degrees. There are approximately 70 US pharmaceutical schools that also award a PharmD which takes approximately 6 years of postgraduate study. The degree was designed for those who want additional clinical, laboratory, and research experience. Areas of graduate study include pharmaceutics and pharmaceutical chemistry, pharmacology (effects of drugs on the body), and pharmacy administration. Many master's and PhD degree holders are hired to perform research or teach at a university.

In 2006, there were nearly 243,000 US active pharmacists with approximately 60% of them working in community pharmacies. Approximately 25% of pharmacists work in hospitals with the remaining 15% working in physician offices, mail order and Internet pharmacies, nursing homes, and the federal government. Median annual wages are $106,000 (BLS, 2008d).

Chiropractors

Chiropractors have a holistic approach to treating their patients. They believe that the body can heal itself without medication or surgery. Their focus is the entire body, emphasizing the spine, without the use of drugs or surgery. They manipulate the body with their hands or with a machine. Chiropractors must be licensed, which requires 2 to 4 years of undergraduate education, the completion of a 4-year chiropractic college course, and passing scores on national and state examinations. In 2007, 16 chiropractic programs and 2 chiropractic institutions in the United States were accredited by the Council on Chiropractic Education. Applicants must have at least 90 semester hours of undergraduate study leading toward a bachelor's degree before entering the program. Chiropractic programs require a minimum of 4200 hours of classroom, laboratory, and clinical experience. During the first 2 years, most chiropractic programs emphasize classroom and laboratory. The last 2 years focus on courses in manipulation and spinal adjustment and clinical experience. Chiropractic programs and institutions grant the degree of Doctor of Chiropractic. In 2006, there were 53,000 chiropractors in the United States. The mean salary for a chiropractor is $105,000 (BLS, 2008a).

Optometrists

Optometrists, also known as Doctors of Optometry or ODs, are the main providers of vision care. They examine people's eyes to diagnose vision problems. Optometrists may prescribe eyeglasses or contact lenses. Optometrists also test for glaucoma and other eye diseases and diagnose conditions caused by systemic diseases, such as diabetes and high blood pressure, and refer patients to other health practitioner. Optometrists often provide preoperative and postoperative care to cataract patients, as well as to patients who have had laser vision correction or other eye surgery.

Optometrists need an OD degree, which requires the completion of a 4-year program at an accredited optometry school. In 2006, there were 16 colleges of optometry in the United States and 1 in Puerto Rico that offered accredited programs. Requirements for admission to optometry schools include college courses in English, mathematics, physics, chemistry, and biology. Because a strong background in science is important, many applicants to optometry school major in a science as undergraduates. Admission to optometry school is competitive. Applicants must take the Optometry Admissions Test, which measures academic ability and scientific comprehension. As a result, most applicants take the test after their sophomore or junior year in college, allowing them an opportunity to take the test again and raise their score. However, most students accepted by a school or college of optometry have completed an undergraduate degree

All states require that optometrists be licensed. Applicants for a license must have an OD degree from an accredited optometry school and must pass both a written National Board examination and a national, regional, or state clinical examination. Many states also require applicants to pass an examination on relevant state laws. Licenses must be renewed every 1 to 3 years and, in all states, continuing education credits are needed for renewal. Optometrists held about 33,000 jobs in 2006. Employment of optometrists is expected to grow in response to the vision care needs of a growing and aging population. Median annual earnings of salaried optometrists were $91,000 in 2006 (BLS, 2008c).

Psychologists

Psychologists study the human mind and human behavior. Research psychologists investigate the physical, cognitive, emotional, or social aspects of human behavior. Psychologists in health service fields provide mental health care in hospitals, clinics, schools, or private settings. Psychologists are employed in applied settings such as business, industry, government, or nonprofit organizations and provide training, conduct research, design organizational systems, and act as advocates for psychology. They usually specialize in one of a number of different areas.

Clinical psychologists—who represent the largest specialty—work most often in counseling centers, independent or group practices, hospitals, or clinics. They help mentally and emotionally distressed clients and may assist medical patients in dealing with illnesses or injuries. Areas of specialization within clinical psychology include health psychology, neuropsychology, and geropsychology. *Health psychologists* study how biological, psychological, and social factors affect health and illness. *Neuropsychologists* study the relation between the brain and behavior. They often work in stroke and head injury programs. *Geropsychologists* deal with the special problems faced by the elderly. Often, clinical psychologists consult with other medical personnel regarding the best treatment for patients, especially treatment that includes medication. Clinical psychologists generally are not permitted to prescribe medication like psychiatrists and other medical doctors may prescribe. However, Louisiana and New Mexico currently allow certain clinical psychologists to prescribe medication with some limitations.

Counseling psychologists use various techniques, including interviewing and testing, to advise people on how to deal with problems of everyday living, including career or work problems and problems faced in different stages of life. *School psychologists* work with students in early childhood and elementary and secondary schools. School psychologists address students' learning and behavioral problems, suggest improvements to classroom management strategies or parenting techniques, and evaluate students with disabilities and gifted and talented students to help determine the best way to educate them.

Industrial–organizational psychologists apply psychological principles and research methods to the workplace in the interest of improving productivity and the quality of work life. *Developmental psychologists* study the physiological, cognitive, and social development that takes place throughout life. Some specialize in behavior during infancy, childhood, and adolescence, or changes that occur during maturity or old age. **Social psychologists** examine people's interactions with others and with the social environment. **Experimental** or **research psychologists** work in university and private research centers and in business, nonprofit, and government organizations.

A doctoral degree usually is required for independent practice as a psychologist. Psychologists with a PhD or Doctor of Psychology (PsyD) qualify for a wide range of teaching, research, clinical, and counseling positions in universities, healthcare services, elementary and secondary schools, private industry, and government. Psychologists with a doctoral degree often work in clinical positions or in private practices, but they may teach, conduct research, or become administrators. A doctoral degree generally requires 5 to 7 years of graduate study, culminating in a dissertation based on original research. The PsyD degree may be based on practical work and examinations rather than a dissertation. In clinical, counseling, and school psychology, the requirements for the doctoral degree include at least a 1-year internship.

Psychologists held approximately 165,000 jobs in 2006. Educational institutions employed about 30% of psychologists in positions such as counseling, testing, research, and administration. About 21% were employed in health care, primarily in offices of mental health. Government agencies at the state and local levels employed psychologists primarily in correctional facilities and law enforcement. Median annual earnings of wage and salary clinical, counseling, and school psychologists in 2006 were $60,000. Median annual earnings of industrial–organizational psychologists in 2006 were $86,000 (BLS, 2008e).

Podiatrists

Podiatrists treat patients for feet diseases and deformities. They are awarded a Podiatric Medicine (PDM) degree upon completion of a 4-year podiatric college program. At least 90 hours of undergraduate education, acceptable scores on either the Medical College Admission Test (MCAT), Dental Admission Test (DAT), or the Graduate Record Exam (GRE) are needed to enter a PDM degree program. In 2007, there were seven colleges of podiatric medicine accredited by the Council on Podiatric Medical Education. Their curriculum is similar to other schools of medicine. Most graduates complete a residency in a hospital, which lasts 2 to 4 years. All states require a license to practice podiatric medicine. Podiatrists may also be board certified in their chosen specialties. All podiatrists must pass a national examination by their National Board. Established in 1912, the American Podiatric Medical Association (APMA) is the premier professional organization representing the nation's Doctors of Podiatric Medicine (BLS, 2009d).

Generally, podiatrists may perform surgeries, prescribe medications and corrective devices such as orthotics, and provide therapies. Many chronic diseases such as arthritis and diabetes exhibit symptoms in patients' feet so podiatrists may coordinate their efforts with other healthcare providers. Podiatrists' specializations include areas of sports medicine, geriatrics, or diabetes and may be board certified in their specialty which requires advanced training. Most podiatrists work in private practice and treat fewer emergencies than other doctors. Some podiatrists serve on the staffs of hospitals and long-term care facilities, teach in schools of medicine, serve as commissioned officers in the armed forces and the US public health service and the Department of Veterans Affairs, and work in state health departments (APMA, 2008). Many operate in solitary practices but recent trends indicate they are forming group practices. According to the BLS 2006 statistics, there are over 12,000 podiatrists nationwide with 2006 median annual earnings of $108,220 (BLS, 2009d).

ALLIED HEALTH PROFESSIONALS

In the early 20th century, healthcare providers consisted of physicians, nurses, pharmacists, and optometrists. As the healthcare industry evolved with increased use of technology and sophisticated interventions, increased time demands were placed on these healthcare providers. As a result, a broader spectrum of healthcare professionals with skills that complemented these primary healthcare providers evolved. These **allied health professionals** assist physicians and nurses in providing care to their patients. The impact of technology has increased the number of different specialties available. They can be divided into four main categories: laboratory technologists and technicians, therapeutic science practitioners, behavioral scientists, and support services (The Association of Schools of Allied Health Professionals, 2009).

Laboratory technologists and technicians or clinical laboratory technologists and technicians have a major role in diagnosing disease, assessing the impact of interventions, and applying highly technical procedures. Examples of this category include radiologic technology and nuclear medicine technology. Therapeutic science practitioners focus on the rehabilitation of patients with diseases and injuries. Examples of this category include physical therapists, radiation therapists, respiratory therapists, dieticians, and dental hygienists.

Behavioral scientists such as social workers and rehabilitation counselors provide social, psychological, and community and patient educational activities (Sultz & Young, 2006). This chapter cannot list all allied health professionals but a list of those allied health careers that have accredited education programs will be discussed.

The Commission on Accreditation of Allied Health Education Programs (CAAHEP) accredits 20 US programs that offer allied health specialties. This section will provide a brief summary of the different accredited allied health educational programs that contribute to providing quality health care. This information was obtained from the CAAHEP Web site (CAAHEP, 2008a).

Anesthesiologist Assistant

Under the direction of an anesthesiologist and as a team member of the anesthesia care component of surgical procedures, this specialty physician assistant assists with implementing an anesthesia care plan. Activities would include performing presurgical and surgical tasks and may also assist in administrative and educational activities. The **anesthesiologist assistant** (AA) primarily is employed by medical centers. In 2006, starting salaries ranged from $80,000 to $85,000 for 40 hours per week. Acceptance into an AA educational program requires an undergraduate premedical education which consists of sciences such as biology, chemistry, physics, and mathematics. The AA program length of duration is 24 to 27 months (CAAHEP, 2008b).

Cardiovascular Technologist

At the request of a physician, this technologist performs diagnostic examinations for cardiovascular issues. Basically, they assist physicians in treating cardiac (heart) and peripheral vascular (blood vessels) problems. They may also review and or record clinical data, perform procedures, and obtain data for physician review. They may provide services in any medical setting but primarily are in hospitals. They also operate and maintain testing equipment and may explain test procedures. These allied health professionals generally work a 5-day, 40-hour week that may include weekends. In 2006, their wages averaged $42,000. Employment of cardiovascular technologists and technicians is expected to increase by 26% through the year 2016. A high school diploma or qualifications in a clinically related allied position is required to enter an education program which may last from 1 to 4 years depending on the background of the student (CAAHEP, 2008c).

Cytotechnologist

Cytology is the study of the how cells function and their structure. **Cytotechnologists**, a category of clinical laboratory technologists, are specialists who collaborate with pathologists to evaluate cellular material. This material is used by pathologists to diagnose diseases such as cancer and other diseases. Cytotechnologists prepare slides of body cells and examine these cells microscopically for abnormalities that may signal the beginning of a cancerous growth. Most cytotechnologists work in hospitals. Employment of clinical laboratory workers such as cytotechnologists is expected to grow 14% by 2016. In 2006, wages for clinical laboratory technologists averaged $47,000 with the cytotechnologists averaging $30,000. In order to enter into their educational program, applicants should have a background in the biological sciences. Applicants must have an undergraduate degree in order to quality for national certification (CAAHEP, 2008d).

Diagnostic Medical Sonographer

Under the supervision of a physician, this specialist provides patient services using medical ultrasound, which photographs internal structures. **Sonography** uses sound waves to generate images of the body for the assessment and diagnosis of various medical conditions. Sonography commonly is associated with obstetrics and the use of ultrasound imaging during pregnancy. This specialist gathers data to assist with disease management in a variety of medical facilities including hospitals, clinics, and private practices. They may assist with patient education. In addition to working directly with patients, **diagnostic medical sonographers** keep patient records. They also may prepare work schedules, evaluate equipment purchases, or manage a sonography or imaging department.

Diagnostic medical sonographers may specialize in obstetric and gynecologic sonography (the female reproductive system), abdominal sonography (the liver, kidneys, gallbladder, spleen, and pancreas), neurosonography (the brain), breast sonography, vascular sonography, or cardiac sonography.

Employment of diagnostic medical sonographers is expected to increase by about 19% through 2016. Sonographers work approximately 40 hours per week but may have weekend and evening hours. In 2006, their salaries averaged $57,000. Colleges and universities offer formal training in both 2- and 4-year programs, culminating in an associate or a bachelor's degree. Applicants to a 1-year educational program must have relevant clinical experience. There are 2-year programs, which are the most prevalent, who will accept high school graduates with an education in basic sciences (CAAHEP, 2008e).

Electroneurodiagnostic Technologist

The **electroneurodiagnostic** (END) **technologist** is involved in the activity of the brain and nervous system. The END technologists work with physicians and other health professionals. The technologist may take medical histories, document the clinical conditions of patients, and be involved in the diagnostic procedures of the patients. They work primarily in neurology departments of hospitals but may also work in private practices of neurosurgeons and neurologists. They generally work 40 hours per week but may be on call for emergencies. In 2006, their salaries averaged $38,000. Their educational programs vary from 12 to 24 months and are often offered at a community college as part of an associate degree. Applicants must have a high school diploma or equivalent to enter the program (CAAHEP, 2008f).

Emergency Medical Technician–Paramedic

People who are ill, have had an accident, or have been wounded often depend on the competent care of **emergency medical technicians (EMTs)** and paramedics. They all require immediate medical attention. EMTs and paramedics provide this vital service as they care for and transport the sick or injured to a medical facility for appropriate medical care.

In general, EMTs and EMT–paramedics provide emergency medical assistance because of an accident or illness that has occurred outside the medical setting. EMTs and paramedics work under guidelines approved by the physician medical director of the healthcare organization to assess and manage medical emergencies. They are trained to provide life-saving measures. EMTs provide basic life support and EMT–paramedics provide advanced life support measures. They may be employed by an ambulance company, fire department, public EMS company, hospital, or a combination thereof. They may be paid or be volunteers from the community. Both EMTs and EMT–paramedics must be proficient in cardiopulmonary resuscitation (CPR). They learn the basics of different types of medical emergencies. EMT–paramedics perform more sophisticated procedures. They also receive extensive training in patient assessment. The work is not only physically demanding but can also be stressful, sometimes involving life-or-death situations. In 2006, their average salaries were approximately $27,000. Firefighters may also be trained as EMTs. EMT training is offered at community colleges, technical schools, hospitals, and academies. EMT training requires 40 hours of training. EMT–paramedics require 200 to 400 hours of training. Applicants for the programs are expected to have a high school diploma or the equivalent. The National Registry of Emergency Medical Technicians (NREMT) certifies emergency medical service providers at five levels: First Responder, EMT-Basic, EMT-Intermediate (which has two levels called 1985 and 1999), and Paramedic. All 50 states require certification for each of the EMT levels (CAAHEP, 2008g).

Exercise Physiologists

Exercise physiologists assess, design, and manage individual exercise programs for both healthy and unhealthy individuals. Clinical exercise physiologists work with a physician when applying programs for patients that have demonstrated a therapeutic benefit for the patient. In 2006, their average wages, depending on geographic area and experience, ranged from $17 to $23 per hour. These allied health professionals may work with fitness trainers, exercise science professionals, or physicians in cardiac rehabilitation in hospital settings. Applicants for their 2-year program should have an undergraduate degree in exercise science (CAAHEP, 2008h).

Exercise Scientist

Exercise scientists can focus on biomechanics, nutrition, sport psychology, and exercise physiology. Exercise scientists work in the fitness and health industry. They perform risk assessments, assess health behaviors, and motivate individuals to change negative behaviors. Their program can be completed in a 4-year undergraduate degree. Applicants must have a high school diploma or equivalent (CAAHEP, 2008i).

Kinesiotherapist

Kinesiotherapy is the application of exercise science to enhance the physical capabilities of individuals with limited functions. The kinesiotherapist provides rehabilitation exercises as prescribed by a physician. They may design programs that will reverse, stabilize, or enhance patients' physical capabilities. They establish, in collaboration with the client, a goal-specific treatment plan to increase their physical functioning. They may be employed in hospitals, rehabilitation facilities, learning disability centers, or sports medicine facilities. In 2006, their salaries averaged $45,000 annually. Applicants for their 4- to 5-year program require a high school diploma or equivalent (CAAHEP, 2008j).

Medical Assistant

Supervised by physicians, this allied health professional must have the ability to multitask. Over 60% of medical assistants work in medical offices and clinics. They perform both administrative and clinical duties. Medical assistants are employed by physicians more than any other allied health assistant. In 2006, their average entry level salary was $27,000. Their educational program consists of an associate degree, certificate, or diploma program (CAAHEP, 2008k).

Medical Illustrator

Medical illustrators are trained artists that portray visually scientific information to teach both the professionals and the public about medical issues. They may work digitally or traditionally to create images of human anatomy and surgical procedures as well as three-dimensional models and animations. Medical illustrators may be self-employed, work for pharmaceutical companies or advertising agencies, or be employed by medical schools. In 2006, salaries varied from $45,000 to $75,000 annually. Applicants must have an undergraduate degree with a focus on art and premedical education. The program is 2 years and results in a master's degree (CAAHEP, 2008l).

Orthotist and Prosthetist

These specialists address neuromuscular/skeletal issues and develop a plan and a device to rectify any issues. The orthotist develops devices called "othoses" that focus on the limbs and spines of individuals to increase function. The prosthetist designs "prostheses" or devices for patients who have limb amputations to replace the limb function. Most of these allied health professionals work in hospitals, clinics, colleges, and medical schools. In 2006, their average salaries ranged from $42,000 to $60,000. Their program may be achieved through a 4-year program or a certificate program which varies from 6 months to 2 years. Applicants for the 4-year program should have a high school diploma. Applicants for the certificate programs must have a 4-year degree (CAAHEP, 2008m).

Perfusionist

A **perfusionist** operates equipment to support or replace a patient's circulatory or respiratory function. Perfusion involves advance life support techniques. They may be responsible for administering blood byproducts or anesthetic products during a surgical procedure. They may be employed by hospitals, surgeons, or group practices. The 2006 salary range was $50,000 to $100,000. The prerequisites for their educational programs vary depending on the length of the program which can range from 1 to 4 years, depending on the individual's experience (CAAHEP, 2008n).

Personal Fitness Trainer

Personal fitness trainers are familiar with different forms of exercise. They have a variety of clients who they serve one-on-one or in a group activity. They may work with exercise science professionals or physiologists in corporate, clinical, commercial fitness, country clubs, or wellness centers. Employment of fitness workers is expected to increase 27% by 2016. In 2006, their average salary was $26,000. Their educational programs consist of 1-year certificate or 2-year associate degree program. Applicants must have a high school diploma or equivalent for program entry (CAAHEP, 2008o).

Polysomnographic Technologist

These allied health professionals perform sleep tests and work with physicians to provide diagnoses of sleep disorders. They monitor brain waves, eye movements, and other physiological activity during sleep and analyze this information and provide it to the patient's physician. They work in sleep disorder centers who may be affiliated with a hospital or operate independently. In 2006, their average wages were $20 per hour. Applicants for their education programs should have a high school diploma or equivalent. Their educational program can range from a 2-year associate degree or a 1-year certificate program (CAAHEP, 2008p).

Respiratory Therapist

There are two levels of respiratory therapists: the certified respiratory therapist and registered respiratory therapist. The entry level respiratory therapist performs basic respiratory care procedures under the supervision of a physician or an advance level therapist. They review patient data, including tests and previous medical history. They implement and monitor any respiratory therapy under the supervision of a physician. They may be involved in the home care of a patient. Entry level therapists are employed in hospitals, nursing care facilities, clinics, sleep labs, and home care organizations. In 2006, their average salaries were $46,000. Applicants are required to have a high school degree or equivalent. Their educational program consists of a 2-year program leading to an associate's degree. An advanced level respiratory therapist participates in clinical decision making such as diagnosing lung and breathing disorders, recommending treatment methods, providing patient education, and developing and recommending care plans in collaboration of physician. The advanced level therapist can be achieved through increased education such as a bachelor's or master's degree (CAAHEP, 2008q).

Specialists in Blood Banking Technology/Transfusion Medicine Specialist

Specialists in blood bank (SBB) technology provide routine and specialized tests for blood donor centers, transfusion centers, laboratories, and research centers. In 2006, their average salaries ranged from $50,000 to $70,000. Applicants for their educational programs must be certified in medical technology and have an undergraduate degree from an accredited educational institution. If they are not certified, they must have a degree from an accredited institution with a major in a biological or physical science and have appropriate work experience. This allied health program ranges from 1 to 2 years (CAAHEP, 2008r).

Surgical Assistant

The **surgical assistant** is a specialized physician's assistant. Their main goal is to ensure the surgeon has a safe and sterile environment to perform. They determine the appropriate equipment for the procedure, select radiographs for surgeon's reference, assist in moving the patient, confirm procedures with the surgeon, and assist with the procedure as directed by the surgeon. Their educational programs range from 10 to 22 months. In 2006, average annual salaries were $75,000. Applicants must have a bachelor of science or higher or an associate degree in an allied health field with 3 years of recent experience, current CPR/basic life support certification, acceptable health and immunization records, and computer literacy (CAAHEP, 2008s).

Surgeon Technologist

Surgeon technologists are key team members of the medical practitioners providing surgery. They are responsible for preparing the operating room by equipping the room with the appropriate sterile supplies and verifying the equipment is working properly. Prior to surgery, they also interact with the patient to ensure they are comfortable, monitor their vital signs, and review patient charts. During surgery, they are responsible for ensuring all surgery team members maintain a sterile environment and providing instruments to the surgeons. Postsurgery, they prepare the room for the next patient. They may also provide follow-up care in the postoperative room. They work in hospitals, outpatient settings, or may be self-employed. In 2006, their average salaries were $36,000 per year. Applicants for their educational programs must have a high school diploma or equivalent. The programs range from 12 to 24 months (CAAHEP, 2008t).

Health Services Administrators

It is important to discuss the importance of health services administrators and their role in health care. They can be found at all levels of a healthcare organization. They may be managing hospitals, clinics, nursing homes, community health centers, etc. At the top of the organization, they are responsible for strategic planning and the overall success of the organization. They are responsible for financial, clinical, and operational outcomes of an organization (Shi & Singh, 2008). Midlevel administrators also play a leadership role in departments and are responsible for managing their area of responsibility. They may manage departments or individual programs. Administrators at all levels work with top administration to achieve organizational goals. As healthcare costs continue to increase, it is important that health services administrators focus on efficiency and effectiveness at all levels of management. Health services administration is taught at both the undergraduate and master's levels. The most common undergraduate degree is a degree in healthcare administration, although most generalist managers require a master's degree. Undergraduate degrees may be acceptable for entry level management positions. Salaries vary by administration level. In 2006, the average salaries were $73,000 but varied depending on level of responsibility and size of organization. Employment is expected to grow 16% by 2016. Approximately 40% of hospitals employ health services administrators.

The most common master's degrees are the Master of Health Services Administration (MHA), Master of Business Administration (MBA) with a health care emphasis, or a Master of Public Health (MPH). The MHA or MBA degree provides a more business-oriented education that health administrators need for managing healthcare organizations. However, having an MPH degree also provides insight into the importance of public health as an integral component of our healthcare system (BLS, 2008b).

CONCLUSION

Healthcare personnel represent one of the largest labor forces in the United States. As a healthcare consumer and potential employee of the healthcare industry, this chapter provided an overview of the different types of employees in the health care industry. Some of them require many years of education; however, some of these positions can be achieved through 1–2 year programs. There are more than 200 occupations and professions among the 13 million health care workers (Sultz & Young, 2006). The healthcare industry will continue to progress as the United States trends in demographics, disease, and public health pattern change and cost and efficiency issues, insurance issues, technological influences, and economic factors continue to evolve. More occupations and professions will develop as a result of these trends. The major trend that will impact the healthcare industry is the aging of the US population. The BLS predicts that half of the next decades' fastest growing jobs will be in the healthcare industry. As of December 2008, the deep economic recession caused millions of US citizens to lose their jobs. When they lost their jobs, they most likely lost their health insurance coverage supplied by their employer. The number of uninsured and underinsured will continue to rise. Healthcare facilities may be providing more charitable care, thereby reducing the profits of their organizations. Government programs that provide healthcare benefits will be maximized and overloaded because of this economic trend. This economic trend will place a huge burden on the healthcare industry. Healthcare personnel may be overworked because of the state of the US economy. As healthcare costs continue to increase, cost-cutting measures will be the focus while continuing to provide quality health care. President Obama stated that healthcare reform is a priority for his administration. As his presidency evolves, it will be interesting to observe what types of healthcare reform can occur during economic strife.

PREVIEW OF CHAPTER SEVEN

This chapter will examine healthcare finance in the United States—who pays for services and what mechanisms are in place for payment. A breakdown of healthcare spending by age and state and type will be discussed, along with a discussion of private and public sources of funding for these expenditures, which includes government funding by Medicare and Medicaid. Reimbursement methods will also be addressed so as a consumer, you will understand why or why not some services are paid for or are partially reimbursed. Tools such as cost sharing (which includes copayments such as coinsurance and deductibles) as part of health insurance programs will be debated as well.

VOCABULARY

Activities of daily living

Advanced practice nurse

Allied health professionals

Allopathic approach

Anesthesiologist Assistant (AA)

Associate degree in nursing (ADN)

Bachelor of Science in Nursing (BSN)

Board certifying or credentialing examination

Cardiovascular technologist

Certified nursing assistants

Certified nurse–midwives

Chiropractors

Clinical psychologists

Counseling psychologists

Cytotechnologists

Dental assistants

Dental hygienists

Dentists

Diagnostic medical sonographer

Doctor of Medicine

Doctor of Osteopathic Medicine

Electroneurodiagnostic technologist

Emergency medical technician–paramedic (EMTs)

Exercise physiologists

Exercise scientists

Experimental psychologists

Generalists

Geographic maldistribution

Health services administrator/manager

Holistic approach

Hospitalists

Industrial–organizational psychologists

Kinesiotherapists

Licensed practical nurse

Medical assistant

Midlevel practitioners

National Practitioner Data Bank

Nonphysician practitioner

Nurse practitioner

Optometrists

Perfusionists

Personal fitness trainer

Pharmacists

Physician assistant

Podiatrists

Polysomnographic technologist

Primary care

Psychologists

Registered nurse

Respiratory therapist

Secondary care

Social psychologists

Specialists

Specialty maldistribution

Surgeon technologist

Surgical assistant

Tertiary care

Transfusion medicine specialist

REFERENCES

American Academy of Nurse Practitioners. (2008). Retrieved November 10, 2009, from http://www.aanp.org/AANPCMS2/AboutAANP.

American Podiatric Medical Association. (2008). Retrieved November 10, 2009, from http://www.apma.org/MainMenu/AboutPodiatry/APMAOverview.aspx.

Association of Schools of Allied Health Professionals. (2009). Retrieved November 10, 2009, from http://www.asahp.org/definition.htm.

Bradley, P. (2008). Nursing: A health care shortage. *Community College Weekly*. Retrieved November 10, 2009, from http://www.ccweek.com/news/templates/template.aspx?articleid=1439&zoneid=7.

Buchbinder, S., & Shanks, N. (2007). *Introduction to health care management*. Sudbury, MA: Jones and Bartlett.

Bureau of Labor Statistics. (2008a). Chiropractors. Retrieved November 16, 2008, from http://www.bls.gov/oco/ocos071.htm.

Bureau of Labor Statistics. (2008b). Medical and health services managers. Retrieved November 16, 2008, from http://www.bls.gov/oco/ocos014.htm.

Bureau of Labor Statistics. (2008c). Optometrists. Retrieved November 16, 2008, from http://www.bls.gov/oco/ocos073.htm.

Bureau of Labor Statistics. (2008d). Pharmacists. Retrieved November 16, 2008, from http://www.bls.gov/oco/ocos079.htm.

Bureau of Labor Statistics. (2008e). Psychologists. Retrieved November 16, 2008, from http://www.bls.gov/oco/ocos056.htm.

Bureau of Labor and Statistics. (2009a). Occupational employment and wages, chiropractors. Retrieved October 28, 2009, from www.bls.gov/oco/ocos097.htm.

Bureau of Labor and Statistics. (2009b). Licensed practical and licensed vocational nurses. Retrieved July 3, 2009, from http://www.bls.gov/oco/ocos102.htm.

Bureau of Labor and Statistics. (2009c). Occupational employment and wages, physician assistants. Retrieved July 3, 2009, from http://www.bls.gov/oes/2008/may/oes291071.htm.

Bureau of Labor and Statistics. (2009d). Occupational employment and wages, podiatrists. Retrieved July 3, 2009, from http://www.bls.gov/oes/2008/may/oes291081.htm.

Bureau of Labor and Statistics. (2009e). Occupational employment and wages, registered nurses. Retrieved July 3, 2009, from http://www.bls.gov/oes/2008/may/oes291111.htm.

Commission on Accreditation of Allied Health Education Programs. (2008a). Anesthesiologist assistant. Retrieved November 25, 2008, from http://www.caahep.org/Content.aspx?ID=20.

Commission on Accreditation of Allied Health Education Programs. (2008b). Cardiovascular technologist. Retrieved November 25, 2008, from http://www.caahep.org/Content.aspx?ID=21.

Commission on Accreditation of Allied Health Education Programs. (2008c). Cytotechnology. Retrieved November 16, 2008, from http://www.caahep.org/Content.aspx?ID=22.

Commission on Accreditation of Allied Health Education Programs. (2008d). Diagnostic medical sonography. Retrieved November 16, 2008, from http://www.caahep.org/Content.aspx?ID=23.

Commission on Accreditation of Allied Health Education Programs. (2008e). Electroneurodiagnostic technology. Retrieved November 16, 2008, from http://www.caahep.org/Content.aspx?ID=38.

Commission on Accreditation of Allied Health Education Programs. (2008f). Emergency medicine technician–paramedic. Retrieved November 16, 2008, from http://www.caahep.org/Content.aspx?ID=39.

Commission on Accreditation of Allied Health Education Programs. (2008g). Exercise physiology. Retrieved November 16, 2008, from http://www.caahep.org/Content.aspx?ID=40.

Commission on Accreditation of Allied Health Education Programs. (2008h). Exercise science. Retrieved November 10, 2008, from http://www.caahep.org/Content.aspx?ID=41.

Commission on Accreditation of Allied Health Education Programs. (2008i). Kinesiotherapist. Retrieved November 10, 2008, from http://www.caahep.org/Content.aspx?ID=42.

Commission on Accreditation of Allied Health Education Programs. (2008j). Medical assistant. Retrieved November 10, 2008, from http://www.caahep.org/Content.aspx?ID=43.

Commission on Accreditation of Allied Health Education Programs. (2008k). Medical illustrators. Retrieved November 10, 2008, from http://www.caahep.org/Content.aspx?ID=44.

Commission on Accreditation of Allied Health Education Programs. (2008l). Orthotist and prosthetist. Retrieved November 10, 2008, from http://www.caahep.org/Content.aspx?ID=45.

Commission on Accreditation of Allied Health Education Programs. (2008m). Perfusionist. Retrieved November 10, 2008, from http://www.caahep.org/Content.aspx?ID=46.

Commission on Accreditation of Allied Health Education Programs. (2008n). Personal fitness training. Retrieved November 10, 2008, from http://www.caahep.org/Content.aspx?ID=47.

Commission on Accreditation of Allied Health Education Programs. (2008o). Polysomnographic technologist. Retrieved November 10, 2008, from http://www.caahep.org/Content.aspx?ID=48.

Commission on Accreditation of Allied Health Education Programs. (2008p). Respiratory therapist. Retrieved November 10, 2008, from http://www.caahep.org/Content.aspx?ID=50.

Commission on Accreditation of Allied Health Education Programs. (2008q). Specialist in blood banking technology/transfusion medicine. Retrieved November 10, 2008, from http://www.caahep.org/Content.aspx?ID=51.

Commission on Accreditation of Allied Health Education Programs. (2008r). Surgical assistant. Retrieved November 10, 2008, from http://www.caahep.org/Content.aspx?ID=52.

Commission on Accreditation of Allied Health Education Programs. (2008s). Surgical technologist. Retrieved November 10, 2008, from http://www.caahep.org/Content.aspx?ID=53.

Health Resources and Services Administration. (2008). HRSA health professions. Retrieved November 10, 2009, from http://www.hrsa.gov/about/default.

Jonas, S. (2003). *An introduction to the U.S. health care system*. New York: Springer.

National Center for Health Statistics. (2008). *Health, United States, 2008, with Chartbook*. Washington, DC: US Government Printing Office. Retrieved December 5, 2008, from http://www.cdc.gov/nchs/data/hus/hus08.pdf.

Pointer, D., Williams, S., Isaacs, S., & Knickman, J. (2007). *Introduction to health care*. New York: Wiley & Sons.

Shi, L., & Singh, D. (2008). *An introduction to health care in America: A systems approach*. Sudbury, MA: Jones and Bartlett.

Sultz, H., & Young, K. (2006). *Health care USA*. Sudbury, MA: Jones and Bartlett.

Yordy, K. (2006). The nursing faculty shortage: Health care crisis. Retrieved November 8, 2009 from http://www.rwjf.org/files/publications/other/NursingFacultyShortage071006.pdf.

NOTES

STUDENT ACTIVITY 6-1

CROSSWORD PUZZLE

Instructions: Please complete the puzzle using the vocabulary words found in the chapter. There may be multiple-word answers. The number in the parenthesis indicates the number of words in the answer.

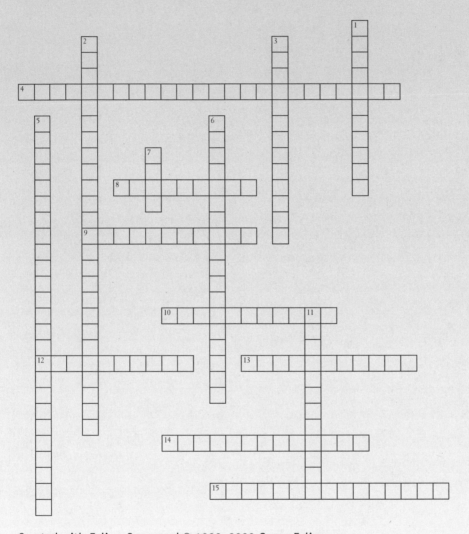

Created with EclipseCrossword © 1999–2009 Green Eclipse

STUDENT ACTIVITY 6-1

Across

4. This concept refers to the increasing number of physician specialists, which has resulted in a reduction of needed primary care physicians. (2 words)

8. This healthcare professional develops devices that focus on the limbs and spines of individuals. (1 word)

9. This care is the essential component of the US healthcare system. (2 words)

10. This term is another word for primary care physicians. (1 word)

12. This technology uses sound waves to generate images of the body for the assessment of disease and conditions. (1 word)

13. This healthcare professional designs devices for individuals who have had limb amputations. (1 word)

14. This type of care focuses on short-term interventions that may require a specialist's intervention. (2 words)

15. This type of nurse is a graduate trained nurse who has been licensed by a state board and has passed the national nursing examination. (2 words)

Down

1. This type of physician provides care solely to hospitalized patients. (1 word)

2. This category assists physicians and nurses in providing care to their patients. (3 words)

3. This category of health provider has a holistic approach to treating patients by emphasizing that the body can heal itself without medicine or surgery. (1 word)

5. This concept applies to the unequal geographic distribution of physicians across the United States. (2 words)

6. This category includes those nonphysician practitioners that provide needed services to patients. (2 words)

7. Emergency medical technicians provide emergency care to individuals outside the healthcare setting. (1 acronym)

11. This type of care is the most complex level of medical care. (2 words)

STUDENT ACTIVITY 6-2

IN YOUR OWN WORDS

Based on Chapter 6, please provide an explanation of the following concepts in your own words. DO NOT RECITE the text.

Doctor of Medicine: _____

_____

_____

Doctor of Osteopathic Medicine: _____

_____

_____

Allopathic approach: _____

_____

_____

Exercise physiologists: _____

_____

_____

Experimental psychologists: _____

_____

_____

Medical illustrator: _____

_____

_____

Kinesiotherapist: _____

_____

_____

Transfusion medicine specialist: _____

_____

_____

Licensed vocation nurse: _____

_____

_____

Certified midwives: _____

_____

_____

Board certification: _____

_____

_____

STUDENT ACTIVITY 6-3

REAL LIFE APPLICATIONS: CASE STUDY

Because of the recent economic downturn, both you and your friend are now unemployed. You have heard that the healthcare industry is a growing industry for employment. You and your friend are unsure of the types of careers available to you and whether you have the educational background to find a job in the healthcare industry. You have decided to either become a nurse or become an allied health professional because there are so many opportunities. You and your friend decide to do research on these opportunities and share your results with each other.

ACTIVITY

You have chosen to explore the area of nursing and have provided the information here regarding nursing opportunities. Your friend has narrowed the allied health career choices to three and has written the responses here. For each of these opportunities, you will provide (1) educational requirements, (2) job responsibilities, and (3) average wages.

Nursing Options

Licensed practical nurse:

_____   _____

_____   _____

_____   _____

Registered nurse:

_____

_____

_____

Allied Health Professionals

Physician assistant:

_____

_____

_____

Cardiovascular technologist:

_____

_____

_____

Health services administrators:

_____

_____

_____

STUDENT ACTIVITY 6-4

INTERNET EXERCISES

Write your answers in the space provided.

- Visit each of the Web sites here.
- Name the organization.
- Locate their mission statement on their Web site.
- Provide a brief overview of the activities of the organization.
- How do these organizations participate in the US healthcare system?

Web Sites

http://www.aanp.org

Organization Name: _____

Mission Statement:

_____

_____

_____

Overview of Activities:

_____

_____

_____

Importance of organization to US health care:

_____

_____

_____

http://www.apma.org

Organization Name: _____

Mission Statement:

_____

_____

_____

Overview of Activities:

_____

_____

_____

STUDENT ACTIVITY 6-4

Importance of organization to US health care:

_____

_____

_____

http://www.caahep.org

Organization Name: _____

Mission Statement:

_____

_____

_____

Overview of Activities:

_____

_____

_____

Importance of organization to US health care:

_____

_____

_____

http://www.ccweek.com

Organization Name: _____

Mission Statement:

_____

_____

_____

Overview of Activities:

_____

_____

_____

Importance of organization to US health care:

_____

_____

_____

STUDENT ACTIVITY 6-4

http://bhpr.hrsa.gov

Organization Name: _____

Mission Statement:

_____

_____

_____

Overview of Activities:

_____

_____

_____

Importance of organization to US health care:

_____

_____

_____

http://www.aapa.org

Organization Name: _____

Mission Statement:

_____

_____

_____

Overview of Activities:

_____

_____

_____

Importance of organization to US health care:

_____

_____

_____

Private and Public Financing of Health Care

LEARNING OBJECTIVES

The student will be able to:

- Discuss the different cost-sharing strategies in health insurance plans.

- Analyze the different types of consumer-driven health plans.

- Discuss the importance of Medicare and Medicaid to health care.

- Identify the different government and private health insurance reimbursement methods.

- Evaluate the different types of health insurance policies.

- Describe PACE, TRICARE, and SCHIP and their importance to health care.

DID YOU KNOW THAT?

- Nearly 60% of Medicare enrollees are female, which corresponds to the longer life expectancy of a US female.

- The state of Massachusetts has the highest per capita of personal healthcare spending at nearly $7000.

- Medicare and Medicaid are the two largest government-sponsored health insurance programs in the United States.

- A lifetime cap of $1,000,000 reimbursement of an enrollee's health services may be established by a private health insurance company.

- Approximately 84% of the US population is covered by some form of health insurance.

INTRODUCTION

As mentioned in several chapters, the percentage of the US gross domestic product (GDP) devoted to health-care expenditures has increased over the past several decades. The Centers for Medicare and Medicaid Services (CMS) projects that health services will consume nearly 20% of the GDP by 2016. According to CMS 2007 statistics, US healthcare expenditures increased 6.1% compared to 6.7% in 2006. Total health expenditures reached $2.2 trillion, which translates to 16.2% of GDP (CMS, 2009a). Since 1970, healthcare spending has grown 2.5% faster than the rest of the US economy. The increase in healthcare spending can be attributed to three causes: (1) When prices increase in an economy overall, the cost of medical care will increase and, even when prices are adjusted for inflation, medical prices have increased; (2) as life expectancy increases in the United States, more individuals will require more medical care, which means there will be more healthcare expenses; and (3) as healthcare technology and research provide for more sophisticated and more expensive procedures, there will be an increase in healthcare expenses (Pointer, Williams, Isaacs, & Knickman, 2007).

There are four areas that account for a large percentage of national healthcare expenditures: hospital care, physician and clinical services, prescription drugs, and nursing and home healthcare expenditures (Longest & Darr, 2008). Unlike countries that have universal healthcare systems, payment of healthcare services in the United States is derived from (1) out-of-pocket payments from patients who pay entirely or partially for services rendered; (2) health insurance plans, such as indemnity plans or managed care organizations; (3) public/government funding such as Medicare, Medicaid, and other government programs; and (4) health savings accounts (HSAs) (Buchbinder & Shanks, 2007; Shi & Singh, 2008; Sultz & Young, 2006). Much of the burden of healthcare expenditures has been borne by private sources—employers and their health insurance programs have borne much of the cost. In 2007, approximately 60% of Americans (180 million) had private health insurance coverage (Davis, 2007). The number of uninsured in the United States has been approximately 47 million; however, with the dramatic increase in unemployed during 2008 and 2009, it is anticipated that the number of uninsured will dramatically increase because they no longer have a relationship with their employer who has provided a large portion of health insurance coverage. Individuals may continue to pay their health insurance premiums through the Consolidated Omnibus Budget Reconciliation Act (COBRA) once they are unemployed but most individuals cannot afford to pay the expensive premiums. Potentially, the government may play a larger role in providing health care. President Barack Obama has named healthcare reform a priority of his administration. There are several healthcare reform bills in the legislature proposed by both political parties that focus on providing affordable health care to more individuals. However, there are major differences on how to implement a policy. It will be interesting to see what type of initiative will be developed to increase the number of individuals who will be able to receive health care.

To understand the complexity of the US healthcare system, this chapter will provide a breakdown of the US healthcare spending by type, age, and state and the major private and public sources of funding for these expenditures. It is important to reemphasize that there are three parties involved in providing health care: the provider, the patient, and the fiscal intermediary such as a health insurance company or the government. Therefore, included in the chapter is also a description of how healthcare providers are reimbursed for their services and how reimbursement rates were developed for both private and public funds.

HEALTHCARE SPENDING BY SERVICE TYPE

In 2007, hospital spending was nearly $700 billion, physician and clinical services was $480 billion, and other professional services such as chiropractors, optometrists, and podiatrists was $62 billion. Dental services were $95 billion and community center and school spending was $66 billion. Home healthcare services were $59 billion, an increase of 11% from 2006. Nursing home spending was $131 billion, prescriptions drug spending was $227 billion, and medical equipment was $61 billion (CMS, 2009a). Hospital spending accounted for the largest percentage of national healthcare expenditures with physician and other services, prescription drugs, and nursing and home health the next three largest.

HEALTHCARE SPENDING BY MAJOR SOURCES OF FUNDS

In 2007, Medicare spending was $431 billion, which was an increase of 7.2% from 2006. Medicaid spending was $329 billion, which was a slight decrease from 2006. Private health insurance premiums grew 6% while benefit payments decreased because of a decline in spending on prescription drugs. Out-of-pocket payments grew 5% in 2007, which was a result of prescription drugs costs, nursing home services, and medical equipment. Out-of-pocket spending accounted for 12% of national health spending in 2007 and has increased over the past 10 years (CMS, 2009a).

HEALTHCARE SPENDING BY AGE AND GENDER

In 2004, spending per persons 65 years and older was $8644; $1245 for children younger than 5 years of age; $1108 for children between 5 and 17 years of age; $1282 for 18 to 24 years of age; and $2277 for 25 to 44 years of age. Average spending for females was $3715 and $2836 for males (Kaiser Family Foundation [KFF], 2007). These numbers correlate with the fact that the longer we age, the more chronic conditions occur that result in higher spending and female life expectancy is longer than male life expectancy.

HEALTHCARE SPENDING BY STATE

In 2004, the state of Massachusetts' per capita of personal healthcare spending was $6683 compared to a low of $3972 in Utah. The highest per capita spending was in Massachusetts, Maine, New York, Alaska, and Connecticut. The lowest per capita spending was in Utah, Arizona, Idaho, New Mexico, and Nevada. Medicare expenditures per beneficiary were the highest in Louisiana ($8659) and lowest in South Dakota ($5640). Medicaid expenditures per enrollee were the highest in Alaska ($10,417) and lowest in California ($3664). California's total personal healthcare spending was the highest at 10.8% with the lowest in Wyoming at 0.1%. All states except Delaware and Wyoming spent at least 10% or greater of GDP (CMS, 2009a).

HEALTH INSURANCE AS A PAYER FOR HEALTHCARE SERVICES

Like life insurance or homeowner's insurance, **health insurance** was developed to provide protection should a covered individual experience an event that required health care. In 1847, a Boston insurance company offered sickness insurance to consumers. During the 19th century, large employers such as coal mining and railroad companies offered medical services to their employees by providing company doctors. Fees were taken from their pay to cover the service. In 1913, a union-provided health insurance was provided by the International Ladies Garment Workers where health insurance was negotiated as part of their employment contract. During this period, there were several proposals for a national health insurance program but the efforts failed. The American Medical Association (AMA) was worried that any national health insurance would impact the financial security of their providers. The AMA persuaded the federal government to support private insurance efforts. Employer-based health insurance grew rapidly post–World War II for three decades with some stability for one decade and an eventual decline in coverage since the late 1980s (Enthoven & Fuchs, 2006). However it is still the major method of providing health care in the United States.

In 1929, a group hospital insurance plan was offered to teachers at a hospital in Texas. This became the foundation of the nonprofit Blue Cross Blue Shield (BCBS) plans. In order to placate the AMA, BCBS initially offered only hospital insurance in order to avoid infringement of physicians' incomes (BCBS, 2009; Starr, 1982). In 1935, the Social Security Act was created and was considered "old age" insurance. During this period, there was continued discussion of a national health insurance program. But with the impact of World War II and the Depression, there was no funding for this program. The government felt that the Social Security Act was a sufficient program to protect consumers. These events were a catalyst for the development of a health insurance program that included private participation. Although a universal health coverage program was proposed during President Clinton's administration in the 1990s, it was never passed. In 2005, Massachusetts proposed mandatory health coverage for all citizens so it may be that universal health coverage may begin at the state level (KFF, 2007). As stated previously, the Obama administration has placed a high priority on healthcare reform, which could include some type of increase in healthcare coverage.

In the 1960s, President Johnson signed Medicare and Medicaid into law which protects the elderly, disabled, and indigent. President Nixon signed into law the Health Maintenance Act of 1973, which focused on effective cost measures for health delivery and was the basis for the current health maintenance organizations (HMOs). Also, in the 1980s, diagnosis-related groups (DRGs) and prospective payment guidelines were established to provide guidelines for treatment. These DRGs were attached to appropriate insurance reimbursement categories for treatment. Also, in the 1980s and 1990s, several consumer laws were passed. COBRA was passed to provide health insurance protection if an individual changes jobs. In 1993, the Family and Medical Leave Act (FMLA) was passed to protect an employee in the event of a family illness. Employees can receive up to 12 weeks of unpaid leave and their health insurance during this period. Also, in 1996, the Health Insurance Portability and Accountability Act (HIPAA) was passed which provided stricter confidentiality regarding the health information of individuals.

TYPES OF HEALTH INSURANCE

Health insurance, particularly employer-provided health insurance, is the primary source of payment of healthcare services in the United States. Unfortunately, employers providing health insurance has become very expensive for businesses. Administrative costs are estimated at $120 billion annually. There are approximately 850 health insurance companies that contract with millions of employers to provide coverage (Emanuel, 2008). There are four types of private insurance: group insurance, individual private health insurance, self-insurance, and managed care plans. **Group insurance** anticipates that a large group of individuals will purchase insurance through their employer and the risk is spread among those paying individuals. If an individual is self-employed, such as small business owner or farmer, they may purchase **individual private health insurance**. Unlike group insurance, the risk is determined by the individual's health. Premiums, deductibles, and copayments are much higher for this type of insurance. Established in the 1970s, **self-funded** or **self-insurance** programs are health insurance programs that are implemented and controlled by the company itself. **Managed care plans** are a type of health program that combines administrative costs and service costs for cost control.

Most group health insurance is provided by employers to their employees (Pointer et al., 2007). Health insurance is a financing mechanism that protects the insured from using their personal funds when expensive care is required. Having insurance also decreases the risks of delays in seeking treatment that may result in costly delays and increased disease (Sultz & Young, 2006). Approximately 84% of the population is covered by some form of health insurance. All insurance plans fall into three categories: voluntary health insurance (VHI), social insurance, and public welfare insurance. **VHI** is a type of private health insurance that is provided by nonprofit and for-profit health plans such as BCBS. **Social insurance** is provided by the government at all levels: federal, state, and local. An example of this type of insurance is Medicare. **Public welfare insurance** is based on financial need. The primary example of public welfare insurance is Medicaid. All insurance plans define a contract between the beneficiaries, the purchasers, which are the employers and government, the health plan organizations, and the providers who deliver the services (Pointer et al., 2007). There are also self-insurance programs that are administered by employers who bear the financial risk of providing their own health insurance to their employees. The funds to operate the program are derived from employee premiums. Reimbursement of health services are taken from this pool of funds rather than from another health insurance company.

There are two forms of payment, fee for service and prepayment, that provide the basis for all health insurance coverage. **Fee for service**, developed by BCBS, is based on the concept of a person purchasing coverage for certain benefits, using the health insurance coverage for these designated benefits, and paying the provider for the services provided. The provider may be paid by the insurance coverage or out of pocket by the patient. In a **prepayment** concept, the individual pays a fixed, predetermined amount for the services rendered. Managed care organizations follow a prepayment model (Sultz & Young, 2006).

COST SHARING OF HEALTH SERVICES

Most insurance policies require a contribution from the covered individual in the form of a copayment, deductible, and/or coinsurance. This concept is called **cost sharing**. Used in both fee-for-service and prepaid plans, **copayments** are costs that the patient must pay at the time they receive the services. It is a designated dollar amount. A type of copayment, **coinsurance**, which is part of a fee-for-service policy, the patient pays a percentage of the cost of the services. A typical coinsurance portion is 20% paid by the individual with the remaining 80% paid by the health insurance plan. **Deductibles** are payments that are required prior to the insurance paying for services rendered in a fee-for-service plan. Deductible amounts vary from individual and family health insurance coverage and cover one calendar year. For example, an individual may have a $250 deductible per calendar year, which means they must pay the $250 before their health insurance covers the services. Unfortunately, the growth in health insurance premiums is an excellent barometer to measure changes in private health insurance costs. Employee premiums have increased between 8 and 14% since 2000. The increase in premium costs has increased the percentage of cost sharing of health insurance on the employee (KFF, 2007). The main issue with the increase in cost sharing is its impact on individuals utilizing healthcare services. A study published in the *New England Journal of Medicine* concluded that adding an additional cost-sharing measure, such as a copayment of $10, reduces the number of women who received a mammography. These results concur with similar studies that examine cost sharing for health screening services (Bach, 2008).

HEALTH INSURANCE LIMITATIONS

Most plans include a stop-loss provision, which is the **maximum out-of-pocket expenditure** that occur in a given year. Once this level has been reached by the individual, the insurance company will pay 100% of the expenses. A **lifetime cap** may be established by a health insurance company, which means the company will usually pay a limit of $1,000,000 or higher for health services rendered. This lifetime cap occurs when an individual incurs high expense levels as a result of a chronic condition (Pointer et al., 2007).

TYPES OF HEALTH INSURANCE POLICIES

Comprehensive health insurance policies provide benefits that include outpatient and inpatient services, surgery, laboratory testing, medical equipment purchases, therapies, and other services such as mental health, rehabilitation, and prescription drugs. Most comprehensive policies have some exclusion attached to their policies. The opposite of comprehensive health insurance policies is **basic** or **major medical policies**, which reimburse hospital services such as surgeries and any expenses related to any hospitalization. There are limits on hospital stays. **Catastrophic health insurance** policies cover unusual illnesses with a high deductible and have lifetime reimbursement caps. There are also specific health insurance policies such as **disease-specific policies** for cancer, etc., and **medigap policies** that provide supplemental insurance coverage for Medicare patients (Shi & Singh, 2008).

TYPES OF HEALTH INSURANCE PLANS

There are two basic types of insurance plans: **indemnity plans** which are fee-for-service plans and managed care plans, which include HMOs, preferred provider organizations (PPOs), and point-of-service (POS) plans. Indemnity plans are contracts between a beneficiary and a health plan but there is no contract between the health plan and providers. The beneficiary pays a premium to the health plan. When the beneficiary receives a healthcare service, the plan will reimburse the beneficiary an established fee for a particular service regardless of the provider's fees. The beneficiary will then reimburse the provider directly (Sultz & Young, 2006).

The managed care plan, which is discussed in depth in Chapter 8, is a special type of health plan that focuses on cost containment of health services. The first type of managed care organization was the HMO, which evolved in the 1970s. As managed care organizations evolved, different types of managed care organizations developed.

Managed care plans combine health services and health insurance functions to reduce administrative costs. For example, an employer contracts with a health plan for services on behalf of their employees. The employer is required to pay a set amount per the enrolled employee on a monthly basis. The contracted health plan has a contract with certain providers to whom it pays a fixed rate per member on a monthly basis for certain services. Enrolled employees may cost share with a copayment. There is no deductible. The enrolled employees have restrictions on their choice of providers or incur larger copayments if they choose a provider out of the network.

A recent trend in health insurance plans is **consumer-driven health plans** (CDHPs) that are tax advantage plans with high deductible coverage. The most common CDHPs are **health reimbursement arrangements** (HRAs) and HSAs. HRAs or **personal care accounts** began in 2001 as a result of an Internal Revenue Service (IRS) regulation. An HRA is funded by the employer but owned by the employees and remains with the company if the employee leaves. This has been an issue because it has no portability (Wilensky, 2006).

An **HSA**, which was authorized by the Medicare Prescription Drug, Improvement, and Modernization Act of 2003, pairs high deductible plans with fully portable employee-owned tax-advantaged accounts. This plan encourages consumers to become more cost conscious when using the healthcare system because they are using their own funds for healthcare services. The HSA, unlike the HRA, is a portable account, which means it can be transferred to another employer when the employee changes jobs. HSAs encourage consumers to understand healthcare service pricing because these accounts are paired with a high deductible. America's Health Insurance Plans (AHIP), an industry trade association, estimates that 4% of firms that offered benefits also offered an HSA or HRA (Wilensky, 2006).

Other types of CDHPs include **flexible spending accounts** (FSAs) and **medical saving accounts** (MSAs). **FSAs** provide employees with the option of setting aside pretax income to pay for out-of-pocket medical expenses. Employees must submit claims for these expenses and are reimbursed from their spending accounts. The drawback is that the amount set aside must be spent within 1 year. Any unspent dollars cannot be rolled over so it is very important to be very specific about the projected medical expenses. Mandated as part of HIPAA, the **MSA** allows workers employed in firms with 50 or less employees, and who have high deductible health insurance plans, to set aside pretax dollars to be used for healthcare premiums and nonreimbursed healthcare expenses (Buchbinder & Shanks, 2007).

As discussed previously, self-funded or self-insurance programs are health insurance programs that are implemented and controlled by the company itself. They retain all of the risk in providing health insurance to their employees by paying any claims from their employees. Both the employee and employer pay into the fund. The employer maintains a trust that is overseen by federal regulation. All claims are paid from the trust. The company will purchase reinsurance from another insurance company to protect themselves from any catastrophic losses. The **reinsurance** sets a **stop-loss measure** that limits the amount the company will pay for claims (Employee Benefit Management Service [EBMS], 2009).

Long-term Care Insurance

As the life expectancy continues to increase in the United States, more people will require more healthcare services for chronic conditions. Unfortunately, Medicare and traditional health insurance policies do not pay for long-term care. Medicaid will pay for long-term care if you qualify for their program. **Long-term care insurance** was developed to cover services such as assistance with activities of daily living as well as care in an organizational setting. The cost of long-term care insurance can vary based on the type and amount of services selected as well as the age at time of purchase and healthcare status. If an individual is already receiving long-term care or is in ill health, a person may not qualify for long-term care insurance. Most long-term care insurance policies are comprehensive, which means they will cover expenses from home health care, hospice, respite care, assisted living, nursing homes, Alzheimer special care, and adult day centers. Long-term care policy costs vary greatly based on age and type of policy. The average annual premium for a policy purchased in 2007 by individual buyers of all ages was $2200 (Department of Health and Human Services [HHS], 2009).

The National Clearinghouse for Long-Term Care Information has provided the following information for purchasing long-term care insurance:

- The policyholder can select a daily benefit amount, which can range from $50 to $500 per day. The policyholder can select how much is paid on a daily basis, depending on the healthcare setting. The type of healthcare setting can also be identified such as home health care or skilled nursing facility.

- The policyholder can select a lifetime amount the policy will provide, which can range from $100,000 to $300,000. More expensive policies will allow unlimited coverage with no dollar limit.

- The policyholder can also select an inflation option, which adjusts the coverage amount as you age.

- Some policies may pay for family/friend long-term care for the policyholder. The policy may also provide reimbursement for equipment or transportation.

There are currently 100 companies that represent 15 insurers that offer long-term care nationally. More employees are now offering long-term care insurance as an option to their employees. Employers do not contribute to the premium cost but may negotiate a better group rate. Long-term care insurance is becoming more popular because individuals are recognizing that their traditional health insurance and Medicare will not pay for long-term care (HHS, 2009).

PUBLIC FINANCING OF HEALTHCARE SERVICES

Since 1965, public financing has played a large role in providing healthcare services to the elderly, disabled, and the indigent. Medicare and Medicaid are the two largest government-sponsored health insurance programs in the United States. Medicare, Title XVIII of the Social Security Act, provides medical care for (1) individuals who are 65 years and older, (2) disabled individuals who are entitled to Social Security benefits, and (3) people who have end-stage renal disease (Shi & Singh, 2008). According to the KKF, in 2006, 88% of Medicare enrollees were 65 years and older, 56% were female, and 41% were considered indigent (KFF, 2007). Medicare is an **entitlement** program because people, after paying into the program for years, are entitled to receive benefits. It is important to emphasize that Medicare and Medicaid have provided access to healthcare services through their programs. The number of uninsured in the United States would be much higher if these programs did not exist (Enthoven & Fuchs, 2006).

Medicare

CMS has oversight of Medicare. There are currently 43 million Medicare enrollees. Projections are expected to increase to 60 million by 2050. Medicare is the healthcare industry's largest payer. Medicare originally was designed as a two-part structure: Part A for hospital insurance and Part B for supplemental or voluntary medical insurance. Recently, two additional parts were added: Part C, Medicare+Choice/Medicare Advantage and Part D, which is a prescription drug plan benefit (CMS, 2009a).

Medicare Part A Hospital Insurance

Medicare Part A is primarily financed from payroll taxes. The employer and employee contribute to the Social Security (Medicare) fund. Employees contribute 1.45% of wages which is matched by employers. Self-employed individuals pay 2.9% of earnings. Part A covers hospital inpatient services, care in a skilled nursing facility, home health visits, and hospice care. The following is a summary of Part A benefits:

- Hospitalization, skilled nursing facility services, some home health, and hospice are available premium free to individuals 65 years or older when they have been receiving Social Security disability benefits for 24 months. Others can utilize these services but must pay a premium and must enroll in Part B. Enrollment for Part A is January to March of each year with benefits beginning July 1 of that year.

- A maximum of 90 days of inpatient hospital care is allowed per episode of illness with a lifetime reserve of 60 additional hospital inpatient days remain when the 90 days has exceeded.

- Medicare patients pay a deductible of one hospital day of care with copayments for each of the 65 to 90 day, equal to 25% of the deductible (CMS, 2009a).

Medicare Part B Voluntary Medical Insurance

Medicare Part B is a supplemental health plan to cover physician services. It is financed 24% from enrollee premiums and 76% from federal treasury funds. The following is a summary of Part B benefits:

- Coverage includes physician care, durable medical equipment, physician-ordered supplies, ambulatory surgical services, outpatient hospital care, outpatient mental health services, and laboratory services. Part B is made available when enrollees sign up for Part A (CMS, 2009a; KFF, 2007).

Medicare Part C Medicare Advantage

Medicare Part C is also referred to as Medicare Advantage. It is required to cover all services in Parts A and B. It is voluntary and available when an individual enrolls in Parts A and B. This program was designed to move Medicare patients into more cost-effective health insurance programs such as HMOs or PPOs. Enrollment is November 15 to December 31 of each year with benefits starting January 1 of the next year. Part C also established antifraud and abuse programs; additional prevention programs for prostate cancer, colorectal screenings, and mammography; rural initiatives; and the establishment of the State Children's Health Insurance Program (SCHIP) for low income children (CMS, 2009a).

Medicare Part D Prescription Drug Benefit

The Medicare Prescription Drug Improvement and Modernization Act of 2003 (MMA), which authorized Medicare Part D, produced the largest additions and changes to Medicare and was projected to cost nearly $750 billion in the first 10 years. Tax revenues of the federal government supports approximately 78% of the program costs, 10% is financed through monthly premiums, 11% is financed by state payments, and 1% from other sources (Buchbinder & Shanks, 2007; Shi & Singh, 2008). Its purpose was to provide relief from costly prescription costs for seniors. Like Part B, it is a voluntary program because enrollees pay a premium for coverage. Effective January 1, 2006, this program developed a prescription drug program for enrollees. The following is a summary of Part D benefits:

- Affordable prescription drug plans were made available for Medicare Advantage plan enrollees and traditional Medicare health plans.

- For seniors who are considered indigent, the MMA established a low income subsidy for the costs of Part D (CMS, 2009a).

Medigap

Medicare covers less than half of total healthcare costs for an enrollee, which leaves them with substantial out-of-pocket expenses. To cover these expenses, Medicare enrollees can receive additional coverage from (1) Medicaid if the Medicare enrollee is eligible, (2) enrollment in

Medicare Advantage which can provide supplemental coverage, (3) employer-sponsored retiree insurance, and (4) purchase supplemental insurance policies from private insurance companies which are called medigap policies (Sultz & Young, 2006).

Medicaid

Medicaid, Title XIX of the Social Security Act, provides health insurance to the medically indigent. It is a welfare program that is administered at the state government level. The program serves 45 million low income Americans. Medicaid spending varies based on the status of the US economy. It is not a federally mandated program; however, all states have Medicaid except Arizona. Managed care enrollment has controlled Medicaid spending. Eligible people include: (1) families with children receiving support under the Temporary Assistance for Needy Families (TANF), (2) people receiving Supplemental Security Income (SSI), and (3) children and pregnant women with income at or below 133% of the federal poverty level, and (4) children whose parents have income too high for Medicaid but too low for private insurance (CMS, 2009a; Shi & Singh, 2008).

All states administer their own program so eligibility varies by state. State programs must match federal funding for their programs and must provide the following services: inpatient and outpatient hospital services, physician care, nursing facility services, home health services, prenatal care, family planning services, health services for children under 21, midwife services, and pediatric and family nurse practitioner services. State programs are responsible for at least 40% of the costs for provider services and must equally share the administrative costs of the Medicaid programs (CMS, 2009a; Sultz & Young, 2006). States have the right to determine the eligibility criteria for Medicaid enrollment, optional services to provide, methods and rates for provider payments, and utilization limits for services (Pointer et al., 2007).

State Children's Health Insurance Program (now Children's Health Insurance Program)

Authorized by the Balanced Budget Act of 1997, and codified as Title XXI of the Social Security Act, **SCHIP**, now CHIP, was initiated in response to the number of children who are uninsured in the United States. The CHIP gave states $40 billion over a decade to provide health care for these children. This program offers additional funds to states to expand Medicaid benefits to children younger than 19 years of age who otherwise may not qualify because the family income exceeds Medicaid levels. This program, like Medicaid, is a federal–state partnership with the federal government paying nearly 75% of the cost. The federal fund was a block grant, which means the funds can expire. In February 2009, President Obama extended the authorization of CHIP funding and increased eligibility for an additional 4 million children (Families USA, 2009).

Program of All-Inclusive Care for the Elderly

Also authorized by the Balanced Budget Act of 1997, Program of All-Inclusive Care for the Elderly (PACE) is a comprehensive healthcare delivery system funded by Medicare and Medicaid. Oversight is provided by CMS, and it is modeled from a San Francisco, CA, senior healthcare center, On Lok Senior Health Services. The PACE model focuses on providing community-based care and services to people who otherwise need nursing home levels of care. Their philosophy is that seniors with chronic care needs are better served in the community when possible. Implemented at the state level, PACE can be offered as a Medicaid option. Participants must be Medicare eligible or 55 years or older with a disability, live in a PACE area, and be certified for nursing home care. An interdisciplinary team assesses the needs of the patient and develops a long-term plan. The PACE model provides services of Medicaid and Medicare but in an integrated manner. They provide both medical and social services as needed. PACE providers are reimbursed from Medicare and Medicaid payments. As of 2008, there were 61 PACE programs operational in 29 states (CMS, 2009b; National PACE Association, 2009).

Worker's Compensation

The employer is financially liable for employees who become injured or ill as a result of working conditions. **Worker's compensation** is a state administered program. Employees may receive cash for lost wages, payment for medical treatment, survivor's death benefits, and indemnification for loss of skills. Although worker's compensation is not a traditional health insurance program, it does provide medical benefits. The main difference between employer health insurance programs and worker's compensation is that the employer must cover the full cost of the benefits (Department of Labor, 2009; Shi & Singh, 2008).

TRICARE

The US Department of Defense operates the Military Health Services System (MHHS) which provides medical services to active duty and retired members of the armed services. As the active duty numbers increased, a special medical care program called **TRICARE** was developed to respond to the growing needs of retired members. TRICARE is regionally managed, structured after managed care, and coordinates the efforts of the Navy, Army, and Air Force. They have an HMO type operation, a PPO type organization, and a traditional fee-for-service program. There are 11 TRICARE regions in the United States with other TRICARE operations in Europe, Latin America, and Pacific (TRICARE, 2009).

Indian Health Service

The Indian Health Service (IHS), a division of HHS, provides comprehensive healthcare services directly to nearly 2 million American Indian and Alaska Native tribes. Their annual budget is approximately $3 billion. This system includes 33 hospitals, 59 health centers, and 50 health stations (IHS, 2009).

REIMBURSEMENT METHODS OF PRIVATE HEALTH INSURANCE PLANS

As healthcare costs have escalated, the government has developed various mechanisms aimed at standardizing reimbursement for healthcare services. Later, insurance companies developed standards for **usual, customary, and reasonable (UCR) services** based on community and state surveys of provider charges. If there was a difference in the reimbursement rates, the provider asked the patient to pay the difference. The problem with fee-for-service reimbursement methods is that it may have become a tool for some physicians to increase the number of services provided to the patient as a way to increase their income (Shi & Singh, 2008).

Insurance companies, managed care organizations, and the government are referred to as **third-party payers**. The other parties are the patient and the healthcare provider. The payment function in healthcare determines the how and how much is reimbursed for the services. Fee for service, which was discussed previously, is the preferred method of reimbursement by providers. Historically, providers set the rate for their services that the government and health insurance companies paid without question. This type of

retrospective reimbursement determines the amount of reimbursement after the delivery of services and provides little financial risk to providers. This type of reimbursement method contributed to the increase in healthcare costs (Feldstein, 2005).

The most common type of reimbursement is a **service benefit plan**. This type of **prospective reimbursement** method was developed and used primarily by managed care organizations. The employer has a contract with a benefit plan and pays a premium for each of its employees. Employees usually pay a portion of the premium to the health plan also. The health plan contracts with certain providers and facilities to provide services to their beneficiaries at a specified rate and makes payments directly to the providers for their services (McLean, 2003).

Beneficiaries/employees and families may have a cost-sharing arrangement with their employer for these services, such as deductibles and coinsurance payments, that provide payment to providers upon the receipt of a service. HMOs are examples of service benefit plans. In a managed care organization, the organization reimburses the provider at a **capitated rate**, which means they receive a set rate for serving enrolled patients regardless of how much care the provider gives. This type of capitation is also used by Medicaid and Medicare for their managed care programs (Pointer et al., 2007).

OTHER PROSPECTIVE REIMBURSEMENT METHODS

Per diem or **per patient day** is a defined dollar amount per day for care is provided. This is the most common form of reimbursement to hospitals. **Cost–plus reimbursement**, a type of retrospective reimbursement, was the traditional method used by Medicare and Medicaid to establish per diem rates for inpatient services. Under this method, reimbursement rates for institutions are based on the total costs incurred in operating the institution which are used to calculate the per diem or per patient day rate. The method is called cost–plus because, in addition to the operating costs, the reimbursement rate allows a portion of the capital costs to determine the rate (Buchbinder & Shanks, 2007; Shi & Singh, 2008; Sultz & Young, 2006).

Other reimbursement methods include:

- **Per diagnosis**: A defined dollar amount is paid per diagnosis. These types of rates are also used for Medicare reimbursements.

- **Bundles for hospital and physician services:** A fixed amount is paid by the managed care organization for patient treatment and is shared by all providers.

- **Fee schedule by current procedural terminology (CPT) code:** The most common method of reimbursement for specialty physicians. The more complex procedure, the higher the rate of reimbursement (CMS, 2009a).

GOVERNMENT REIMBURSEMENT METHODS FOR HEALTHCARE SERVICES

The federal government has sought to control healthcare expenditures through programs such as DRGs, ambulatory patient groups (APGs), ambulatory payment categories (APCs), home health resource groups (HHRGs), resource utilization groups (RUGs), and resource-based relative value scales (RBRVSs). States also used regulatory efforts such as certificate of needs (CONs) to control expenditures. Also, Medicaid growth costs have been limited by hospital preadmission screening, limiting hospital stays, reducing per diem rates, increasing copayments, and decreasing service coverage. Reducing Medicaid reimbursements creates issues of **cost shifting**. Healthcare organizations must find other ways to be reimbursed or they will not be profitable so they raise the prices to privately insured patients to offset the small reimbursement charges of Medicaid and Medicare (Feldstein, 2005).

Hospital Reimbursement

In 1982, Congress passed the **Tax Equity and Fiscal Responsibility Act** (TEFRA) and the **Social Security Amendments of 1983** to manage Medicare cost controls. There was a mandate to hospitals for a **prospective payment system** (PPS) to establish reimbursement rates for certain conditions. CMS reimburses hospitals per admission and per diagnosis which is based on a **DRG**—a prospective payment system for hospitals established through the Social Security Amendments of 1983. Each DRG group represents similar diagnoses of diseases that are expected to have similar use of hospital services. The amount of reimbursement is set per discharge of a patient. Hospitals that can provide services at lower costs may keep the difference in the reimbursement rates (Longest & Darr, 2008).

Resource-based Relative Value Scale

Under the Omnibus Budget Reconciliation Act of 1989, Medicare developed a new initiative of **RBRVS** to reimburse physicians according to a relative value assigned to a service. This reimbursement is divided into three components: physician work, practice expenses, and malpractice insurance. Medicare pays a flat fee for physician visits and is based on the Healthcare Common Procedure Coding System which is used to code professional services. The RBRVS, implemented in 1992, has become a standard Medicare Part B reimbursement method. This system increased reimbursement for family and general practice by about 15%. Also, physicians who had not signed a Medicare participation agreement, meaning they do accept Medicare reimbursement as the full payment for services, were prevented from **balance billing** so the physician is not able to bill the patient the difference between Medicare payments and the physician charges. The statute limited the amount the physician could balance bill the patient (Longest & Darr, 2008).

Ambulatory Patient Groups/Ambulatory Payment Categories

APGs were developed in the 1980s and are a system of codes that explained the number and types of services used in an ambulatory visit. Similar to the DRG classification, patients per APG had similar clinical classifications, resource use, and costs.

Implemented in August 2000, **APCs** were adapted from the APGs. The APC divides all outpatient services into 300 procedural groups/classifications based on similar clinical content such as surgery, medical, and ancillary services. Each APC is assigned a payment weight based on the median cost of services within the APC. The rates are also adjusted for wage differential by location. This type of rate is a bundled rate established by Medicare (CMS, 2009a).

Resource Utilization Groups

This type of prospective payment systems for skilled nursing facilities, used by Medicare, provides for a per diem based on the clinical severity of patients. A classification system called **RUG**, a type of DRG, was designed to differentiate patients based on how much they use the resources of the facility. As the patient's condition changes, the rate of reimbursement changes. A per diem rate was established using these classifications (Longest & Darr, 2008; Shi & Singh, 2008).

Home Health Resource Groups

Implemented in October 2000, the **HHRG**, which is a prospective payment used by Medicare, pays a fixed predetermined rate for each 60-day episode of care, regardless of the services. All services are bundled under a home health agency. The HHRG uses 80 distinct groups to classify patients' conditions (Longest & Darr, 2008).

HEALTHCARE FINANCIAL MANAGEMENT

Although for-profit and not-for-profit healthcare organizations have different missions, both types of organizations have financial objectives to achieve. The most common are: (1) generating a reasonable net income to continue effective operations, (2) setting prices for services, (3) contracting management of third-party payers such as Medicare and Medicaid and health service providers, (4) analyzing information for cost control, (5) adhering to governmental regulations such as reimbursement methods, and (6) minimizing financial risk (Buchbinder & Shanks, 2007). To ensure these objectives are met, many healthcare organizational structures include the following positions to supervise the financial management function. The **chief financial officer** (CFO) supervises the **comptroller** who is charged with accounting and reporting functions. The CFO may also supervise the **treasurer** who is responsible for cash management, banking relations, accounts payable, etc. An **internal auditor** who reports to the CFO ensures that accounting procedures are performed in accordance with appropriate regulations (McLean, 2003). All of these positions ensure that the organization is focusing on its mission to provide quality healthcare services. If there is no strong financial management system in place, the organization will fail.

FUNDS DISBURSEMENT

After services are delivered, the agency has to verify and pay the claims received from the providers. Disbursement of funds, which is often called **claims processing**, is carried out in accordance of the administrative procedures of the program. Most insurance companies and managed care organizations have a claims department to process payments. Self-funded insurance programs often hire a third-party administrator to process claims. Medicare and Medicaid contract with commercial insurance companies to process claims for them (Pointer et al., 2007).

CONCLUSION

As healthcare expenditures continue to increase, the major focus of the healthcare industry is cost control in both the public and private sector. For years, healthcare costs were unchecked. The concept of **retrospective reimbursement methods** for healthcare services, which means that a provider submitted a bill to a health insurance company that automatically reimbursed the provider, had no incentive to control costs in health care. This type of reimbursement method contributed to expensive health care for both the healthcare insurance companies and the individual who was paying out of pocket for their services. The establishment of a prospective reimbursement system for Medicare, which means a reimbursement system was developed based on care criteria for certain conditions regardless of providers costs, was an incentive system for providers to manage how they were providing services. The DRGs, RUGs, and RBRVs are examples of this type of reimbursement method. The focus now is efficiency and quality.

Also, the implementation of managed care organizations has focused on cost control. Although healthcare spending decreased in the 1990s, healthcare costs have continued to increase since. The implementation of CDHPs have assisted individuals with controlling healthcare costs by providing opportunities to save money for health care while obtaining a tax advantage. However, with the economic recession, there will be an increased number of individuals for a period of time that will have no health services because they are unemployed. This is a potential healthcare crisis because a large percentage of individuals historically have received their health care through their employer. This problem may further burden the government at all levels as individuals become eligible for public programs. The current administration has indicated that health care is a priority for implementing new public policy so any new initiatives may attempt to rectify this serious situation.

PREVIEW OF CHAPTER EIGHT

Managed care organizations revolutionized how healthcare services were delivered. Their focus was cost control as a result of the continued increasing cost of national healthcare expenditures. Managed care organizations developed a network of providers who belonged to the organization. HMOs were the original model for managed care organizations. The consumer had to choose these providers for their care. This model was an adjustment to both providers and patients. Providers were threatened by loss of income and consumers felt they lost control of the ability to choose their own provider. As the model has evolved, there have been modifications on how managed care has focused on consumer preferences while still maintaining cost control measures. Depending on the managed care model, providers were allowed to care for both managed care consumers and their own private patients. PPOs allowed consumers to choose their provider although they were required to pay an additional cost share if their physician was not within their network. Over the past decade, other models have been developed to address continued physician and consumer concerns. Chapter 8 will discuss the history of managed care organizations, the different models of managed care, issues regarding managed care, and how it has impacted traditional healthcare services. As a consumer it is very important for you to understand the managed care models because many of you either are participating in a managed care organization or will be using a managed care organization for your primary care.

VOCABULARY

Ambulatory patient groups (APGs)

Ambulatory payment categories (APCs)

Balance billing

Bundles for hospital and physician services

Capitated rate

Catastrophic health insurance

Chief financial officer (CFO)

Children's Health Insurance Program (CHIP)

Claims processing

Coinsurance

Comprehensive health insurance policies

Comptroller

Consumer-driven health plans

Copayments

Cost–plus reimbursement

Cost sharing

Deductibles

Diagnosis-related group (DRG)

Entitlement program

Fee for service

Fee schedule for CPT code

Flexible spending accounts (FSAs)

Group insurance

Health insurance

Health reimbursement arrangements (HRAs)

Health savings accounts (HSAs)

Home health resource group (HHRG)

Indemnity plans

Individual private health insurance

Internal auditor

Lifetime cap

Major medical policies

Managed care plans

Maximum out-of-pocket expenditures

Medical saving accounts (MSAs)

Medicare Part A

Medicare Part B

Medicare Part C

Medicare Part D

Medicare Prescription Drug Improvement and Modernization Act of 2003

Medigap policies

National Clearinghouse for Long-Term Care Information

Out of pocket

Per diem

Prepayment

Program of all-inclusive care for the elderly (PACE)

Prospective reimbursement

Public welfare insurance

Reinsurance

Resource-based relative value scales (RBRVs)

Resource utilization group (RUG)

Retrospective reimbursement

Self-insurance/self-funded insurance programs

Service benefit plan

Social insurance

Stop loss measure

Third party payer

Treasurer

TRICARE

Usual, customary, and reasonable services (UCR)

Voluntary health insurance

Worker's compensation

REFERENCES

Bach, P. (2008). Cost sharing for health care: Whose skin? Which game? *New England Journal of Medicine*, *358*, 4, 411–413.

Blue Cross Blue Shield Association. (2009). Retrieved November 9, 2009, from http://www.bcbs.com/careers/about-bcbsa/history-of-the-blues.html/.

Buchbinder, S., & Shanks, N. (2007). *Introduction to health care management*. Sudbury, MA: Jones and Bartlett.

Centers for Medicare and Medicaid Services. (2009a). *National health expenditure fact sheet*. Retrieved May 25, 2009, from http://www.cms.hhs.gov/NationalHealthExpendData/25_NHE_FACT_SHEET.asp.

Centers for Medicare and Medicaid Services. (2009b). *Program for all inclusive care for the elderly*. Retrieved May 26, 2009, from http://www.cms.hhs.gov/PACE/.

Davis, K. (2007). Uninsured in America: Problems and possible solutions. *British Medical Journal*, *334*, 336.

Department of Health and Human Services. (2009). *Long-term care insurance*. Retrieved May 27, 2009, from http://www.longtermcare.gov/LTC/Main_Site/Paying_LTC/Private_Programs/LTC_Insurance/index.aspx.

Department of Labor. (2009). *Office of Worker's Compensation Programs*. Retrieved May 26, 2009, from http://www.dol.gov/esa/owcp/dfec/regs/compliance/wc.htm.

Emanuel, E. (2008). *Health care, guaranteed*. New York: Public Affairs.

Employee Benefit Management Services, Inc. (2009). *Self funding overview*. Retrieved may 22, 2009, from http://www.ebms.com/Default.aspx?cID=33.

Enthoven, A., & Fuchs, V. (2006). Employment-based health insurance: past, present and future. *Health Affairs*, *25*, 6, 1538–1547.

Families USA. (2009). *SCHIP 101: What is the state's children's health insurance program, and how does it work?* Retrieved May 26, 2009, from http://www.familiesusa.org/assets/pdfs/SCHIP-101.pdf.

Feldstein, P. (2005). *Health care economics*. Clifton Park, NY: Thomson/Delmar Learning.

Indian Health Services. (2009). Retrieved November 9, 2009, from http://www.ihs.gov/index.cfm?module=About.

Longest Jr., B., & Darr, K. (2008). *Managing health services organizations and systems*. Baltimore: Health Professions Press.

Kaiser Family Foundation. (2007). *Health care costs: A primer. Key information on health care costs and their impact*. Retrieved May 27, 2009, from http://www.kff.org/insurance/upload/7670.pdf.

McLean, R. (2003). *Financial management in health care organizations* (pp. 12–19). Clifton Park, NY: Thomson/Delmar Learning.

National PACE Association. (2009). *NPA shared services program*. Retrieved November 9, 2009, from http://www.npaonline.org/website/article.asp?id=5.

Pointer, D., Williams, S., Isaacs, S., & Knickman, J. (2007). *Introduction to U.S. health care*. Hoboken, NJ: Wiley Publishing.

Shi, L., & Singh, D. (2008). *Delivering health care in America* (4th ed.). Sudbury, MA: Jones and Bartlett.

Starr, P. (1982). *The social transformation of American medicine*. Cambridge, MA: Basic Books.

Sultz, H., & Young, K. (2006). *Health care USA: Understanding its organization and delivery* (5th ed.). Sudbury, MA: Jones and Bartlett.

TRICARE. (2009). Retrieved November 9, 2009, from http://tricare.mil/tma/AboutTMA.aspx.

Wilensky, G. (2006). Consumer driven health plans: Early evidence and potential impact on hospitals. *Health Affairs*, 25, 1, 174–186.

NOTES

STUDENT ACTIVITY 7-1

CROSSWORD PUZZLE

Instructions: Please complete the puzzle using the vocabulary words found in the chapter. There may be multiple-word answers. The numbers in the parenthesis are the number of words in the answers.

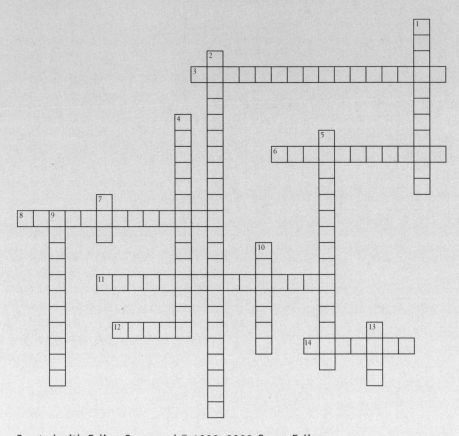

Created with EclipseCrossword © 1999–2009 Green Eclipse

STUDENT ACTIVITY 7-1

Across

3. The disbursement of funds to pay for submitted bills for healthcare services. (2 words)

6. This health insurance concept requires a contribution from a covered individual, which may be a copayment or deductible. (2 words)

8. This retrospective type of reimbursement method paid for services as they were submitted by healthcare providers. Did not focus on cost control. (3 words)

11. Medicare is this type of insurance. (2 words)

12. Type of reimbursement divided into three components: physician work, practice expenses, and malpractice insurance. (1 acronym)

14. This program, implemented by the Department of Defense, is structured after managed care and is a coordinated effort of the Army, Navy, and Air Force. (1 word)

Down

1. This procedure occurs when a company has a self-funded insurance program and wants to protect themselves from any catastrophic losses. (1 word)

2. This tool provides employees with the option of setting pretax income aside to pay for out-of-pocket expenses. Funds must be spent within 1 year. (3 words)

4. Also called fee-for-service plans. (2 words)

5. In a self-funded insurance program, this tool will limit the amount a company will pay for claims. (3 words)

7. Reimbursement system that was developed based on categories of similar disease diagnoses. (1 acronym)

9. Medicare is this type of program because employees pay into this program for years and can claim benefits. (1 word)

10. This type of reimbursement is a defined dollar amount per day for care. (2 words)

13. This newly implemented pilot health program is a comprehensive program funded by Medicare and Medicaid and is modeled from a California senor healthcare center. (1 acronym)

STUDENT ACTIVITY 7-2

IN YOUR OWN WORDS

Based on Chapter 7, please provide an explanation of the following concepts in your own words. DO NOT RECITE the text.

Reinsurance: _____
_____
_____

Flexible spending accounts (FSAs): _____
_____
_____

Prospective reimbursement: _____
_____
_____

Diagnosis-related group (DRG): _____
_____
_____

Resource utilization group: _____
_____
_____

Coinsurance: _____
_____
_____

Consumer-driven health plans: _____
_____
_____

Cost sharing: _____
_____
_____

Entitlement program: _____
_____
_____

STUDENT ACTIVITY 7-3

REAL LIFE APPLICATIONS: CASE STUDY

Your grandmother just turned 65 and is very confused about Medicare. She doesn't understand why there are four parts to this health insurance program. She has asked you to help her with enrolling in Medicare.

ACTIVITY

(1) List the different parts of Medicare and (2) explain what each part is and why it may be important to your grandmother.

RESPONSES

_____

_____

_____

_____

_____

_____

_____

_____

_____

_____

_____

_____

STUDENT ACTIVITY 7-4

INTERNET EXERCISES

Write your answers in the space provided.

- Visit each of the Web sites listed here.
- Name the organization.
- Locate their mission statement on their Web site.
- Provide a brief overview of the activities of the organization.
- How do these organizations participate in the US healthcare system?

Web Sites

http://www.tricare.mil

Organization Name: _____

Mission Statement:

_____

_____

_____

Overview of Activities:

_____

_____

_____

Importance of organization to US health care:

_____

_____

_____

http://www.npaonline.org

Organization Name: _____

Mission Statement:

_____

_____

_____

Overview of Activities:

_____

_____

_____

Importance of organization to US health care:

_____

_____

_____

http://www.familiesusa.org

Organization Name: _____

Mission Statement:

_____

_____

_____

Overview of Activities:

_____

_____

_____

Importance of organization to US health care:

_____

_____

_____

www.cms.hhs.gov

Organization Name: _____

Mission Statement:

_____

_____

_____

Overview of Activities:

_____

_____

_____

Importance of organization to US health care:

_____

_____

_____

STUDENT ACTIVITY 7-4

http://www.schip-info.gov

Organization Name: _____

Mission Statement:

_____

_____

_____

Overview of Activities:

_____

_____

_____

Importance of organization to US health care:

_____

_____

_____

http://www.ebms.com

Organization Name: _____

Mission Statement:

_____

_____

_____

Overview of Activities:

_____

_____

_____

Importance of organization to US health care:

_____

_____

_____

Impact of Managed Care on Healthcare Delivery

LEARNING OBJECTIVES

The student will be able to:

- Define managed care.
- Describe the network-based types of managed care organizations (MCOs).
- Discuss the history of managed care.
- Discuss four major goals of managed care.
- Assess the relationship of managed care with providers.
- Identify four cost control methods of MCOs.

DID YOU KNOW THAT?

- The concept of managed care has been evolving since the early 1930s.
- The oldest form of managed care is the health maintenance organization (HMO).
- From 2000 to 2007, healthcare premiums rose 98% while wages only rose 23%, despite the prevalence of managed care models that focus on cost control.
- Carve outs are healthcare services that will not be paid by MCOs and could include experimental treatment, drug costs, and behavioral health costs.

- The Health Plan Employer Data and Information Set (HEDIS) is a data set of healthcare plan's service activities and is used to evaluate healthcare plans. Although there is a voluntary submission process, nearly 100% of all health plans submit their data to HEDIS.
- According to *Fortune* magazine's analysis of industries, managed care had the highest growth rate of the five major healthcare sectors.

INTRODUCTION

Managed care refers to the cost management of healthcare services by controlling who the consumer sees and how much the service cost. MCOs were introduced 40 years ago, but became more entrenched in the healthcare system when the Health Maintenance Organization Act of 1973 was signed into law by President Nixon (Buchbinder & Shanks, 2007; Shi & Singh, 2007; Sultz & Young, 2006). Healthcare costs were spiraling out of control during that period. Encouraging the increase in the development of HMOs, the first widely used managed care model, would help to control the healthcare costs. MCOs' integration of the financial industry with the medical service industry resulted in controlling the reimbursement rate of services, which allowed them more control over the health insurance portion of health care (Sultz & Young, 2006).

Physicians were initially resistant to managed care models because they were threatened by loss of income. As the number of managed care models increased, physicians realized they had to accept this new form of healthcare delivery and, if they participated in a managed care organization, it was guaranteed income. Managed care became very popular in the 1990s. Enrollment increased from 27% in 1988 to 95% in 2002 ("Managed care organizations," 2007). For a period, healthcare costs decreased during the 1990s as a result of the influence of MCOs. However, the influence was short-lived and healthcare costs continued to increase. From 2000 to 2007, healthcare premiums rose 98% while wages only rose 23% (Wunker & Duncan, 2009). Projections for 2009 indicated that there will be an increase of 10.6% for HMOs as compared to the 2008 increase of 10.9%. Prescription drug costs will increase 9.2%, which is below the 2008 9.5 increase ("Health costs decelerate," 2008).

This chapter will discuss the history of the evolution of managed care and why it developed, the different types of managed care, the MCO assessment measures used for cost control, the issues regarding managed care, and how managed care has impacted the delivery of healthcare services.

HISTORY OF MANAGED CARE

As discussed in Chapter 1, the delivery of health care evolved around the individual relationship between the provider and patient/consumer. The payment was either provided by a health insurance company or paid out of pocket by the consumer. This **fee-for-service (FFS)** system or **indemnity plan** increased the cost of health care because there were no controls on how much to charge for the provider's service. As healthcare costs continued to spiral out of control throughout the decades, more experiments with contract practice and prepaid service occurred randomly throughout the US healthcare system (Shi & Singh, 2007; Sultz & Young, 2006).

According to Shi and Singh (2007), from 1850 to 1900, railroad, mining, and lumber companies provided their employees with healthcare services. The companies contracted with a physician to provide services to their employees at a rate per worker (which is a capitation rate because it limits the amount the provider will be

paid for per service). The reason these companies had to contract with a physician was because of the remote areas of work locations. When group health insurance programs were formed in the 1940s, it reduced the power of the corporations over managing the healthcare coverage and increased the power of the health insurance companies. The health insurance companies and providers had no incentives to control the costs of services. The concept of contractual practices and capitation were not adopted nationwide, which pleased the American Medical Association (AMA) because providers could increase their income with a traditional FFS practice. As a result of this system, healthcare costs continued to increase dramatically.

The concept of managed care has been evolving seriously since the early 1930s. The Committee on the Costs of Medicare Care recommended in 1932 that health care should be reorganized into a type of prepaid formula to control costs of services (Committee on the Costs of Medical Care, 1932). The FFS system was recognized even then as inefficient because there was no coordination of care of the patient between the primary care provider and other providers. There was also no focus on minimizing cost of services.

In the early 1930s and 1940s, several health plans adopted the concept of prepaid practice plans: the Group Health Association of Washington, the Group Health Cooperative of Puget Sound, the Health Insurance Plan of Greater New York, and the Group Health Plan of Minneapolis and the Kaiser Permanente Medical Care program, which became the model for HMOs (Shi & Singh, 2007). According to the Kaiser Permanente Web site, the Kaiser Permanente Plan was developed in 1933 as a result of providing care to construction, shipyard, and steel workers for Kaiser Industries, which they owned during this period. Dr. Sidney Garfield, a surgeon, recognized the potential to provide care to the thousands of workers involved in extensive projects so he built a hospital and set up a practice to care for these workers. Unfortunately, he often did not receive pay for his services because the insurance companies were not timely in their reimbursement and some workers were uninsured. Harold Hatch, an insurance agent, developed the prepaid concept of medical care. Dr. Garfield would receive insurance remuneration up front per day for each worker. This system worked extremely well and was used for several different industrial projects until 1945 when many of these large projects were completed. Kaiser Permanente opened this type of managed care system to the public in 1945. Membership increased to 300,000 members as a result of union membership. Kaiser Permanente, located in Oakland, CA, has continued this type of concept successfully. It is the largest nonprofit health plan today with 8.6 million members (Kaiser Permanente, 2009).

Legislative Influence on Managed Care Development

In 1973, President Nixon signed into law the HMO Act. This Act authorized $375 million in funding (loans and grants) for HMO expansion of existing facilities, which rewarded them for focusing on cost control. The Act also required that any business that had 25 or more employees offer an HMO option if available. According to a 2004 report by AMA's Council on Medical Services on managed care, over the next 30 years, several legislative acts were passed that impacted how managed care developed (Hoven, 2004).

The HMO Act of 1973 was amended in 1976 and 1978, which relaxed requirements for HMOs and restricted funding for HMO assistance programs for 2 years. In 1988, the HMO Act was amended to allow employees to contribute less to HMO plans than to traditional FFS plans. In 1982, the Tax Equity and Fiscal Responsibility Act cut more federal funding for health care, including HMOs. The Balanced Budget Act of 1997 established Medicare+Choice (M+C; Part C) which developed different structures for managed care plans. In 2003, the Medicare Prescription Drug, Improvement and Modernization Act of 2003 replaced M+C with Medicare Advantage (Hoven, 2004).

Over three decades, MCOs' strategies increased their exposure. More companies and health insurance companies became interested in controlling healthcare costs. The federal government decided to use HMOs for their army veterans. In the 1990s, the growth rate of MCOs was 10% per year. The peak enrollment of MCOs was 1999 with a total membership of nearly 90 million. There are currently 78 million members enrolled in MCOs (Simoner, 2007).

MANAGED CARE CHARACTERISTICS

Regardless of the type of MCO, all MCOs have five common characteristics:

- They all establish relationships with organizations and providers to provide a designated set of services to their members.

- They all establish criteria for their members to utilize the MCO.

- They all establish measures to estimate cost control.

- They all provide incentives to encourage health service resources.

- They all provide and encourage utilization of programs to improve the health status of their enrollees (Knight, 1998).

The MCO provides comprehensive services that include primary, secondary, and tertiary care. Depending on the type of MCO, physicians may work exclusively for the MCO or may be under contract with the MCO. MCOs will also contract with hospitals and outpatient clinics to ensure they provide comprehensive services.

Different Types of Managed Care Models

There are six organizational structures of MCOs.

1. **Health maintenance organizations (HMOs):** HMOs are the oldest type of managed care. Members must see their primary care provider first in order to see a specialist. There are four types of HMOs: staff model, group model, network model, and the independent practice association.

   - The **staff model** hires providers to work at a physical location.

   - The **group model** negotiates with a group of physicians exclusively to perform services.

   - The **network model** is similar to the group model but these providers may see other patients who are not members of the HMO. There is a negotiated rate for service for members to see providers who belong to the network.

   - The **independent practice associations** (IPAs) contract with a group of physicians who are in private practice to see MCO members at a prepaid rate per visit. The physicians may sign contracts with many HMOs. The physicians may also see non-HMO patients. This type of HMO was a result of the HMO Act of 1973.

2. **Preferred provider organizations (PPOs):** These providers agree to a relative value-based fee schedule or a discounted fee to see members. They do not have a gatekeeper like the HMO so a member does not need a referral to see a

specialist. The PPO does not have a copay but does have a deductible. This plan was developed by providers and hospitals to ensure that non-members could still be served while providing a discount to MCOs for their members. A member may see a provider not in the network but they may pay more out of pocket for their services. The bill could be as much as 50% of the total bill. They are currently the most popular type of plan (American Heart Association, 2009; Sultz & Young, 2006).

3. **Exclusive provider organizations (EPOs):** They are similar to PPOs but they restrict members to the list of preferred or exclusive providers members can use.

4. **Physician hospital organizations (PHOs):** These organizations include physician hospitals, surgical centers, and other medical providers that contract with a managed care plan to provide health services (Judson & Harrison, 2006).

5. **Point-of-service (POS) plans:** The POS plans are a blend of the other MCOs—a type of HMO/PPO hybrid (American Heart Association, 2009). They encourage but do not require that plan members to use a primary care provider who will become the gatekeeper of services. Members will receive lower fees if they use a gatekeeper model. They may also see an out-of-network provider at any time but will be charged a higher rate. This type of plan was developed as a result of complaints about the inability of a member to choose their provider (Anderson, Rice, & Kominski, 2007).

6. **Provider-sponsored organizations (PSOs):** These organizations are owned or controlled by healthcare providers. This is an emerging term that describes provider organizations that are formed to directly contract with purchasers to deliver healthcare services. PSOs are formed by organizations such as IPAs. However, unlike IPAs, they assume insurance risk for their beneficiaries (Longest & Darr, 2008).

THE MANAGED CARE ORGANIZATION PAYMENT PLAN

Depending on the type of MCO structure, their financing structure with providers may differ as well.

There are three major types of provider remuneration: capitation, discounted fees, and salaries. With a **capitation policy** or per member per month policy the provider is paid a fixed monthly amount per employee, often called a PMPM payment. This member fee is given to the provider regardless of how often the members use the service and the types of services used. The provider is responsible for providing all services deemed necessary.

Discounted fees are a type of FFS but are discounted based on a fee schedule. The provider provides the service and then can bill the MCO based on the fee schedule. Each service can be billed separately. The provider anticipates a large referral pool from the MCO so they will accept the discounted rates.

Salaries are the third method of payment. In this instance, the provider is actually an employer of the MCO. Annually, a type of bonus is distributed among the providers based on how often services have been used by members. So although they receive a salary, they will be rewarded by additional performance measures (Centers for Medicare and Medicaid Services [CMS], 2009).

COST CONTROL MEASURES OF MANAGED CARE ORGANIZATIONS
Restriction on Provider Choice

Members of an MCO often have restrictions on their choice for a provider. As the types of MCOs have evolved over the years, the restrictions have lessened, but there is a financial penalty such as a higher copayment or higher deductible for choosing a provider out of the network.

Gatekeeping

In some MCOs, the primary care provider is the gatekeeper of all of the care for the patient member. Any secondary or tertiary care would be coordinated by the gatekeeper. The primary care provider is responsible for the case management of a member patient. If additional medical services are needed, the primary care provider must refer the member patient for additional services. Some members do not like having a gatekeeper and would prefer to make these decisions themselves. As a result of this model, some MCOs require a preauthorization of services by the MCO. Many MCOs have clinical guidelines to determine service approval (Buchbinder & Shanks, 2007).

Services Review

Utilization review evaluates the appropriateness of the types of services provided. According to Shi and Singh (2007), there are three types of utilization reviews: prospective, concurrent, and retrospective. **Prospective utilization review** is implemented before the service is actually performed by having the procedure authorized by the MCO, having the primary care provider decide to refer the member for the service, or assessing the service based on the clinical guidelines. **Concurrent utilization reviews** are decisions that are made during the actual course of service such as length of inpatient stay and additional surgery. **Retrospective utilization review** is an evaluation of services once the services have been provided. This may occur to assess treatment patterns of certain diseases. This type of review may include a financial review to assure accuracy of billing. **Practice profiling**, an offshoot of retrospective utilization review, examines specific provider patterns of practice. This is a type of employee performance review because the focus is to determine which provider also fits in with the organizational culture of the MCO.

MEDICARE AND MEDICAID MANAGED CARE

Medicare Managed Care

As stated previously, the M+C program was created as a result of the Balanced Budget Act of 1997. Implemented in 2000, the purpose of M+C was to encourage Medicare enrollees to use managed care services. Medicare offered risk plans and cost plans for their enrollees. **Risk plans** pay a premium per member that is based on the member's county of residence. Members could use both in-network and out-of-network providers. The risk plans covered all Medicare services and vision and prescription care. **Medicare cost plans** reimburse the MCOs on a preset monthly basis per enrollee based on a forecasted budget. The cost plans allowed members to pursue care outside the network. In 2000, the program's enrollment was at a high of over 6 million members (CMS, 2009; Shi & Singh, 2007).

In 2003, the Medicare Prescription and Drug Improvement and Modernization Act (MMA) renamed the program **Medicare Advantage (MA)** and allowed PPOs as an option. It also allowed enrollees to participate in private fee-for-service (PFFS) plans as part of the MA. CMS evaluated the administration of the MA program and, based on that evaluation, they developed strategies to recruit more MCO participation. Despite these improvements, managed care enrollment initially dropped nearly 2 million in 2004. With changes in MA, 2006 enrollment surpassed the M+C enrollment (CMS, 2009). As a result of the MMA, the newly revamped MA program has been a financial boost to MCOs. Prior to the passage of the MMA, many providers refused Medicare and Medicaid patients because the reimbursement rates were low. As a result of the MMA, the top MCOs—Aetna Healthcare, Wellpoint, and United HealthCare—received reimbursements from the federal government for nearly $80 billion in 2007, which was an increase from nearly $25 billion in 2003 (Trombetta, 2008). The MA program is slated to cost $100 billion this year and critics say that about $15 billion of that is excess. Analysts estimate that in 2009, CMS will pay MA plans an estimated 14 to 18% more than comparable PFFS costs (Wechsler, 2009). The Obama administration anticipates introducing healthcare reforms that will target MA for cost reductions.

Medicaid Managed Care

According to CMS, of the total Medicaid enrollment in 2004, approximately 60% were receiving Medicaid managed care benefits. All states except Alaska and Wyoming have Medicaid managed care. Managed care plans use the gatekeeper model, HMOs, and prepaid health plans. **Carve outs** are services that Medicaid is not obligated to pay for under an MCO contract. Carve outs have occurred because the MCO cannot provide the service or it is too expensive. Unfortunately, mental health services and substance abuse treatment services are often categorized as carve out services (CMS, 2009).

A recent study performed by the Urban Institute indicated that MCOs had an impact on access to care for some of the Medicaid beneficiaries. Supplemental security income (SSI) beneficiaries, a subgroup of Medicaid, who were located in urban areas were less likely to have had a healthcare visit within a 12-month period than those Medicaid beneficiaries enrolled in FFS programs. In rural areas, SSI beneficiaries were more likely to have made a healthcare visit within the past 12 months although they also used the emergency room as their healthcare provider (Coughlin & Young, 2004).

ASSESSMENT OF MANAGED CARE MODELS

National Committee on Quality Assurance

From a health consumer perspective, when an organization's top priority is cost control, there may be concerns about losing a level of quality. As discussed in Chapter 1, the iron triangle of cost, access, and quality can be applied to manage care. When an organization focuses on cost, quality and access may suffer. As managed care was integrated into Medicaid and Medicare, the government also became more involved in the evaluation of managed care providers. Also, as competition increased in the managed care arena, there was fear that more services would be reduced to maintain lower premiums (Sultz & Young, 2006). As a result of these issues, the **National Committee on Quality Assurance** (NCQA) was established to maintain the quality of care in health plans.

NCQA was established in 1990 to monitor health plans and improve healthcare quality. Their focus is to measure, analyze, and improve healthcare programs. The NCQA accredits MCOs and, although a voluntary review process, the process includes surveys completed by managed care experts and physicians. They evaluate access and service and quality of the MCO's providers, primary prevention activities, and case management for the chronically ill. An organization can be accredited at three levels: excellent, commendable, and accredited. This accreditation, although voluntary, has alleviated concerns of the MCOs' focus on cost control. The NCQA has developed a report card of accredited health plans that consumers can access on their Web site. In the past, the NCQA had developed different criteria for the different types of MCOs. As of 2009, the NCQA developed standards and guidelines for all MCOs regardless of their organizational structure. The NCQA also has a physician directory that recognizes quality practices. There are 40 states that recognize NCQA accreditation and believe that the organization improves the quality of care provided by health plans. As the MCO industry has become very competitive, it is to the benefit of an MCO to become accredited (NCQA, 2009).

Health Plan Employer Data and Information Set

HEDIS was established by the NCQA in 1989. It is used by nearly 100% of all health plans to measure service and quality of care. The reported data is available to MCOs and physicians. HEDIS uses 71 measures from different areas of health care. Because so many health plans submit data to this HEDIS database and because the measures are so specifically defined, comparisons of health plans' performance can be performed. Health plans also use HEDIS results to assess performance (NCQA, 2009).

HEDIS measures health issues such as medication use patterns, breast cancer rates, rates of chronic diseases such as diabetes, childhood health issues, high blood pressure issues, heart disease and mental health disease, and health plans' treatment of these major health issues. Healthcare plans and providers use this database for performance assessment and consumers may use this information by using the State of the Health Care Quality Report, which analyzes the healthcare system. The Committee on Performance Measurement has members which represent the consumers, providers, health plans, employers, and other stakeholders who decide what type of data should be collected by the HEDIS and what type of measures should be used. There are four standards that are the focus of a NCQA review: quality management, utilization standards, members' rights and responsibilities, and services. The following are the focal points of these four areas. This information is a summary of evaluation criteria developed by the NCQA (NCQA, 2009).

Members' Rights and Responsibilities

Members' Written Information

- Written plan that outlines the members' rights and responsibilities and how written information is distributed to members
- Written plan that outlines the benefits, charges, and complaint process to members
- Directory for members to access necessary telephone numbers
- Written policy of MCO's protection of members from violation of their medical privacy

Member Services

- Resource accessibility for members to submit claims
- Efficiency measurement of claims processing
- Technology to improve access to and processing of claims
- Accessibility of pharmaceutical benefits and member responsibility

- The Web site's ease of use for member services
- Assurance of member information accuracy
- Member health risk appraisal using different Web educational tools
- Health information availability 24 hours a day
- Member assessments for wellness programs
- Member incentives to develop healthy behaviors

Accessibility of Services/Practitioners Availability/Member Satisfaction will focus on:

- Access to medical care for emergency and after-hours care
- Mental health services accessibility and performance measures to ensure quality of care
- Coordination between mental health and general medical care
- NCQA review of MCO to determine member accessibility to MCO physicians in the designated areas
- MCO is culturally sensitive to its patients, such as resolving language barriers
- Adequate number of both specialty and general practitioners available to MCO members
- Measures performed to ensure quality performance of providers
- MCO has a system in place to address members' complaints and if there are periodic member satisfaction surveys to assess quality of care
- Plan in place for how the MCO will take steps to rectify any quality issues

Complex Case/Disease Management/Clinical Practice Guidelines Review will focus on:

- Does the MCO to have a system in place to recognize members who have more complex medical issues that require case management?
- Is there a system to place to ensure that case management is done efficiently and effectively?
- Services offered to chronically ill patients and how the patient is managed.
- Review the clinical practice guidelines and, if they are changed periodically, distributed to the providers.
- Review medical record policies to ensure all care is documented and any policies in place to improve medical documentation.

Denials and Appeals of Medical Care

- Obtaining appropriate clinical information for medical decisions
- Denial plan for medical care requests
- Appeal plan for denial of care decisions
- Written notification plan of denials to members
- Written notification of any overturned decisions to members

Additional Procedures for Pharmaceutical/Mental Health Care

- Written plan for drug coverage
- Policy for patient safety
- Routine review of the policy
- Are mental health patients appropriately referred and managed by mental health practitioners?

Quality Management and Improvement

Program structure/operations reviews will focus on the following:

- MCO's written quality assurance program that is updated annually and has specific measures regarding behavioral health.
- Assessment whether quality assurance program has a quality improvement (QI) committee that manages the program with a physician involved.
- Is there is a work plan so quality assurance activities can be updated?
- How active is the QI committee in reviewing the program and is the QI program known to the providers of the MCO?
- If the QI committee takes action, review if there are issues regarding QI.
- Review if providers are cooperating with the QI committee and ensure access to medical records and other information is made available while maintaining provider–patient confidentiality.

Utilization Management

Structure/criteria for utilization of services/physician participation review will focus on the following:

- Written procedure for managing care
- Designation of appropriate physician to type of care

- Evaluation of the program on a timely basis
- Use of evidence-based clinical criteria for denying and approval of care
- Physician participation in developing criteria
- Evaluation plan of the criteria used
- Quality of healthcare professionals who review denials of care
- Use of consultants to assess medically necessary determinations
- Time frames for clinical decisions
- Notification process for members regarding clinical decisions

ISSUES WITH MANAGED CARE

According to AMA's 2003 survey, the *Portrait of Physicians*, physicians who contract with several MCOs are concerned with providing quality care to their patients because the MCOs' focuses are on cost. As a result of their focus on cost, the physician's ability to practice without close monitoring of their healthcare choices can be limited. Surveys indicate that the more managed care networks the physician contracts with, the less satisfied they are with managed care. However, if providers are provided an orientation regarding managed care during their education, they are more receptive to MCOs (AMA, 2009).

Physicians are also concerned with **physician network rentals** or **silent PPOs**, which are unauthorized third parties outside the contract between the MCO and the physician that gain access to the MCO discount rates. Examples of these network rentals are automobile insurers or workmen's compensations insurers. They obtain the physician's rates from a database. The main insurer who has the contract with the physician does not provide the information to the physician and the third parties continue to benefit from the discounted rates. There are currently 14 states that prohibit these silent PPOs (Berry, 2008; Carroll, 2009). This scheme takes money from the physicians because they are obtaining discounts fraudulently. Physicians have pursued legal action against MCOs because of issues with reimbursement such as the abuse of these discounted rates by unauthorized users.

As a result of these issues, the AMA has developed a **Private Sector Advocacy Unit** which addresses issues with managed care such as those identified here. They have provided guidance to physicians on contract development, claims management, complaint processes, and HIPAA compliance forms. The AMA has also been a strong lobbyist for legislation to protect physicians from silent PPOs (Hoven, 2004).

The concept of **medical loss ratio** or the minimum amount of dollars a healthcare plan spends on providing care rather than administration has been targeted by the California Medical Association, which has been lobbying state government to require healthcare plans to spend at least 85% of their profits on reimbursement claims (Carroll, 2008). This cap would limit the continued increase in premiums that healthcare consumers continue to pay year after year. The healthcare plans feel that if that cap would occur, there would be less focus on providing quality customer service. This long running battle is a result of annual Rand Reports that give medical loss ratio (MLR) statistics on healthcare plans. For example, Great-West Healthcare of California's MLR is 69.4%, a decrease from 86% in 2003. This indicates that more funds are being targeted to operational rather than quality healthcare services. It is important to note that the MLR will be different between nonprofit and for-profit organizations because their missions are different (Carroll, 2008). As a result of the varying differences in MLRs of health organizations, some states have passed MLR laws to ensure that a minimum amount is being spent on delivering quality healthcare services to their patients.

Recently United HealthCare paid a $350 million settlement because their subsidiary, Ingenix, had underestimated (as much as 28%) the schedule of **usual and customary fees**, which are the standardized rates assessed for reimbursement of both in-network and out-of-network healthcare services. This underestimation resulted in increased out-of-pocket expenses for their members. There were 100 million beneficiaries that were assessed out-of-pocket expenses based on this database. As part of this settlement, United HealthCare was also required to develop a new database that would be developed by an independent contractor (Miller, 2009).

CONCLUSION

The managed care model for healthcare delivery was developed for the primary purpose of containing healthcare costs. By administering both the healthcare services and the reimbursement of these services, and therefore eliminating a third party health insurer, the industry felt that this model would be very cost-effective. Both the consumer or patient and the physician's concerns were the same—worry about providing quality care while focusing predominantly on cost. The consumer was also worried about loss of freedom of choice of their primary care provider. The physician was worried about loss of income.

As managed care evolved, more managed care models evolved that allowed more choice for both the consumer and the physician. Eventually, there were models such as PPOs and POS plans that allowed a consumer to more freely choose their provider. However, there was a financial disincentive to use a provider outside the network of the MCO. The provider was also able to see non-MCO patients, which increased their income. The provider also received a financial disincentive because any MCO patient was given health care at a discounted rate.

Critics of MCOs have said that although they have eliminated the health insurer from the equation of providing care, the MCOs have absorbed that savings into their organization. With the passage of the MMA, MA MCOs have been reimbursed by the government at very high rates. In 2007, United HealthCare and Humana earned 66% and 11% respectively of their net income from MA reimbursements (Trombetta, 2008).

There also have been reimbursement issues with how MCOs have reimbursed the physicians. As discussed in the chapter, the issue with silent PPOs has financially hurt the physicians. Physicians have also had problems with timely reimbursement from MCOs. As also discussed in the chapter, there were issues with fraudulent reimbursement rates of out-of-network services, which resulted in members paying exorbitant out-of-pocket expenses.

Many MCOs have been very profitable for years. The recent CEO of United HealthCare retired with a $1.2 billion package. The most profitable HMO in the Unite States is Coventry Health Care of Bethesda, Maryland. Their MLR is approximately 80%. Kaiser Permanente, a nonprofit MCO, has an MLR of 99%—that means that nearly all of their premiums are returned to the members for their care (Carroll, 2008). With the economic issues that have been and will be facing the United States, with the number of uninsured Americans rising daily as more people lose their jobs, it seems almost unethical that some MCOs' MLRs are so low.

PREVIEW OF CHAPTER NINE

Chapter 9 discusses the tremendous impact of information technology (IT) on health care. Health information technology's (HIT) goal is to manage health information that can be used by all stakeholders in the industry which includes the consumer, the providers, the health insurance companies, employees, and pharmaceutical companies. HIT has allowed the documentation of every transaction to be more quickly documented, which has resulted in the increased efficiency of healthcare data. HIT allows different systems to share patient data which will increase the quality and efficiency of health care. From a consumer standpoint, HIT has impacted the ability for a patient to access more data via electronic sources. There have also been electronic initiatives to provide basic healthcare online.

The Obama administration is committed to a national computerized system of patient data that will focus on increased efficiency and quality of care and has budgeted nearly $20 billion to accelerate the development of computerizing physician's offices by creating regional IT centers. This chapter will discuss the history of HIT, the different applications, and the barriers for the implementation of IT in health care and the impact of IT on you as a healthcare consumer.

VOCABULARY

Capitation policy

Carve outs

Concurrent utilization reviews

Discounted fees

Exclusive provider organizations

Fee-for-service plans

Gatekeeper

Group model

Health maintenance organization (HMO)

Health Plan Employer Data and Information Set (HEDIS)

Indemnity plan

Independent practice associations

Managed care

Medical loss ratio

Medicare Advantage

Medicare cost plans

National Committee on Quality Assurance (NCQA)

Network model

Physician hospital organizations

Point-of-service plans

Practice profiling

Preferred provider organizations (PPO)

Private Sector Advocacy Unit

Prospective utilization review

Retrospective utilization review

Risk plans

Salaries

Silent PPOs

Staff model

Usual and customary fees

Utilization review

REFERENCES

American Heart Association. (2009). *Managed health care plans*. Retrieved February 7, 2009, from http://www.americanheart.org/presenter.jhtml?identifier=4663.

Anderson, R., Rice, T., & Kominksi, G. (2007). *Changing the U.S. health care system*. San Francisco, CA: Jossey-Bass.

Berry, E. (2008). Model law banning silent PPOs could serve as draft for legislatures. *American Medical News*, December. Retrieved February 7, 2009, from http://www.ama-assn.org/amednews/2008/12/29/bisa1229.htm.

Buchbinder, S., & Shanks, N. (2007). *Introduction to health care management*. Sudbury, MA: Jones and Bartlett.

Carroll, J. (2008). Doctors seek to limit health plan profitability. *Managed Care*, September, 5–6.

Carroll, J. (2009). Silent PPOs spur doctor push back. *Managed Care*, January, 6–7.

Centers for Medicare and Medicaid Services. (2009). Retrieved November 9, 2009, from http://www.cms.hhs.gov/HealthCareFinancingReview/Downloads/02fallpg1.pdf.

Committee on the Costs of Medical Care. (1932). *Medical care for the American people: The final report*. Chicago: University of Chicago Press.

Coughlin, T., & Young, S. (2004). *Final report: Estimating the impacts of Medicaid managed care on Medicaid SSI beneficiaries: A national study*. Washington, DC: The Urban Institute.

Health costs decelerate, yet still climb fast. (2008). *Managed Care*, September, 52.

Hoven, A. (2004). Impact of the health maintenance act of 1973. *Report of the Council on Medical Services*, CMS Report 4-A-04.

Judson, K., & Harrison, C. (2006). *Law & ethics for medical careers*. New York: McGraw-Hill.

Kaiser Permanente. (2009). *About Kaiser Permanente*. Retrieved October 29, 2009, from http://xnet.kp.org/newscenter/aboutkp/historyofkp.html.

Knight, W. (1998). *Managed care: What it is and how it works*. Gaithersburg, MD: Aspen Publishers.

Longest, B., & Darr, K. (2008). *Managing health services organizations and systems*. Baltimore: Health Professions Press.

Managed care organizations. (2007). *The Next Generation: An Introduction to Medicine*, *4*, 1. Retrieved January 28, 2009, from http://www.nextgenmd.org/vol4-1/managed_care_organizations.html.

Miller, J. (2009). Troubling times have insurers in the hot seats. *Managed Healthcare Executive*. Retrieved February 5, 2009, from http://managedhealthcareexecutive.modernmedicine.com/mhe/Business+Strategy/Troubling-times-have-insurers-in-the-hot-seat/ArticleStandard/Article/detail/577624.

National Committee for Quality Assurance. (2009). *UM standards and guidelines*. Retrieved Feburary 6, 2009, from http://www.ncqa.org/tabid/851/Default.aspx.

Shi, L., & Singh, D. (2007). *Essentials of the U.S. health care delivery system*. Sudbury, MA: Jones and Bartlett.

Simoner, D. (2007). Managed care in the USA: Origins, HMO strategies and the marketing of health services. *Journal of Public Affairs*, 7, 357–571.

Sultz, H., & Young, K. (2006). *Health care USA: Understanding its organization and delivery* (5th ed.). Sudbury, MA: Jones and Bartlett.

Trombetta, B. (2008). A remedy for managed care. *Marketing Health Services*, Summer.

Wechsler, J. (2009). Congress hopes to cut MA excess. *The Managed Healthcare Executive*. Retrieved February 7, 2009, from http://managedhealthcareexecutive.modernmedicine.com/mhe/Politics+and+Policy/Congress-hopes-to-cut MA-excess/ArticleStandard/Article/detail/573821?searchString=Congress hopes to cut MA.

Wunker, S., & Duncan, D. (2009). Health plans: Disrupt and prosper. *Managed Care*, January, 26 29.

CROSSWORD PUZZLE

Instructions: Please complete the puzzle using the vocabulary words found in the chapter. There may be multiple-word answers. The numbers in the parenthesis are the number of words in the answers.

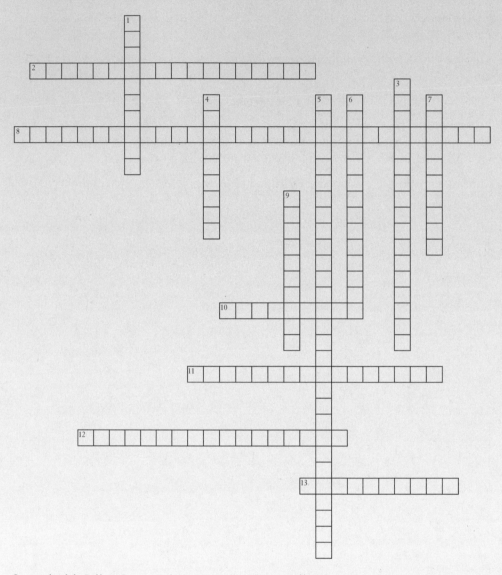

Created with EclipseCrossword © 1999–2009 Green Eclipse

STUDENT ACTIVITY 8-1

Across

2. This model is a combination of a HMO/PPO model. (4 words)

8. This organization contracts with a group of private practice physicians to see MCO members at a prepaid rate per visit. (3 words)

10. Offered by Medicare, these pay a premium per member, which is based on a county of residence so the members can use both in network and out-of-network providers. (2 words)

11. This calculation looks at the minimum amount of dollars a healthcare plan spends on providing care rather than administrative costs. (3 words)

12. This is a type of review which looks at physician patterns of practice. (2 words)

13. The provider is paid a fixed monthly amount per member regardless of how often the member uses the services. (1 word)

Down

1. This type of HMO model hires physicians to work at a physical location. (2 words)

3. This type of Medicare plan allows enrollees to participate in private fee-for-service plans. (2 words)

4. These are services that Medicaid is not obligated to pay under an MCO contract. (2 words)

5. This model is the oldest type of MCO. (3 words)

6. These charges are a type of fee for service but are reduced based on a fee schedule. (2 words)

7. The primary care provider of an MCO acts as a coordinator for all of the member's healthcare services. (1 word)

9. These are unauthorized parties outside the contract of an MCO and their members that gain access to MCO rates. (2 words)

STUDENT ACTIVITY 8-2

IN YOUR OWN WORDS

Based on Chapter 8, please provide an explanation of the following concepts in your own words. DO NOT RECITE the text.

Managed care:

_____

_____

_____

Health maintenance organizations:

_____

_____

_____

Preferred provider organizations:

_____

_____

_____

Point-of-service plans:

_____

_____

_____

Indemnity plan:

_____

_____

_____

Carve outs:

_____

_____

_____

Fee-for-service plans:

_____

_____

_____

Usual and customary fees:

_____

_____

_____

Medical loss ratio:

_____

_____

_____

Silent PPOs:

_____

_____

_____

STUDENT ACTIVITY 8-3

REAL LIFE APPLICATIONS: CASE STUDY

A friend, who had been a dependent on her parents' insurance, recently graduated from college and was offered a full-time healthcare management position. When she started to complete her human resource (HR) application, the HR manager asked her what type of healthcare plan she chose. She had no idea because she had always been treated under her parents' policies and never thought about what she may need. Her new employer offered several different healthcare plans: fee-for-service, HMO, PPO, and POS plans. She was very confused and was not clear on which plan she should select. She asked you to explain the differences between the different plans.

ACTIVITY

(1) Describe the characteristics of these healthcare plans and (2) identify the differences between the different plans. Answer these questions using the information from the text.

RESPONSES

_____

_____

_____

_____

_____

_____

_____

_____

_____

_____

_____

_____

_____

_____

INTERNET EXERCISES

Write your answers in the space provided.

- Visit each of the Web sites listed here.
- Name the organization.
- Locate their mission statement/values statement on their Web site.
- Provide a brief overview of the activities of the organization.
- How do these organizations participate in the US healthcare system?

Web Sites

http://www.ncqa.org

Organization Name: _____

Mission Statement:

_____

_____

_____

Overview of Activities:

_____

_____

_____

Importance of organization to US health care:

_____

_____

_____

http://www.nextgenmd.org

Organization Name: _____

Mission Statement:

_____

_____

Overview of Activities:

_____

_____

_____

STUDENT ACTIVITY 8-4

Importance of organization to US health care:

_____
_____
_____

http://www.americanheart.org

Organization Name: _____

Mission Statement:

_____
_____
_____

Overview of Activities:

_____
_____
_____

Importance of organization to US health care:

_____
_____
_____

http://www.managedhealthcareexecutive.modernmedicine.com

Organization Name: _____

Mission Statement:

_____
_____
_____

Overview of Activities:

_____
_____
_____

Importance of organization to US health care:

_____
_____
_____

STUDENT ACTIVITY 8-4

http://www.managedcare.com

Organization Name: _____

Mission Statement:

_____

_____

_____

Overview of Activities:

_____

_____

_____

Importance of organization to US health care:

_____

_____

_____

http://www.amednews.com

Organization Name: _____

Mission Statement:

_____

_____

_____

Overview of Activities:

_____

_____

_____

Importance of organization to US health care:

_____

_____

_____

The Influence of Information Technology

LEARNING OBJECTIVES

The student will be able to:

- Define and discuss health information technology, health information systems, and health/medical informatics.

- Evaluate the importance of the Office of the National Coordinator for Health Information Technology to health care.

- Assess the importance of the National eHealth Collaborative to health information technology policy.

- Discuss the importance of Dr. Octo Barnett to healthcare technology.

- Evaluate the impact of information technology on healthcare stakeholders.

- Discuss the difference between an EMR/EHR and an EHR.

DID YOU KNOW THAT?

- Both President Bush and President Obama have supported an initiative for electronic health records.

- E-prescribing is a form of a clinical decision support system.

- In an American Medical Association 2004 survey, approximately 25% of physicians reported that they communicated with their patients via email.

- The Veterans Health Administration's health information technology system is one of the best in the nation.

- In 2006, Centers for Medicare and Medicaid Services developed the largest data enterprise warehouse in history to gather hospital, prescription, and physician data to analyze the claims data for Medicare and Medicaid.

INTRODUCTION

The general term of **informatics** refers to the science of computer application to data in different industries. **Health** or **medical informatics** is the science of computer application that supports clinical and research data in different areas of health care. It is a methodology of how the healthcare industry thinks about patients and how their treatments are defined and evolved. For example, **imaging informatics** applies computer technology to organs and tissue (Coiera, 2003; Open Clinical, 2009). **Health Information systems** are systems that store, transmit, collect, and retrieve these data (Anderson, Rice, & Kominski, 2007). **Health** information technology's (HIT) goal is to manage the health data that can be used by patients/consumers, insurance companies, healthcare providers, healthcare administrators, and any stakeholder that has an interest in health care (Goldstein & Blumenthal, 2008).

HIT impacts every aspect of the healthcare industry. All of the stakeholders in the healthcare industry use HIT. Information technology (IT) has had a tremendous impact on the healthcare industry because it allows documentation of every transaction to be more quickly documented. When an industry focuses on saving lives, it is important that all activity has a written document that describes the activity. Computerization of documentation has increased the management efficiency of healthcare data. The main focus of HIT is the national implementation of an electronic patient record. Both Presidents Bush and Obama have supported this initiative. This is the foundation of many IT systems because it will enable different systems to share the patient information which will increase the quality and efficiency of health care. This chapter will discuss the history of IT, different applications of IT to health care, and discuss the evolution of the electronic medical records/electronic health records and the barriers for implementation.

HISTORY OF INFORMATION TECHNOLOGY IN THE HEALTHCARE INDUSTRY

Computers' first widespread use was in the 1960s as a result of the implementation of Medicaid and Medicare. Healthcare providers were inundated with forms to complete for both programs. In order to receive reimbursement from both programs, services needed to be tracked and forms needed to be completed and submitted to these programs. As a result, computers were used to assist with the financial management of these programs (Buchbinder & Shanks, 2007). As a result of computer integration, more healthcare providers recognized the efficiency of computers to manage programs. Hospitals particularly recognized the efficiency of electronic billing. During the 1960s, hospitals developed their own computer systems that housed their financial information. The hospitals were responsible for the maintenance of these systems. These systems, which were large mainframe systems, required a large staff to maintain their operations. All of the hospitals' data was stored on these mainframe computers. Computer

programs were developed by the hospitals to extract data reports. These mainframe computers were very expensive. They were eventually replaced in the 1970s with minicomputers which were more efficient, more cost-effective, and easier to maintain. These minicomputers were connected to a main computer that stored all of the data. These minicomputers were also used to enter information. Eventually, specific computer systems were developed for laboratories and clinics. It is important to mention Dr. G. Octo Barnett, who is a Professor of Medicine at Harvard Medical School and the senior director at the Laboratory of Computer Science at Massachusetts General Hospital (Appleby, 2008). He developed the first computer program for healthcare applications, called MUMPS, in 1964 that became the basis of very sophisticated programs used today.

During the 1980s and 1990s, the development and widespread use of personal computers (PCs) revolutionized information systems and technology. PCs were not reliant on a main computer for analyses. They were able to generate more sophisticated reports. PCs were often linked as a network to share information among different departments in hospitals. The development of a PC also enabled more computerization of physician practices, etc. The establishment of a chief information officer (CIO) in healthcare organizations emphasized how important information systems and technology had become to healthcare organizations. The US healthcare system has been the world leader for developing cutting-edge technology in health care. It has impacted how diagnostic procedures are performed, how data is collected and disseminated, how medicine is delivered, how providers treat their patients, and how surgeries are performed. There are several healthcare stakeholders that are impacted by technology. Consumer, providers, employers, researchers, all governmental levels, nonprofit and for-profit healthcare organizations, and insurance payers have all been impacted by technology (What is A Chief Information Officer?, 2009). Technological advances have been blamed, in part, for the continued rise of healthcare expenditures, but the results of technological advances cannot be disputed.

The Institute of Medicine (IOM) has published a series of reports over the past several years that focus on improving the quality of health care in the United States. In 2001, they published the report "Crossing the Quality Chasm: A New Health System for the 21st Century," which stresses the importance of improving the IT infrastructure. IOM emphasized the importance of an electronic health record (EHR), an electronic record of patient's medical history. The report also discussed the importance of patient safety by establishing data standards for collecting patient information (IOM, 2009).

In 2004, President Bush established the **Office of the National Coordinator for Information Technology** within the Department of Health and Human Services (HHS). In 2005, the **American Health Information Community** (AHIC) was chartered to develop recommendations on how to increase HIT use in our healthcare system. They focused on surveillance, consumer awareness, chronic health care, and EHRs. This federal advisory board concluded their work in 2008 and was established as a public–private corporation. In 2008, this initiative was renamed the **National eHealth Collaborative**. This organization has already met with President Obama regarding HIT. During his tenure, President Bush indicated that most US citizens should have an electronic patient record by 2014. President Obama has also supported this issue and has budgeted $19 billion to accelerate the use of computerized medical records in physicians' office by creating regional HIT extension centers (HHS, 2009). The deadline could be a challenge. According to a *New England Journal of Medicine* 2008 study, only 17% of US physicians use computerized patient records (Lohr, 2009).

ELECTRONIC PATIENT RECORDS

History

In 1991 and 1997, the IOM issued reports that focused on the impact of computer-based patients' records as important technology for improving health care (Vreeman, Taggard, Rhine, & Wornell, 2006). There are two concepts in electronic patient records that are used interchangeably but are different—the **electronic medical record** (EMR/EHR) and the **electronic health record** (EHR). The **National Alliance for Health Information Technology** (NAHIT) defines the EHR as the electronic record of health-related information on an individual that is accumulated from one health system and is utilized by the health organization that is providing patient care while the EMR accumulates more patient medical information from many health organizations that have been involved in the patient care. Simply, the EHR is an EMR that can be integrated with other systems (NAHIT, 2009). The IOM has been

urging the healthcare industry to adopt the electronic patient record but initially costs were too high and the health community did not embrace the recommendation. This discussion will focus on the EHR.

As software costs have declined, more healthcare providers have adopted the use of the EHR system. In 2003, HHS began to promote the use of HIT including the use of the EHR. The IOM was asked to identify essential elements for the establishment of an EHR. The IOM broadly defined the definition of an EHR to include:

- The collection of longitudinal data on a person's health
- Immediate electronic access to this information
- Establishment of a system that provides decision support to ensure the quality, safety, and efficiency of patient care (IOM, 2009)

Benefits of Electronic Medical Record/ Electronic Health Record

Several studies have been performed to assess the impact of the EHR on healthcare delivery. Administrators of several healthcare delivery systems reported many benefits to the implementation of an EHR. Many administrators cited the capability of more comprehensive reporting that integrated both clinical and administrative data. It also provided an opportunity to analyze and review patient outcomes because of the standardization of the clinical assessments. Also noted was the development of electronic automated reports that improved the discharge of a patient. The reports also provided an opportunity for the administrator to assess the workload of a department. The EHR also improved operational efficiency. The EHR had excellent capabilities to process and store data. Administrators also reported that the computerized documentation took 30% less time than the previous handwritten notes (Shields et al., 2007). However, it is difficult to develop an electronic record that can integrate with other medical systems. It is important that standards are developed for the EHR to ensure standard data elements are collected and to ensure that the software will be integrated into other systems.

Several studies indicated there was an improvement in interdepartmental communication. The EHR provided aggregate data in the patient records to other departments and the information about the patient was legible. The actual design and implementation of an

EHR system contributed to the development of a more interdisciplinary approach to patient care (Ventres & Shah, 2007; Whitman & David, 2007). The implementation of an EHR system led to improved data accuracy because it reduced the need to replicate data. The EHR system also provided a platform for routine data quality assessments which was important to maintain the accuracy of the EHR data. The EHR system provides an opportunity for future research. The data captured in the database could be used to analyze outcomes and develop baseline data for future research.

BARRIERS TO ELECTRONIC HEALTH RECORD IMPLEMENTATION

A major issue with any national implementation of an EHR system is the development of data standards that should be used nationally. The American National Standards Institute's HL7 has released a version of an EHR functionality specification. The American Society for Testing and Materials also released specifications for patient information exchange for continuity of care. The consistency of standards will play a major role in the national use of EHRs (Sriram & Fenves, 2009).

From a user perspective such as a physician's office, a major issue with EHR implementation is the cost of the implementation of the system. Software purchases, hardware, network upgrades, training, and computer personnel must be considered in the purchase of the system. Estimates vary from $15,000 to $30,000 per physician and can be amortized over a period of 5 years (Adler, 2004). Estimates should also include annual costs of $5000 to $15,000 over the first 5 years. According to Lowes (2007), Barbara Drury (President of Pricare, an HIT consulting firm) recently compared several bids of five EHR vendors; the bids were for upgrading a physician's practice computer system to include the EHR components. The vendor quotes varied from $58,000 to $13,000 for similar practices. These quotes also do not include any hardware upgrades for their systems. Therefore, it is very important for a provider to understand what they are receiving from a vendor and comparison shop for the most appropriate system for the best price.

For example, a 13-surgeon practice in Reno, Nevada, started phasing out their paper system and adopting an electronic health system in January 2006. Over a 3-year period, they were able to trim 10 staff positions including medical and front desk staff at an annual cost savings of $250,000, they saved an estimated annual transcription cost of $72,000, and they no longer had to rent storage space for their paper records for a savings of $50,000. The transition into automation was easier for a surgical practice because most surgeons are technologically advanced because of their specialty. Prior to the implementation of an EHR system, they had heard horror stories about the barriers to EHR implementation so they gradually phased in the system over a 6-month period when the providers ceased all paper charts. They scanned the patient information into the system but, per state regulations, they maintained 10 years of patient data in an offsite storage unit. There have been many reports of the barriers to implementing automation in health care but this is an excellent example of a successful transfer to technology because they gradually phased in the system. They had an in-house trainer to guide them. Also, the surgeons' attitudes were very receptive because they recognized the value of technology (Anderson, 2009).

Silver Cross hospital, a 306-bed hospital located in Illinois that had 450 doctors with privileges at their hospital, understood these issues and developed a strategy to successfully implement an EHR system ("Community EHR: Myth or reality," 2007). The main reason they were successful was because they provided opportunities for providers to actively participate in the implementation plan. They selected the system that would be used, they formed task forces to discuss the implementation, and shared the cost of the system purchase with the providers. They treated the providers as business partners. The entire process was transparent which enabled the providers and their staff to voice their concerns. They also designed trainings for both the providers and the staff to ensure they would be comfortable with the EHR system. As a result of this approach, the hospital reached an 80% penetration usage rate with the providers that worked with the hospitals.

In 2006, the American Hospital Association surveyed more than 1500 community hospitals which represents 31% of all community hospitals nationally. Results indicated that nearly 70% of hospitals had full or partial EHR records. Approximately 50% shared electronic patient data with others in 2005 and 2006 (Shields et al., 2007). Large urban hospitals used more HIT. Hospitals' spending on IT is increasing annually and, therefore, cost is often cited as a barrier to adoption.

JKL Healthcare System is a not-for-profit organization that operates three acute care hospitals with five satellite ambulatory locations, a research component, a network of 50 local physician offices, and a home care services company. In 2001, they decided to implement an EHR and physician order entry system. Their goal was to implement the system quickly to ensure that physicians did not redirect prospective patients to competitors.

The challenge was to train over 1500 employees and 450 physicians on this system to avoid any adverse patient outcomes and to improve quality of care. In order for it to be cost-effective, the compliance would need to be 100% by all physicians. The anticipated cost of the system was $35 million (O'Brien, 2007). Nine months after the system's implementation, the physicians surveyed indicated they would not want to return to a paper system. Nearly 90% of the physicians surveyed said that the system made it easier for them to work. Nearly all medication errors caused by illegibility and transcription were eliminated. Patient satisfaction for overall care also increased as a result of the systems. Staff felt their jobs became more efficient because many staff could be reviewing the same information from different systems. Because JKL Healthcare was one of the first to successfully implement an EHR system, it will serve as a consultation site for other healthcare systems (O'Brien, 2007).

According to Valerius (2007), migrating from a hard copy system to an electronic system, requires several components, including a physician order communication/results retrieval, electronic document/control management, point-of-care charting, electronic physician order entry and prescribing, clinical decision support system, provider patient portals, personal health records, and population health. When an organization implements an electronic system, there are changes in the workflow because much of the process was previously manual. Training is required for both healthcare professionals and staff to fully utilize the system.

When purchasing a system for patient electronic records, it was found that there were equipment or software inadequacies which created a processing of the data much slower. If the system failed, it created frustration for healthcare professionals and administrators. Both of these problems emphasized the need for adequate training for both the providers and staff. Much of the initial training required overtime for the staff. Most of the training lasted approximately 4 months. Continued training was also required for maintenance of the system (Valerius, 2007).

In October 2008, Microsoft announced their HealthVault Web site (HealthVault, 2009) that enables patients to develop EHRs free of charge. It is up to the individual as to how much medical information the person wants to store online with this Web site. The Web site also has links to several health Web sites that can assist with exercise programs, heart issues, drug reactions, software that allows users to share their medical information with their providers, etc. In November 2008, the Cleveland Clinic agreed to pilot data exchanges between HealthVault and the Cleveland Clinic's personal health record system. The Clinic has enrolled 400 patients in the areas of diabetes, hypertension, and heart disease to test the system. They will be testing their health status at home using blood pressure monitors, weight scales, heart rate monitors, and glucometers. The patients will test themselves and the reports will be uploaded to the Clinic using the HealthVault. They will also be able to access health education material on HealthVault regarding their diseases. This is the first pilot study in the country to assess this tool (Cleveland Clinic, 2009).

PRIMARY CARE INFORMATION PROJECT IN NEW YORK CITY MODEL

In 2008, the New York City Department of Health and Mental Hygiene (DOHMH), as part of a $27 million Mayoral initiative to improve the quality and efficiency of health care in New York City, developed the **Primary Care Information Project** (PCIP) to support the adoption and use of prevention-oriented EHRs primarily among providers who care for the city's underserved and vulnerable populations. DOHMH will work with a vendor, eClinicalWorks—a leading provider of integrated end-to-end EHRs and practice management systems for multilocation, multispecialty medical practices. PCIP involved primary care practices located in underserved communities (including family medicine, pediatrics, internal medicine, and obstetrics/gynecology). In order to participate in the project and receive the eClinicalWorks software, physicians were required to contribute $4000 and a commitment to bring their technology and infrastructure up to market standards. The project recruited more than 1600 physicians who serve 200,000 patients in New York City that included outpatient clinics, community health centers, small group physician practices, and a women's jail. It is a difficult process because it is a major change, but it has been cost-effective and efficient (New York City DOHMH, 2009).

LEGAL AND ETHICAL ISSUES OF AN EMR/EHR/EHR SYSTEM

Computerized information systems that are seen in finance, manufacturing, and retail have not achieved the same penetration in health care. EHRs have captured the attention of politicians, insurance companies, and practitioners as a way to improve patient safety because patient information will be more complete and standardized which will enhance the decision-making process of a practitioner (Murer, 2007). Major barriers to EHR implementation have been discussed including training and financial impact of an organization as the system becomes integrated with daily operations. However, legal and ethical issues are also a concern. As with any technological development, regulations often lag behind implementation. A major legal barrier is the sharing of the patient information electronically with other providers. Does this violate any Health Insurance Portability and Accountability Act (HIPAA) regulations pertaining to privacy and confidentiality? Does the patient have to consent this sharing of information each time their information is electronically shared with other providers (Christman, 2007)? Recent surveys have indicated that nearly 50% of US adults polled indicated that they had concerns about privacy and security of their information but felt that a computerized system like EHRs would outweigh the risks. The remaining 50% of those polled indicated that the EHR systems do not outweigh the risks of privacy and security (Swartz, 2005).

The issue of provider and organizational liabilities has also been discussed. As part of an EHR system, a provider may electronically prescribe medication to a patient. Are there any violations under state and federal fraud laws regarding electronic prescriptions of drugs? The Centers for Medicare and Medicaid Services (CMS) issued regulations in 2005 that established legal exceptions and safe harbors related to the use of e-prescribing and EHR technology. If these exceptions are more widely publicized, this may increase the usage of EHR adoptions (Murer, 2007).

REGIONAL HEALTH INFORMATION ORGANIZATIONS/NATIONAL HEALTH INFORMATION NETWORK

As part of the **Office of the National Coordinator for the Health Information** that was discussed previously in the chapter, as part of the EHR initiative, **Regional Health Information Organizations** (RHIOs) would be developed that would allow healthcare providers to access and share patient electronic information that is stored locally. These RHIOs would become part of the **National Health Information Network** (NHIN). In September 2008, a live demonstration of the NHIN occurred, using laptops, and different hypothetical medical incidents were managed using the NHIN. The network enabled the providers to access patient information immediately. The basis of both the regional and national networks is the EHR. Once that becomes established in 2014, both the RHIO and NHIN will be implemented (Traynor, 2008).

CLINICAL DECISION SUPPORT SYSTEMS

Artificial intelligence (AI) is a field of computerized methods and technologies created to imitate human decision making. A technique of AI is **expert systems** (ESs) which were developed to imitate experts' knowledge in decision making (Coiera, 2003). **Electronic clinical decision support systems** (CDSSs) are systems that are designed to integrate medical information, patient information, and a decision-making tool to generate information to assist with cases. They are a type of knowledge-based system. The key functions of a CDSS are (1) administrative, (2) case management, (3) cost control, and (4) decision support. Administrative protocols consist of clinical coding and documentation for procedure approval and patient referrals if necessary. Case management control focuses on the management of patients to ensure they are receiving timely interventions. Cost control is a focus because the system monitors orders for tests and medication which reduces unnecessary interventions (Perreault & Metzger, 1999).

Specifically, ESs can be used to alert and remind healthcare providers of a patient's condition change, or to have a laboratory test performed or have an intervention performed. An ES can also assist with a diagnosis using the system's database. The system can expose any weaknesses in a treatment plan or check for drug interactions and allergies. A system can also interpret imaging tests routinely to flag any abnormalities. It is important to note that the more complex duties of a system require the integration of an EMR/EHR system so the system can interface with the patient data (Coiera, 2003).

Some of the first decision support systems were developed in the 1970s. The INTERNIST I was developed at the University of Pittsburgh in 1974 to support diagnoses in internal medicine. It developed a large medical database using patient observations to assess potential diseases. These systems never progressed to commercial use because physicians were not accepting of these new systems during this period. Although several decision support systems were developed, no systems were commercialized until the 1980s, such as **Dxplain**, which used lab data and symptoms to produce a ranked list of potential diagnoses. The following is a chronological list of different types of CDSSs that have been developed over the last 20 years.

- **Dxplain** is in use at a number of hospitals and medical schools for medical education.

- Developed in 1977, the **PUFF** system was developed to interpret pulmonary function tests. It is still routinely used in hospitals.

- **HELP** was also developed in 1980 and was used for hospital management as well as a CDSS. It is used in hospitals routinely. ESs were also successfully developed for laboratory management.

- **APACHE I** was developed in 1981 for use in intensive care units. **APACHE II** and **APACHE III** upgrades were implemented in 1985 and 1991, respectively. It was developed for commercial use and is routinely used.

- In the 1990s, **GIDEON** was developed for diagnosis and treatment of infectious diseases. It became a commercial product.

- **IBROB** was developed in 1995 for use in obstetrics and is in routine use.

- **ATHENA** was developed in 2002 for management of hypertension and is in routine use.

- In 2002, **LISA** was developed for leukemia management and is in use today.

Research over the past several years has indicated that CDSSs have many potential benefits that can be classified into three categories: (1) improved patient safety, (2) improved quality of care, and (3) improved efficiency in healthcare delivery. Although the barriers to implementation were identified previously, the benefits for many institutions have outweighed those barriers so they have found ways to utilize these CDSSs. More CDSSs are being developed to provide information for various types of diseases (Open Clinical, 2009).

COMPUTERIZED PHYSICIAN ORDER ENTRY

Computerized physician order entry (CPOE) systems are CDSSs that enable a patient's provider to enter a prescription order or order for a lab or diagnostic test in a computer system. The order entry has four components: (1) information can be entered from a handheld device, laptop, or desktop computer; (2) it enables the provider to order a test, prescription, or procedure; (3) it is connected to a decision support system that alerts the provider to any problems with their orders; and (4) it can be integrated into the overall computer system of the organization. The CPOE first appeared in 1971 when NASA Space Center and Lockheed Corporation developed a system for a hospital in California. Although it improves quality assurance in patient care, thus reducing medical errors, 2003 estimates showed that only 5% of hospitals were using CPOE (Ash, Gorman, Seshardri, & Hersch, 2004). Similar to the EMR/EHR, barriers to implementing a CPOE system are the initial financial investment, the customization requirement with the current organization's computer system, medical and administrative training to use this system, and staff's fear of change. These barriers can be addressed before successful implementation of a CPOE.

E-prescribing, a form of CPOE, focuses on electronic prescription ordering by a provider for their patient. It also focuses on improving patient safety. Medication ordering and the administration of these medications can be incorrectly given to a patient because of similar sounding names, similar dosages, similar labeling. E-prescribing can be performed on a desk computer, laptop, or handheld device that will record physicians' prescription orders, which eliminates having an individual read a handwritten prescription. CPOE also includes a decision support system that includes possible drug interactions, dosage information, etc., that assist with the physician making the best decision possible for a patient. In January 2009, Medicare and some private healthcare plans began paying a bonus to physicians who e-prescribe to their Medicare patients. Medicare will also penalize physicians who do not e-prescribe by 2012 by reducing their reimbursement rates by 1%. IT companies are providing free software to physicians to encourage them to electronically prescribe. The number of physicians who are e-prescribing has risen over the past year. It is estimated between 12 and 16% of all office-based physicians are e-prescribing. E-prescribing encourages patients to fill their prescriptions because it reduces waiting times at the drugstore. A limitation with e-prescribing is that federal laws prohibit electronic prescribing of any type of controlled substance prescription, which could include sleeping pills or antidepressant drugs, but there are many drugs that are not controlled substances (Landro, 2009). This system can be used alone but it is best used with the EHR system because it integrates the information from the patient's EHR into its decision making.

More of these systems are being integrated into the EHR rather than kept a standalone system. The CDS Expert Review Panel and colleagues recommended that the e-prescribing system contains the following database elements: patient payer and plan data, patient medications and their status, patient demographic information, patient allergies to drugs, diagnoses, lab tests, and pharmacy information. The Panel also recommended that user should (1) be able to select dosage, strength, and duration; (2) be made aware of any drug alerts regarding drug interactions; (3) be able to view patient instructions; (4) be able to view weight-based dosing; (5) be able to view food interactions with drugs; (6) be notified when the prescription is due for renewal; and (7) be notified if the patient does not refill the prescription (Teich et al., 2005).

PHARMACY BENEFIT MANAGERS

Technology-based tools provide exceptional value to the prescription benefits of a health insurance program. E-prescribing will become more commonplace with the mandates of Medicare. In order to manage this technology effectively and efficiently, a **Pharmacy Benefit Manager** (PBM) uses technology-based tools to assess and evaluate the management of the prescription component so it can be customized to address the needs of the organization. PBMs are companies that administer drug benefits for employers and health insurance carriers. They contract with managed care organizations, self insured employers, Medicaid and Medicare managed care plans, federal health insurance programs, and local government organizations. Approximately 95% of all patients with drug coverage received benefits through a PBM. They manage approximately 70% of more than 3 billion prescriptions in the United States each year. The PBM integrates medical and pharmacy data of the population to determine which interventions are the most cost-effective and clinically appropriate (Federal Trade Commission, 2009).

DRUG–DRUG INTERACTIONS

Drug–drug interactions (DDIs) are used by software programs to alter pharmacists and clinicians about potential drug interactions. These alerts can be notifying the provider that two drugs may interact or there may be management strategies provided regarding the DDIs. In a January 2009 article, a group of experts developed a list of 25 important DDIs and management strategies that should be used in when prescribing in an ambulatory setting. Interactions within acute care settings were not included. Alert messaging was developed for these 25 DDIs for e-prescribing and pharmacy systems. Detailed information was also provided about why the DDIs occurred and what management strategies could be used for these problems. This type of additional information will educate providers regarding potential issues while prescribing (Murphy et al., 2009).

TELEHEALTH, TELEMEDICINE, AND E-HEALTH

Telehealth is the broad term that encompasses the use of IT to deliver education, research, and clinical care. An important activity of telehealth is the use of email between providers and their patients. In an American Medical Association 2004 survey, approximately 25% of physicians reported that they communicated with their patients via email. Telehealth also includes communication between healthcare providers. **E-health** refers to the use of the Internet by both individuals and healthcare professionals to access education, research, and products and services. There are several Web sites such as WebMD and Healthline that provide consumers with general healthcare information. A 2008 study that examined why consumers access the Internet found that consumers perceived the Internet as an alternative source for health information. Consumers used the Internet as a way to avoid visiting a provider and to increase their access to health care. It also provided a way of obtaining information discreetly and anonymously. It also provided a source of support groups. It is important to emphasize that consumers must be conscious of the quality of the Web sites they access to ensure the information they are receiving is accurate (Leung, 2008).

Telemedicine refers to the use of IT to enable healthcare providers to communicate with rural care providers regarding patient care or to communicate directly with patients regarding treatment. The basic form of telemedicine is a telephone consultation. Telemedicine is most frequently used in pathology and radiology because images can be transmitted to a distant location where a specialist will read the results. Telemedicine is becoming more common because it increases healthcare access to remote locations such as rural areas. It is also a cost-effective mode of treatment. As EMR/EHRs are used more frequently, it will be possible to provide more comprehensive services. A limitation may be how to reimburse a provider for providing an electronic consultation. Another limitation may also be if there are issues with reimbursement across state lines (Anderson et al., 2006).

CHIEF INFORMATION OFFICER

As more healthcare services are delivered electronically, many healthcare organizations have designated a **chief information officer** (CIO) to manage the organization's information systems. Some organizations may also refer this position as a **chief technology officer (CTO)** or they may have both. Normally, the CIO is a vice president of the organization and the CTO reports to that position. The CIO also integrates HIT into the organization's strategic plan. The CIO must have knowledge of current information technologies as they apply to the healthcare industry and how new technology can apply to the organization. The CIO is also responsible for motivating employees whenever there is any technological change (Oz, 2006). C. Martin Harris, who is the CIO of the Cleveland Clinic, feels that the challenge of the CIO (who he believes is a change agent) is to move from the implementing of the EHR to continuing to provide quality care to the patient by developing an integrated system model regardless of the size of the organization or the location of the organization. As more health care is being delivered by technology, it will be the responsibility of the CIO to develop a model that is patient oriented rather an operations oriented (Harris, 2008).

COUNCIL FOR AFFORDABLE QUALITY HEALTH CARE

The Council for Affordable Quality Health Care (CAQH), a nonprofit organization, consists of alliances of health plans and trade associations that discuss efficiency initiatives to streamline healthcare administration by working with healthcare plans, providers, the government, and consumers. As part of their initiative, they have created a **Committee on Operating Rules for Information Exchange** (CORE) that borrows from the banking industry's standards for one of the largest electronic payment systems in

the world. Based on stakeholder input, CORE has set up standards and operating rules for streamlining processes between providers and healthcare plans. This system allows for real-time access to patient information pre- and postcare. Aetna became certified to use the CORE standards in 2007 and required all of their data-exchange business partners to become CORE certified (Thomashauer, 2008). Established by HHS, the Health Information Technology Standards Panel (HITSP) utilized the CORE platform in its first set of data standards. HITSP is working toward the national integration of both public and private healthcare data standards for sharing among all organizations (Thomashauer, 2008).

OTHER APPLICATIONS

Enterprise Data Warehouse

Enterprise data warehouses (EDWs) are developed to provide information that helps organizations in strategic decision making. Data warehousing requires an integration of many computer systems across an organization. Older systems, often referred to as **legacy systems**, are difficult to integrate but worthwhile because they further supported strategic decision making. Business EDWs collect numeric data to assess trends. Retail, banking, and manufacturing use EDWs because these industries usually have repetitive actions that can be easily categorized. For example, banks have savings accounts, CDs, Roth IRAs, money markets, etc. It is very easy to analyze that type of data. Healthcare transactions can occur in the hospital, in community health centers, and in physicians' offices and each transaction is unique. Other patient healthcare data may not be numeric (Immon, 2007). There is written information that needs to be integrated into a system such as a physician's prognosis. Therefore, a healthcare EDW must be developed that acknowledges these differences. One of the first healthcare systems to utilize an EDW was the Veteran's Health Administration (VHA).

Veteran's Health Administration's Enterprise Data Warehouse

IOM has indicated that the VHA's HIT system is one of the best in the nation. VHA's system was once considered inefficient. VHA's Office of Health Information (OHI) supports veterans, doctors, nurses, and other healthcare providers by defining the requirements and direction of the Department of Veterans Affairs' (VA) electronic healthcare system known as VistA (VA, 2009). It uses an IT-based system that is used for clinical management, e-prescriptions, patient and drug information, and decision support. This system, which is comprised of 128 independent VistA systems in use at VA hospitals and clinics, implemented an EWD in 2005, which served as a central data repository. The EDW has been instrumental in providing effective services to over 5 million veterans on an annual basis (Bates & Turano, 2006).

The Centers for Medicaid and Medicare Services Enterprise Data Warehouse

In 2006, CMS, as a pilot study, developed the largest EDW in history to gather hospital, prescription, and physician data to analyze the claims data for Medicare and Medicaid. They initially integrated claims from 2005 and 2006. They felt that the integration of their data would enable them to analyze the number of claims submitted by providers. It also assisted in identifying any potential fraud and abuse. It is to be analyzed to determine its effectiveness before phasing out any legacy programs (Havenstein, 2006).

Radio Frequency Identification

Radio frequency identification (RFID) chips transmit data to receivers. Each of these chips is uniquely identified by a signal indicating where it is located. RFID has been used in the business industry for inventory management by placing a chip on each of the pieces of inventory. Wal-Mart was one of the first retailers to use RFID technology to manage their massive inventory. Recently, RFID technology has been targeted to be used in the healthcare industry. For example, RFID can be used for the following:

- Tracking pharmaceuticals as they are shipped from the manufacturer to the customer
- Tracking costly medical equipment to ensure easy access
- Identifying providers in hospitals to ensure efficiency in care
- Identifying laboratory specimens to reduce medical errors
- Tracking patients, including infants, while they are hospitalized
- Tracking hazardous materials that pose a public health threat (Crounse, 2005)

In 2006, the market for RFID healthcare systems was $90 million. It is anticipated that the market will increase to $2.1 billion in 2014. It is currently used extensively in hospitals. Currently, approximately 25% of healthcare RFID tags are used to identify people to ensure they are given the appropriate medication and interventions. Approximately 16% of RFID tags are used for expensive equipment, 13% are used for pharmaceuticals, and 4% are used for blood identification to reduce medical errors (ID TechEx, 2009).

It is anticipated that over the next 10 years, RFID will be used primarily on labels of drugs to eliminate any drug counterfeiting by providing the full custody information on the RFID tag of the drug. They have already been used in Wal-Mart to control and monitor their drug supply for their pharmacies. The barriers to limitation are the cost of the systems, the fear of change from the staff, and lack of training. As with any other IT, all of these barriers can be addressed.

APPLIED HEALTH INFORMATION TECHNOLOGY

The PhreesiaPad

Chaim Indig and Evan Roberts, both younger than 30 years old, spent a year examining the healthcare market. They felt, as entrepreneurs, that the healthcare industry was the best entry for them to start a business. They realized that patient check-in at doctors' offices was a problem. Backed by venture capital firms and with advice from medical professionals, they developed PhreesiaPad, a wireless digital device with a touch screen keyboard that allows a patient to enter their demographic information and the reason they are visiting the doctor. This new technology eliminates the patient's need to replicate their information each time they pay a visit to the doctor. The system is currently being used in 49 states and thousands of doctors' offices (Scotti, 2009). When the patient is finished, a report is automatically generated for the doctor to review before seeing the patient. This increases office efficiency, shortens visit rates, and reduces error rates. This information can also be uploaded to an EHR.

However, it is important to note that the patient information is also sent to the Phreesia server that, in turn, displays on the patient's screen a pharmaceutical advertisement appropriate for their condition.

In exchange for the advertisement, the physician receives the technology for free. If the practice opts not to advertise, they can purchase the system for $5000. The controversial issue with Phreesia is the direct advertising of medications to patients at a time when they may have to make a decision about prescriptions (Phreesia, 2009).

Healthy Advice Network

The **Healthy Advice Network** provides education to patients electronically while in the waiting room or an exam room. Health education information is customized with brand advertising messages displayed on digital flat screens in physicians' waiting rooms. There are 25-minute loops of brand materials that focus on prevention and management of disease. In 2009, this information was provided to 118.4 million annual patient visits. There are different educational packages that include large pharmaceutical or specialty pharmaceutical manufacturers and consumer packaged goods companies (Healthy Advice, 2009). From 2001 to 2008, the Network won several national consumer health information awards. The brand company sponsors the educational messages so there is no fee to the provider because it provides a direct opportunity to encourage the patient to use the company's product. This type of education can be examined in two ways. It provides important information to the patient regarding their health. However, it also is manipulating the patient to ask the provider for the advertiser's product that has been sponsoring the 25-minute loop in the waiting room. From a business perspective, it is an excellent opportunity for the company to market their brand to both the physician and patient simultaneously without taking up the provider's time. According to studies, there is close to a 10% new prescription increase from consumer patients watching the sponsored educational loops in the waiting room. A recent physician survey indicated that 93% of those surveyed thought the loops increased the education of the patients as healthcare consumers (Healthy Advice, 2009). The other issue is whether the patients are being manipulated by the loops because they may under the assumption that the physician specifically supports the brand and they will ask for that brand because of that assumption.

MedBillManager

Founded in 2006, **Change:healthcare** is a progressive technology firm that is dedicated to educating healthcare consumers regarding the US healthcare system.

They have developed products for individuals who are interested in understanding the healthcare system. They also have products for employers to help employers understand what type of healthcare benefits they are providing to their employees. They also have developed a medical bill management tool which analyzes how consumers and employers can save money. Their tool focuses on the cost of healthcare. It also enables the consumers to see what others are paying for services (Change:Healthcare, 2009).

IntelliFinger

Developed by eMedicalFiles, the IntelliFinger (patent pending) is **biometric authentication technology** that authenticates the identification of a patient by their fingerprint that is scanned when they enter an office for a medical visit, presurgery visit, at check out, or at the pharmacy when they are picking up controlled substances. The technology translates the fingerprint into a numeric combination that is matched with the patient's medical information. This prevents fraudulent use of insurance cards and should reduce Medicaid and Medicare fraud. The IntelliFinger can be added to any EHR system. It sells for approximately $500 to $1200 per unit (Future Healthcare, 2009). Because the patient's fingerprint is scanned at the check-in desk and the fingerprint is matched by a number code to the patient's computer information, check-in is expedited and insurance information verified. This eliminates fraudulent activity because patients cannot use someone else's insurance card (Future Healthcare, 2009).

DocketPort Scanner

In 2002, the innovative Card Scanning, Inc. was started by a physician because he wanted to develop a user-friendly scanner—the DocketPort Scanner, which uses imaging software to scan a patient's insurance card and transfer the information to the patient form within 30 seconds. It eliminates copying costs and the staff time that it would normally take to copy the card and put it in the patient file. This scanner can be integrated into an EHR system. Scanner prices range from $349 to $479. The software is priced at $150. This can be used in provider offices or other sites (Innovative Card Scanning, Inc., 2009).

Acuson P10

Siemens has introduced a pocket-sized ultrasound, Acuson P10, that can be used for traditional applications of diagnostic and screening tests. It can be used in outpatient areas, intensive care units, and rescue helicopters to provide instant information to make a diagnosis. Priced at $9499, the device can be used for chest, pelvis, stomach, and obstetrics ultrasounds. The results can be viewed on the screen but can also be uploaded to a computer. It can store 30,000 still images or 500 moving image sequences. This technology eliminates the need for the provider to send the patient to an imaging center (Siemens AG, 2009).

Piccolo Xpress Chemistry Analyzer

The size of a shoebox, the $16,000 Piccolo xpress is a compact, portable chemistry analyzer that delivers blood test results quickly. The provider places blood, etc., on a small disc and slides the disc into the Piccolo xpress. The provider requests tests to be performed using its touch screen display which prints out a hardcopy report in approximately 12 minutes, or the information can be transferred to an EHR. This technology expedites the provider's ability to diagnose a patient. (Abaxis, 2009).

THE IMPORTANCE OF HEALTH INFORMATION TECHNOLOGY

A 2009 study focused on the implementation and management of IT in the hospital setting. Szydlowski and Smith (2009) interviewed six hospital CIOs (or their equivalents) and nurse managers to assess why they used HIT. The CIOs indicated they used HIT to streamline administrative processes in the organization. They all recognized the substantial cost to invest in HIT but they recognized that the investment was long term and that it would ultimately be very cost-efficient. The nurse managers focused on the ability to reduce medical errors as a result of HIT. They also indicated that having electronic patient data ultimately contributed to more efficient and effective clinical decision making. The barriers to successful implementation identified by both the CIOs and the nurse managers were inadequate training on HIT and the amount of time needed to become familiar with HIT.

CONCLUSION

The healthcare industry has lagged behind utilizing IT as a form of communicating important data across healthcare systems nationally. Despite that fact, there have been specific applications developed for HIT such as e-prescribing, telemedicine, e-health, and specific applied technology such as the Intellifinger, Docketscanner, the Phreesia Pad, Accuson P10, and the Piccolo xpress, which were discussed in this chapter. Healthcare organizations have recognized the importance of IT and have hired CIOs and CTOs to manage their data. However, the healthcare industry needs to embrace an electronic patient record across all of its health systems. This will enable patients to be treated effectively and efficiently nationally. Having the ability to access a patient's health information could assist in reducing medical errors. As a consumer, utilizing a tool like HealthVault could provide you with an opportunity to consolidate all of your medical information so, if there are any medical problems, the information will be readily available.

PREVIEW OF CHAPTER TEN

Healthcare services is one of the most heavily regulated industries. Those who provide services, receive and pay for services, and regulate services are impacted by the law. Chapter 10 will discuss how healthcare providers legally organize their businesses, the contractual relationship between the healthcare provider and the healthcare consumer, pertinent laws and regulations that impact health care, and trends in legislation that may impact the healthcare industry.

VOCABULARY

Artificial intelligence

Biometric authentication technology

Chief information officer

Computerized physician order entry

Drug–drug interactions

Dxplain

E-health

Electronic clinical decision support systems

Electronic health record

Electronic medical record

Enterprise data warehouse

E-prescribing

Expert system	Legacy systems
Health information technology	Medical informatics
HealthVault	Primary Care Information Project
Healthy Advice Network	Radio frequency identification
Informatics	Telehealth
Information technology (IT)	Telemedicine

REFERENCES

Abaxis. (2009). Retrieved November 2, 2009, from http://www.abaxis.com/medical/piccolo.html.

Adler, K. (2004). Why it's time to purchase an electronic health record system. *Family Practice Medicine*, *11*, 10, 43–46.

Anderson, H. (2009). A go-slow EHR approach: A surgical group that spent six months phasing out paper to reaping tangible savings. *Health Data Management*, *17*, 2, 44.

Anderson, R., Rice, T., & Kominksi, G. (2007). *Changing the U.S. health care system*. San Francisco, CA: Jossey-Bass.

Appleby, C. (2008). IT visionary: G. Octo Barnett, MD. *Most Wired Magazine*, March. Retrieved October 30, 2009, from http://www.hhnmostwired.com/hhnmostwired_app/jsp/articledisplay.jsp?dcrpath=HHNM.

Ash, J., Gorman, P., Seshadri, V., & Hersh, W. (2004). Computerized physician order entry in U.S. hospitals: results of a 2002 survey. *Journal of the American Medical Informatics Association*, *11*, 2, 95–99.

Bates, J., & Turano, A. (2006). An introduction to data warehouse and business intelligence. Government information technology issues: a view to the future. *Government Information Technology Executive Council*, 113–135.

Buchbinder, S., & Shanks, N. (2007). *Introduction to health care management*. Sudbury, MA: Jones and Bartlett.

Change:Healthcare. (2009). Retrieved November 10, 2009, from https://www.changehealthcare.com/home/about.

Christman, K. (2007). Will electronic medical records doom your practice? *Journal of American Physicians and Surgeons*, *11*, 3, 67–69.

Cleveland Clinic. (2009). Cleveland Clinic pilots Microsoft HealthVault. Retrieved March 5, 2009, from http://my.clevelandclinic.org/news/2008/cleveland_clinic_pilots_microsoft_healthvault.aspx.

Coiera, E. (2003). *The guide to health informatics* (2nd ed.). London: Hodder Arnold.

Community EHR: Myth or reality webinar. (November 2, 2007). Retrieved November 10, 2009, from http://www.healthdatamanagement.com/web_seminars/-25128-1.html.

Crounse, B. (2005). RFID: Increasing patient safety, reducing health care costs. Retrieved October 30, 2009, from http://www.microsoft.com/industry/healthcare/providers/businessvalue/housecalls/rfid.mspx.

Department of Health and Human Services. (2009). Health information technology. Retrieved Feburary 16, 2009, from http://www.hhs.gov/healthit/onc/background/.

Department of Veterans Affairs. (2009). Retrieved November 10, 2009, from http://www1.va.gov/houston_va_rd/docs/va_warehouse.doc.

Federal Trade Commission. (2009). Retrieved November 10, 2009, from http://www.ftc.gov/opa/2004/07/healthcarerpt.shtm.

Future Healthcare. Patient identification. Retrieved November 10, 2009, from http://www.futurehealthcareus.com/?mc=Patient_Identification&page=its-viewarticle.

Goldstein, M., & Blumenthal, D. (2008). Building an information technology infrastructure. *Journal of Law, Medicine & Ethics*, 709–715.

Harris, C. (2008). C. Martin Harris, CIO, Cleveland Clinic. *Health Management Technology*, *29*, 7, 10.

Havenstein, H. (2006). Health agency plans massive data warehouse. Retrieved March 8, 2009, from http://www.computerworld.com/s/article/9004370/Health_agency_plans_massive_data_warehouse.

HealthVault. (2009). Retrieved November 10, 2009, from http://www.healthvault.com/personal/websites-overview.html.

Healthy Advice. (2009). Retrieved November 10, 2009, from http://www.healthyadvicenetworks.com/etp/about-healthy-advice.html.

ID TechEx. (2009). Retrieved November 10, 2009, from http://www.idtechex.com/research/topics/rfid_000003.asp.

Innovative Card Scanning, Inc. (2009). Retrieved November 10, 2009, from http://www.scansharp.com/s.nl/sc.10/category.28/.f.

Institute of Medicine of the National Academies. (2009). Retrieved February 16, 2009, from http://www.iom.edu/CMS/8089.aspx.

Immon, B. (2007). Data warehousing in a health care environment. *The Data Administration Newsletter*. Retrieved March 5, 2009, from http://tdan.com/print/4584.

Landro, L. (2009). Incentives push more doctors to e-prescribe. Retreived October 30, 2009, from http://online.wsj.com/article/SB123249533946000191.html.

Leung, L. (2008). Internet embeddedness: Links with online health information seeking, expectancy value/quality of health information websites, and Internet usage patterns. *Cyber Psychology & Behavior*, *11*, 5, 565–569.

Lohr, S. (2009). How to make electronic medical records a reality. Retrieved October 30, 2009, from http://www.nytimes.com/2009/03/01/business/01unbox.html.

Lowes, R. (2007). Avoiding EHR sticker shock. *Medical Economics*, *84*, 20, 41–45.

Murer, C. (2007). EHRS: Issues preventing widespread adoption. *Rehab Management*, *20*, 38–39.

Murphy, J., Malone, D., Olson, B., Grizzle, A., Armstrong, E., & Skrepnek, G. (2009). Development of computerized alerts with management strategies for 25 serious drug-drug interactions. *American Journal of Health-System Pharmacists*, *66*, 38–44.

National Alliance for Health Information Technology. (2009). Retrieved November 10, 2009, from http://www.medicalnewstoday.com/articles/101878.php.

New York City Department of Health and Mental Hygiene. (2009). HER expansion initiative. Retrieved March 5, 2009, from http://www.nyc.gov/html/doh/html/pcip/pcip-ehr-app.shtml.

O'Brien, M. (2007). Implementation of the EPIC electronic medical record physician order-entry system. *Journal of Health care Management*, *51*, 5, 338–343.

Open Clinical. (2009). Health informatics. Retrieved February 17, 2009, from http://www.openclinical.org/health-informatics.html.

Oz, E. (2006). *Management information systems*. Mason, OH: Thomson Southwestern.

Perreault, L., & Metzger, J. (1999). A pragmatic framework for understanding clinical decision support. *Journal of Health care Information Management*, *13*, 2, 5–21.

Phreesia. (2009). Retrieved March 5, 2009, from http://www.phreesia.com/news.asp.

Scotti, C. (2009). Young guns: Phreesia tries to revolutionize doctor's visits. Retrieved October 30, 2009, from http://www.foxbusiness.com/story/small-business/young-guns-phreesia-tries-revolutionize-doctors-visits/.

Shields, A., Shin, P., Leu, M., Levy, D., Betancourt, R., Hawkins, D., et al. (2007). Adoption of health information technology in community health centers: Results of a national survey. *Health Affairs*, *26*, 3, 1373–1383.

Siemens AG. (2009). Retrieved November 10, 2009, from http://www.medicalnewstoday.com/articles/114511.php.

Sriram, R., & Fenves, S. (2009). Health care information systems are essential medicine. *Industrial Engineer*, February, 35–39.

Swartz, N. (2005). Electronic medical records' risks feared. *Information Management Journal*, *39*, 3, 9.

Szydlowski, S., & Smith, C. (2009). Perspectives from nurse leaders and chief information Officers on health information technology implementation. *Hospital Topics: Research and Perspectives on Healthcare*, *87*, 1, 3–9.

Teich, J., Osheroff, J., Pifer, E., Sittig, D., Jenders, R., & CDS Expert Review Panel. (2005). Clinical decision support in electronic prescribing: Recommendations and an action plan. *Journal of the American Medical Informatics*, *12*, 4, 365–378.

Thomashauer, T. (2008). Symphony of collaboration. *Health Management Technology*, *29*, 10, 26–28.

Traynor, K. (2008). National health information network passes test. *American Journal of Health-System Pharmacists*, *15*, 2086–2087.

Valerius, J. (2007). The electronic health record: What every information manager should know. *The Information Management Journal*, *4*, 1, 56–59.

Ventres, W., & Shah, A. (2007). How do EHRs affect the physician-patient relationship? *American Family Physician*, *75*, 9, 1385–1390.

Vreeman, D., Taggard, S., Rhine, M., & Worrell, T. W. (2006). Evidence for electronic health record systems in physical therapy. *Physical Therapy*, *86*, 3, 434–446.

What is a Chief Information Officer? (2009). Retrieved November 10, 2009, from http://www.ejobdescription.com/CIO_Job_Description.html.

Whitman, J. C., & David, S. (2007). Effectively integrating your EMR/EHR initiative. *The Physician Executive*, *33*, 5, 56–59.

CROSSWORD PUZZLE

Instructions: Please complete the puzzle using the vocabulary words found in the chapter. There may be multiple-word answers. The numbers in the parenthesis indicate the number of words in the answer.

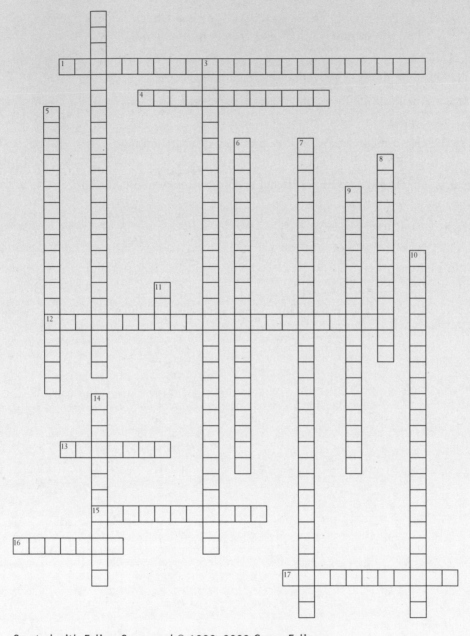

Created with EclipseCrossword © 1999–2009 Green Eclipse

STUDENT ACTIVITY 9-1

Across

1. Electronic patient medical information that is accumulated in one health system and is used by the providers who treat the patient. (3 words)

4. Use of information technology to enable healthcare providers to communicate with patients that may not be able to visit them physically because they are in a rural area. (1 word)

12. Computerized techniques that imitate human decision making. (2 words)

13. Use of information technology to deliver education, research, and clinical care. (1 word)

15. Science of computer application to data in different industries. (1 word)

16. A decision support system that uses lab data and symptoms to produce a ranked list of diagnoses. (1 word)

17. Microsoft Web site that enables patients to maintain their medical information and access health education. (2 words)

Down

2. This person in the organization is responsible for managing the organization's information systems. (3 words)

3. Electronic system that enables a physician to order prescriptions, lab tests, etc. (4 words)

5. Computer application to tissues and organs. (2 words)

6. Systems that electronically transforms data that can be used in organizations to be used for decision making. (2 words)

7. Systems that are designed to integrate medical information, patient information, and a decision making tool to generate information to assist with cases. (4 words)

8. These are older systems in an organization. (2 words)

9. Science of computer application that supports clinical and research data in different areas of health care. (2 words)

10. An integration of data from several different sources that supports strategic decision making. (3 words)

11. This software program alerts physicians and clinicians about potential drug–drug interactions. (1 acronym)

14. Physicians electronically prescribe medicine for their patients. (1 word)

STUDENT ACTIVITY 9-2

IN YOUR OWN WORDS

Based on Chapter 9, please provide an explanation of the following concepts in your own words. DO NOT RECITE the text.

Health information technology: _____

_____

_____

Expert systems: _____

_____

_____

Electronic health records: _____

_____

_____

Legacy systems: _____

_____

_____

Enterprise data warehouse: _____

_____

_____

Radio frequency identification: _____

_____

_____

Healthy Advice Network: _____

_____

_____

Biometric authentication technology: _____

_____

_____

Phreesia Pad: _____

_____

_____

STUDENT ACTIVITY 9-3

REAL LIFE APPLICATIONS: CASE STUDY

You were just hired as the office manager of a six-physician office. As part of your responsibilities, one of the physicians asked you to investigate the possibility of an electronic health record (EHR) system. He is interested in this but the other physicians are reluctant to change to the system. They had heard that the federal government was going to mandate this by 2014 and wanted to be proactive. The physician asked you to prepare a presentation to all of the physicians regarding the issues of implementing an EHR system.

RESPONSES

_____

_____

_____

_____

_____

_____

_____

_____

_____

_____

_____

_____

_____

_____

_____

_____

_____

_____

STUDENT ACTIVITY 9-4

INTERNET EXERCISES

Write your answers in the space provided.

- Visit each of the Web sites listed here.
- Name the organization.
- Locate their mission statement on their Web site.
- Provide a brief overview of the activities of the organization.
- How do these organizations participate in the US healthcare system?

Web Sites

http://www.openclinical.org

Organization Name: _____

Mission Statement:

_____

_____

_____

Overview of Activities:

_____

_____

_____

Importance of organization to US health care:

_____

_____

_____

http://www.healthyadvicenetworks.com

Organization Name: _____

Mission Statement:

_____

_____

_____

Overview of Activities:

_____

_____

_____

STUDENT ACTIVITY 9-4

Importance of organization to US health care:

_____
_____
_____

http://www.healthdatamanagement.com

Organization Name: _____

Mission Statement:

_____
_____
_____

Overview of Activities:

_____
_____
_____

Importance of organization to US health care:

_____
_____
_____

http://www.nationalehealth.org

Organization Name: _____

Mission Statement:

_____
_____
_____

Overview of Activities:

_____
_____
_____

Importance of organization to US health care:

_____
_____
_____

STUDENT ACTIVITY 9-4

http://www.phreesia.com

Organization Name: _____

Mission Statement:

_____

_____

_____

Overview of Activities:

_____

_____

_____

Importance of organization to US health care:

_____

_____

_____

http://www.healthvault.com

Organization Name: _____

Mission Statement:

_____

_____

_____

Overview of Activities:

_____

_____

_____

Importance of organization to US health care:

_____

_____

_____

Chapter 10

Legal Aspects of Healthcare Delivery

LEARNING OBJECTIVES

The student will be able to:

- Describe the legal relationship between patient and provider.
- Identify six types of legal structures for health organizations.
- Identify six health laws and their importance to healthcare providers and consumers.
- Apply civil and criminal liability concepts to healthcare providers and consumers.
- Discuss the importance of contracts to health care.
- Describe tort reform and identify four measures for tort reform.

DID YOU KNOW THAT?

- In 2006, nearly 500 hospitals were fined for Medicare fraud.
- The **False Claims Act**, passed in 1863 during the Civil War, was enacted because defense contractors at the time sold the US government inferior mules which were used to transport goods for soldiers battling the war.
- The **Physician Referral Laws** were passed because providers were referring patients to medical services in which they or family members had a financial interest.
- Torts, which are legally wrongful acts by healthcare providers, are derived from the French language, meaning *wrong*.
- **Qui tam** provisions, a concept used in antitrust law, is Latin for *he who sues*. This provision enables individuals to sue providers for fraudulent activity against the federal government, recovering a portion of the funds returned to the government.

INTRODUCTION

Law is a body of rules for the conduct of individuals and organizations that is often interpreted differently and may change over time. Law is created so there is at least a minimal standard of action required by individuals and organizations. There is law created by federal, state, and local governments. As the judiciary system interprets previous legal decisions regarding a case, they are creating **common law** (Buchbinder & Shanks, 2007). The minimal standard for action is federal law although state law may be stricter. Legislature creates laws that are called **statutes**. Both common law and statutes are then interpreted by administrative agencies by developing **rules and regulations** that interpret the law. Healthcare services is one of the most regulated industries. Those who provide, receive, pay for, and regulate healthcare services are affected by the law. Therefore, it is important to understand basic legal principles that impact healthcare decisions (Miller, 2006). This chapter will discuss how healthcare providers legally organize their businesses, the contractual relationship between the healthcare provider and the healthcare consumer, civil and criminal healthcare law, antitrust law, and major federal pieces of legislation and regulations that impact healthcare providers and consumers.

LEGAL STRUCTURE OF HEALTHCARE ORGANIZATIONS

There are five common types of legally formed structures that may be used in the healthcare industry: nonprofit and for-profit corporations, partnerships, limited liability companies, sole proprietorships, and joint ventures (Longenecker, Moore, Petty, & Palich, 2008; Miller, 2006).

A **corporation** is a legal entity, separate from the owners. This means that it can file suit, be sued, hold and sell property, and engage in business. Corporations are established through a corporate charter, or articles of incorporation, established in the state of their main headquarters. Corporations are usually formed to protect the stockholders or owners from unlimited liability. Their liability is limited to their investment in the corporation. Stockholders are normally not required to use their personal assets to protect the corporation (Longenecker et al., 2008; Miller, 2006). However, in smaller corporations, if they are seeking additional financing from financial institutions, the lender may require the stockholders to pledge their personal assets as collateral for any financial agreements. Corporations can be for-profit or nonprofit. There are also simple C, subchapter S, and professional corporations. Taxation is dependent on the type of corporation selected. Most large corporations are C, or simple corporations. Many smaller organizations may structure themselves as subchapter S or professional corporations. A PC or PA affixed to a dentist, doctor, or attorney means their practice has been set up as a **professional corporation**. Although state definitions vary, the term implies that the owner requires a license to practice. Although this corporation does not protect the owner from malpractice or liability, the corporation protects the owners from each others' liabilities. Many states require this type of organization before a practice can be established (Longenecker et al., 2008).

For-profit and **not-for-profit organizations** are common legal structures for the healthcare industry; most physician practices and skilled nursing facilities are traditionally structured **for profit**. They are privately owned by investors, provide goods and services to maximize profits, and pay taxes. They have limited obligation to provide care for the needy. Nonprofit corporations may also use the term "charity" for their organization. Their profits cannot be given to individuals. Many **nonprofit** corporations are tax exempt and must demonstrate their charitable purposes. There are two types of not-for-profit healthcare organizations: business-oriented (private) and government-owned organizations and public corporations. They are required to provide care to the needy. The **business-oriented not-for-profits** are private with no ownership interests. They operate based on fees from services and goods. Many religiously affiliated hospitals are structured as not-for-profit. **Government-owned** hospitals are often tax exempt and often have federal or state funding. They often serve the uninsured and have a research and training component. Public health clinics are also legally structured as a nonprofit organization (Buchbinder & Shanks, 2007).

The **sole proprietorship** is the simplest method of establishing a business. The business, for example, a single practice office, is owned solely by the individual. The individual owns all of the assets but assumes responsibility of all losses. The sole proprietorship of a business would have **unlimited liability**, which means the liability extends beyond the scope of their business. Their personal assets can be attacked as well. It would be unusual for a healthcare provider to establish his or her practice as a sole provider because of the unlimited liability issue (Small Business Association [SBA], 2008). The **partnership** is a legal entity formed by two or more individuals to operate a business. Two physicians may form a partnership to operate a practice. It is a simple structure to implement that eliminates many legal procedures which are needed to establish a corporation. However, like a sole proprietorship, the liability to the partners is unlimited. There may also be issues with the partnership that could include personality conflicts, opposing views on how to manage the business, and differing views on the mission of the business. Although partnerships can be very successful, there is the issue of unlimited liability which means the owners, like the sole proprietorship, would be responsible for all debts and problems of other partners. It would be unusual for healthcare providers to establish a simple partnership because of the unlimited liability issues (SBA, 2008). **Limited partnerships** have one or more general partners who have unlimited liability but other partners who have limited partnerships, which means they have limited liability (Longest & Darr, 2008).

The **limited liability company** is a fairly new type of organization that is popular because it offers the liability protection of a corporation but is easy to form like a sole proprietorship. There can be an unlimited number of owners or a single owner. Owners are taxed on the percentage of income received from the company. The LLC designation is included after the name of the company. This type of organization would be a possibility for providers to establish their practice under. It does protect the providers more from liability issues (Longenecker et al., 2008; SBA, 2008).

Joint ventures are legal structures formed between two separate structures such as two healthcare organizations or a physician's practice and a hospital that **contractually form** an organization to achieve a common goal. The original entities share the revenues, costs, and control of the joint venture (Longest & Darr, 2008).

THE RELATIONSHIP BETWEEN THE PROVIDER AND CONSUMER

The most important relationship in the healthcare system is the relationship between the patient—the healthcare consumer—and their provider, which could be a physician or an organization such as a clinic or hospital where the physician has a relationship. A physician can establish a relationship with a patient in three ways: (1) establishing a **contractual relationship to care for a designated population**, (2) establishing an **express contract** with a patient under mutual agreement, and (3) establishing a relationship under an **implied contract** (Miller, 2006).

In order for a contract to exist, there must be four components of the contract: (1) agreement between two parties, (2) both parties must be competent to consent to the agreement, (3) the agreement must be of value, and (4) the agreement must be legal. If any of these components are missing, the parties are not bound by the agreement to comply with the terms. It is important to emphasize that the agreement does not have to be formally written (Buchbinder & Shanks, 2007). This chapter will discuss several types of contracts as they pertain to health care.

A **contract to care for a designated population** is indicative of a health maintenance organization (HMO) or managed care contract. A physician is contractually required to care for those member patients of a managed care organization. They may sign contracts to provide care for hospitals, schools, or long-term care facilities that have designated populations (Miller, 2006).

An **express contract** is a simple contract—merely a mutual agreement of care between the physician and patient. The physician may define the limitations of the contract, including the parameters of their care. They may only decide to practice in a certain geographic area or, if they are a specialist, they would only provide services in that area of specialty. An **implied contract** can be implied from a physician's actions. If a physician gives advice regarding medical treatment, there is an implied contract. The relationship between a patient and hospital, a **contractual right to admission**, can be considered a contract if a hospital has contracted to treat certain members of an organization, like a managed care organization; if so, the hospital is required to treat those members. A second example of this type of contractual right to admission is if governmental hospitals, such as county hospitals, are required to provide care for patients regardless of ability to pay (Miller, 2006).

How Does a Relationship with a Provider End?

If a patient withdraws from the relationship with the provider, then the physician no longer has a duty to provide follow-up. That is one way to end a provider relationship. Also, if medical care is no longer needed, the relationship naturally is completed. If a patient is transferred to another provider, the provider then establishes a relationship with the new patient. However, a physician could withdraw from a relationship by giving sufficient notice of their withdrawal or providing their patient with a referral. However, if a physician withdraws from a relationship without sufficient reason, the provider may be liable for breach of contract (Miller, 2006).

CIVIL AND CRIMINAL LAW AND HEALTH CARE

There are civil and criminal laws that impact the healthcare industry. **Civil law** focuses on the wrongful acts against individuals and organizations based on contractual violations. **Torts**, derived from the French word for *wrong*, is a category of wrongful acts, in civil law, which may not have a preexisting contract. To prove a civil infraction, you do not need as much evidence as in a criminal case. **Criminal law** is concerned with actions that are illegal based on court decisions. In order to convict someone of a criminal activity, it has to be proven without a reasonable doubt of guilt. Examples of criminal law infractions would be Medicare fraud, illegal abortions, etc. (Miller 2006).

As stated earlier, torts are wrongdoings that occur to individuals or organizations regardless of whether a contract is in place. There are several different types of violations that can apply to health care. There are two basic healthcare torts: (1) **negligence**, which involves the unintentional act or omission of an act that would contribute to the positive health of a patient, and (2) **intentional torts**, such as assault and battery or invasion of privacy (Buchbinder & Shanks, 2007).

In the healthcare industry, negligence must be proven by (1) the person found negligent of action or lack of action who must have had a duty to the other party, (2) there must be a lapse of breach of duty, (3) damages occurred as a result of the person, or (4) there must be a causal link established between the parties (Buchbinder & Shanks, 2007). An example of negligence would be if a provider does not give the appropriate care or withholds care that results in damages to the patient, such as poor health, and that there was a proven causal relationship between the physician's decision and the patient's worsened health status. In the healthcare industry, intentional torts such as assault and battery would be a surgeon performing surgery on a patient without their consent (Miller, 2006). Invasion of privacy would be the violation of patients' health records. Privacy issues relating to patient information is a major issue in the healthcare industry. These activities are categorized under the term medical malpractice.

According to the *American Heritage Dictionary*, **medical malpractice** is the "Improper or negligent treatment of a patient by a provider which results in injury, damage or loss" (p. 1060). According to the Institute of Medicine's (IOM) landmark report *To Err is Human*, medical malpractice results in approximately 80,000 to 100,000 deaths per year. Disputes over improper care of a patient have hurt both the providers and patients. Patients have sued physicians because they feel their provider has not provided them the level of care compared to the standard of care in the industry. Studies have indicated that patients on average wait 5 years to receive payment from malpractice cases; most patients are not compensated as a result of a medical error (Emanuel, 2008). As a result, providers pay increasingly huge malpractice insurance premiums. From 2000 to 2004, malpractice insurance premiums increased 120% (Emanuel, 2008). As a result of the increase in malpractice insurance premiums, the concept of **defensive medicine** has been introduced which means that providers often order more tests and provide more services than necessary to protect themselves from malpractice lawsuits (Shi & Singh, 2008).

TORT REFORM DISCUSSION

As a result of the number of malpractice claims in the United States, malpractice insurance premiums have increased, resulting in some states no longer offering malpractice insurance, which means there are fewer physicians in needed areas. Some states have tried to facilitate the unavailability of malpractice insurance by developing a state system of subsidizing a portion of the premiums (Miller, 2006). Historically, however, there have been continued malpractice insurance crises during the 1970s, 1980s, and, most recently, the beginning of this century (Danzon, 1995). The issues in the 1970s led to joint underwriting measures that required insurance companies to offer medical malpractice if the physician purchased other insurance. In some states, compensation funds were established to offset large award settlements. The level of malpractice suits lessened but the amount of awards were still huge. During the mid-1980s, the premiums were rising again—nearly 75%. It was determined that any initiatives established in the 1970s were not effective (Rosenbach & Stone, 1990). A third malpractice insurance crisis has occurred in the 2000s. Issues with obtaining medical malpractice insurance in several states have increased, forcing physicians to turn to joint underwriting associations which can charge exorbitant premiums.

As a result of the recent malpractice insurance crisis, more states have adopted statutory caps on monetary damages that a plaintiff can recover in malpractice claims. States felt that a cap on monetary damages would have less impact on malpractice insurance premiums because the less an insurance company has paid out in insurance claims, the less the insurance company would have to raise insurance rates. According to the National Conference of State Legislatures, in 2005, there were 48 states that considered malpractice reform legislation with 30 states adopting law (Waters, Budetti, Claxton, & Lundy, 2007). For example, Nevada adopted a cap of $350,000 on noneconomic damages in medical malpractice cases. However, some state appellate courts have declared caps as unconstitutional (Nelson, Morrisey, & Kilgore, 2007). Studies have been contradictory regarding the positive impact caps on claims have on reducing malpractice insurance rates. States have also developed other several tort reform measures that relate to filing claims, standard of care, attorney fees, statute of limitations on claims, and alternatives to the court system to resolving disputes.

Many legal factors have contributed to the increase in claims. Voluntary hospitals are no longer exempt from malpractice suits. The fact that employers now have to take responsibility for their employees' wrongdoing has also increased claims. The concept of informed consent for the patient has expanded and therefore increased claims. The acceptable standard of care, which used to be strictly based on a locality rule, has now become a state or national standard, which has also resulted in increased claims (Miller, 2006). Statutes specifying the acceptable standard of care in a malpractice suit in a local setting were replaced by a national or state standard. This increased the ability to locate expert witnesses that would testify at a trial regarding the standard of care given to the plaintiff.

Expert witness qualifications are also specified to ensure that the witness is indeed an expert in their field. Clinical practice guidelines, which are developed to ensure an acceptable standard of care, are also used (Miller, 2006). The informed consent of a patient to receive care was also expanded in the 1970s to become a patient-friendly standard that specifies what information must be given to the patient to ensure they are making an informed decision regarding their care (Office of Technology Assessment [OTA], 1993). This will be discussed further in the informed consent portion of this chapter.

Some physicians are leaving private practice because they can no longer afford the premiums—they are now in administrative positions at all levels of government, are academicians, or teaching at medical universities.

The malpractice insurance issues have forced many states to review their malpractice guidelines. Some states' tort reform, which has imposed limits on the amount awarded, continues to cause controversy. However, recent federal studies have indicated that imposing caps on awards may be an effective method to reduce malpractice costs and to discourage frivolous lawsuits. Also, the US Supreme Court ruled that any awards must be included in an individual's taxed income (Miller, 2006).

RECOMMENDATIONS FOR SYSTEM REFORM

Because trial costs can be lengthy and costly, other resolutions have been recommended such as (1) alternative dispute resolution methods, (2) neo-no-fault insurance, and (3) the Model Medical Accident Compensation System. Each of these solutions will be discussed (Anderson, Rice, & Kominski, 2007).

Alternative dispute resolution (ADR) is a nonjudicial process that has been employed over the last 30 years in employment claims and has become favored as an alternative to costly litigation in the court system. ADR can be accomplished through different methods such as conciliation, mediation, and arbitration. **Conciliation** consists of bringing the two parties together to discuss their situation, mediation is bringing the two parties together and suggesting possible solutions, and arbitration, which is the most formal, consists of holding a hearing where the cases are presented and an award is made (Carroll & Buchholtz, 2006). **Arbitration** can be a binding decision, which means the parties have to legally abide by the decision.

There are advantages and disadvantages to ADR. It is less costly than litigation. It may protect the reputation of both parties because the processes are quietly performed. However, a major issue with arbitration is the selected arbitrator. The arbitrator may be selected by the defendant not the plaintiff and the arbitrator may be sympathetic to either side. It is important that an independent arbitrator be assigned in these cases.

Neo-no-fault insurance is to encourage early out-of-court settlement for the actual losses by using the money for litigation and related expenses to pay for adequate compensation. If this does not work, traditional litigation may be pursued (Anderson, Rice, & Kominski, 2007).

The **Model Medical Accident Compensation Act** applies worker compensation principles to medical injury compensation. This administrative process focuses on prompt and limited compensation for an increased number of injured individuals. A greater proportion of the money would go directly to the individual. This process would occur on an individual basis, apply the standards of care, and examine the medical errors associated with the case. Funds are provided by a state fund (Anderson, Rice, & Kominski, 2007).

HEALTHCARE CONSUMER LAWS

Other legislative acts will be discussed thoroughly throughout the text; however, these acts directly impact how health care is provided to consumers.

Hill-Burton Act

The **Hill-Burton Act of 1946** was passed because the federal government recognized the lack of hospitals in the United States during the 1940s. They passed the Hospital Survey and Construction Act, more commonly known as the Hill-Burton Act. Federal grants were provided to states for hospital construction to ensure there were 4.5 beds per 1000 people (Shi & Singh, 2008). This Act had a huge influence on creating more hospitals nationally. If a hospital received federal funds from the Hill-Burton Act, they agreed to a community service requirement, so any person residing in the area of the hospital cannot be denied treatment in the portion of the hospital financed by the Hill-Burton Act (exceptions: lack of needed services, unavailability of the services needed, or the patient's ability to pay). Nursing homes are also eligible for Hill-Burton funding so the regulations also apply to them. Inability to pay cannot be a basis for denial when the person needs emergency services that the hospital can provide. There are several exclusions to these regulations:

- If hospitalization is not medically necessary, there is no right to admission.
- Scope of services: If the hospital does not provide the services needed by the patient, they do not have to admit the patient.
- Capacity: If space or staffing is not available, they do not have to admit a patient; however, they have to stabilize them for transport to another facility (Shi & Singh, 2008).
- The facilities must provide free care to people in the amount of 10% of the amount of grants received or 3% of their annual operating costs (National Health Law Program, 2008).

Hospitals that are under the Hill-Burton Act are required to post notices about the program in their area of admission. These notices must be easy to read and in languages appropriate to the community.

Emergency Medical Treatment and Active Labor Act

Emergency Medical Treatment and Active Labor Act of 1986 (EMTALA), enforced by the Centers for Medicare and Medicaid Services (CMS) and the Office of Inspector General (OIG), require Medicare participants to receive emergency care from a hospital or medical entity that provides dedicated emergency services. This was passed as part of the Consolidated Omnibus Budget Reconciliation Act of 1985 (COBRA). This requirement is a type of fiduciary duty that means the healthcare provider or organization is obligated to provide care to someone who has placed their trust in them (CMS, 2008). This law is also called the "antidumping" statute because, prior to the enactment of this law, many hospitals dumped Medicare patients. Penalties for violating EMTALA include monetary fines, impact on their Joint Commission accreditation status, license suspension, and damage to their reputation (Ringholz, 2005). The original act was amended in 2000. CMS issued guidelines in 2003 and 2004 that further explained the Act. This legislation protects the consumer to ensure they receive appropriate emergency care when they present themselves to regulated hospitals and medical organizations (Lipton, 2005).

Employee wellness programs, which can include promotion of exercise, health risk appraisals, disease management, healthcare coaching, have become a popular employee benefit. A survey of 1100 companies indicated that over 60% of the companies offered an employer health awareness/workplace wellness program (Moran, 2008). However, there have been legal issues surrounding the implementation of wellness programs in the workplace because they discriminate based on the health conditions of employees. The Health Insurance Portability and Accountability Act (HIPAA) states that wellness programs that are part of a group health plan must be designed to promote health and cannot be a subterfuge discriminating against an employee based on a health condition. Many wellness programs also offer incentives for wellness program performance. The incentive program must be designed so that all employees may participate in the incentive program regardless of health conditions, which means the incentive/rewards program must be flexible to adapt to employees who want to participate but may be restricted based on a health condition (Department of Labor [DOL], 2008).

Children's Health Insurance Program

The **Children's Health Insurance Program** (CHIP) was enacted under the Balanced Budget Act of 1997, is Title XXI of the Social Security Act, and is jointly financed by federal and state funding and administered by the states. Administered by CMS, the purpose of this program is to provide coverage for low-income children younger than the age of 19 who live above the income level requirements of Medicaid. They cannot be eligible for Medicaid or be covered by private health insurance (National Health Law Program, 2008). Approximately 10 million children who are uninsured and ineligible for public assistance are positively impacted by this program. Children who are eligible for state health benefit plans are not eligible for CHIP. CHIP provides a capped amount of funds to states on a matching basis for federal fiscal years (FY) 1998 through 2007. Studies have indicated that this program has improved access to insurance for children (Shone, 2005). Legislation was passed that extended the funding for the CHIP program until 2013.

Benefits Improvement and Protection Act

The **Benefits Improvement Act of 2000** (BIPA), formally called the Medicare, Medicaid, and SCHIP Benefits Improvement and Protection Act, modifies Medicare payment rates for many services. It also adds coverage of preventive and therapeutic service. It increases federal funding to state programs. From a healthcare consumer aspect, it protects Medicare beneficiaries by granting them the ability to appeal provider termination of services (Congressional Budget Office, 2008). It requires providers to issue a written notice to the patient that coverage has been terminated, giving an end date for the termination. The patient has the right to appeal the decision.

EMPLOYMENT-RELATED HEALTH LEGISLATION

The **Employee Retirement Income Security Act of 1974** (ERISA) regulates pension and benefit plans for employees, including medical and disability benefits.

It protects employees because it forbids employers from firing an employee so that they cannot collect under their medical coverage. An employee may change the benefits provided under their plan, but employers cannot force an employee to leave so that the employer does not have to pay the employee's medical coverage any longer.

The **Pregnancy Discrimination Act of 1978** is an amendment to Title VII of the Civil Rights Act of 1964. This act protects female employees that are discriminated against based on pregnancy-related conditions, which constitutes illegal sex discrimination. The Equal Employment Opportunity Commission (EEOC) is responsible for monitoring and enforcing any violations of this law. This law applies to employers with 15 employers or more, employment agencies and labor organizations, and the federal government (EEOC, 2008).

COBRA, an amendment to ERISA, was passed to protect employees who lost or changed employers to they could keep their health insurance if they paid 102% of the full premium (Anderson, Rice, & Kominski, 2007). The Act was passed because, at the time, people were afraid to change jobs, resulting in the concept of **job lock** (Emanuel, 2008). Although it does provide an opportunity to keep coverage while changing jobs, there may be individuals who cannot afford the premiums so they may end up uninsured anyway. COBRA also included provisions that require hospitals to provide care to everyone who presented in an emergency department, regardless of their ability to pay. Fines were accrued if it was determined that hospitals were refusing treatment (Sultz & Young, 2006). This component was very important because many individuals were refused treatment because they could not pay for the services or were uninsured.

HIPAA was passed to promote patient information and confidentiality in a secure environment. The amount of information released is controlled by the consumer. HIPAA was an amendment to the ERISA and the Public Health Service Act (PHSA) to increase the access to healthcare coverage when employees changed jobs. HIPPA made it illegal to obtain personal medical information for reasons other than healthcare activities, which also includes genetic information. The Department of Health and Human Services (HHS) was required to develop a unique health identifier for each individual, employer, health plan, and provider (Shi & Singh, 2008). It also guaranteed that individuals could purchase health insurance for a preexisting condition if they (1) have been covered by a previous employer program for a minimum of 18 months, (2) have exhausted any coverage through COBRA, (3) are ineligible for other health insurance programs, and (4) were uninsured for no longer than 2 months. HIPAA also prohibited employers from stating pregnancy as a preexisting condition. Employers cannot charge higher premiums to employees according to health status (Anderson, Rice, & Kominski, 2007). Other provisions include (1) small businesses with 2 to 50 employees cannot be refused insurance, (2) self-employed individuals are allowed an increased tax deduction (30 to 80% by 2006) for health insurance premiums, and (3) employers or insurance companies cannot drop individuals for high usage of their medical plans (Shi & Singh, 2008).

The **HIPAA National Standards to Protect Patient's Personal Medical Records of 2002** further protected medical records and other personal health information maintained by healthcare providers, hospitals, insurance companies, and health plans. It gives patients new rights to access of their records, restricts the amount of patient information released, establishes new restrictions to researchers' access, and increased criminal and civil sanctions for improper use (Department of Energy Office of Science, 2008).

It is important to discuss the landmark legislation of the **Americans with Disabilities Act of 1990** (ADA), which focused on individuals who are considered disabled in the workplace. This Act applies to employers who have 15 employers or more. According to the law, a disabled person is someone who has a physical or mental impairment that limits the ability to hear, see, speak, or walk. The Act was passed to ensure that those individuals who had a disability but who could perform primary job functions were not discriminated against. According to the Act, disabilities included learning, mental, epilepsy, cancer, arthritis, mental retardation, AIDS, asthma, and traumatic brain injury (DOL, 2008). Alcohol and other drug abuses are not covered under ADA. If an employer can make reasonable accommodations for a disabled individual, without suffering financial hardship, they are requested to hire disabled individuals. From a healthcare standpoint, a nursing home cannot refuse to admit a person with AIDS that requires a nursing service if the hospital has that type of service available.

The **Family Medical Leave Act of 1993** (FMLA) requires employers with 50 or more employees within a 75-mile radius who work more than 25 hours per week and who have been there more than 1 year to provide up to 12 work weeks of leave, during any 12-month period to provide care for a family member or the employee itself. Family members include the employee, child, spouse, or parent. A serious medical condition is any physical or mental condition that involves inpatient care or continuing treatment by a healthcare provider. This benefit can also include post-childbirth or adoption. The employer must provide healthcare benefits although they are not required to provide wages. This benefit does not cover the organization's 10% highest paid employees. The employer is also supposed to provide the same job or a comparable position upon the return of the employee (Noe, Hollenbeck, Gerhart, & Wright, 2009). The 2008 National Defense Authorization Act of 2008 expanded the FMLA to include families of military service members, which means that an employee may take up to 12 weeks of leave if a child, spouse, or parent has been called to active duty in the armed forces Additionally, if a service member is injured or ill as a result of active duty, the employee may take up to 26 weeks of leave in a single 12-month leave year (Hickman, Gilligan, & Patton, 2008). National Caregiver Support Program (NCSP) is similar to the FMLA but considered more consumer friendly. It was established in 2000 through the Older Americans Act (OAA) which provides services to individuals older than 60 years of age. Limited Funding restricts NCSP's ability to make more costly services available (Anderson, Rice, & Kominski, 2007).

The **Mental Health Parity Act of 1996** defines the equality or parity between lifetime and annual limits of health insurance reimbursements on both mental health and medical care. Unfortunately, the Act did not require employers to offer mental health coverage, it did not impose limits on deductibles or coinsurance payments, nor did it cover substance abuse. However, it did highlight the issue of parity coverage between mental health issues and traditional medical care. This federal legislation spurred several states to implement their own parity legislation (Anderson, Rice, & Kominski, 2007).

In 2000, President Clinton signed an executive order, or directive, prohibiting every federal department and agency from using genetic information in any hiring or promotion. Although the directive is not a law, it allows the President to provide a directive to the executive portion of the federal government to adhere to certain actions. The federal government would not be allowed to request any genetic test as a condition of hiring. They could not use any protected genetic information of employees to deprive them of any promotion. They also could not deny employees any overseas positions because they have a predisposition to any illness (Department of Energy Office of Science, 2008).

The **Genetic Information Nondiscrimination Act of 2008** prohibits US insurance companies and employers from discriminating on the basis of information derived from genetic tests. Specifically, it forbids insurance companies from discriminating through reduced coverage or price increases. It also prohibits employers from making adverse employment decisions based on a person's genetic code, nor can employers or insurance companies demand a genetic test (National Human Genome Research Institute, 2009).

ANTITRUST LAWS

The purpose of **antitrust law** is to protect the consumer by ensuring there is a market driven by competition so the consumer has a choice for their health care. In a sense, antitrust laws protect the competition so the consumer has a choice. Antitrust laws apply to most healthcare organizations. Federal antitrust laws focus on interstate and foreign commerce but the term "interstate commerce" has been interpreted by the US Supreme Court to include local activities that have impact on interstate commerce (Miller, 2006).

There are both federal and state antitrust laws. Examples of antitrust issues would be large mergers that would encourage monopolies in healthcare and price fixing among competitors. There are four main antitrust federal laws that will be discussed in this chapter: the Sherman Antitrust Act, Clayton Act, the Federal Trade Commission Act, and the Robinson-Putnam Act (the amendment to the Clayton Act). These acts are important to know because they were developed to ultimately protect the healthcare consumer and those who provide healthcare services.

There are two federal agencies that enforce antitrust violations: the Federal Trade Commission and the Department of Justice. The **Federal Trade Commission** (FTC), established in 1914 by the **Federal Trade Commission Act**, is one of the oldest federal agencies and is charged with the oversight of commercial acts and practices. Two major activities of the FTC are to maintain free and fair competition in the economy and

to protect consumers from misleading practices. They may issue "cease and desist orders" to companies to ensure they stop their practices until a court decides what the company may do (Carroll & Buchholtz, 2006). The **Department of Justice** (DOJ), headed by the US Attorney General, was established in 1870 to handle the US legal issues, including the enforcement of federal laws (DOJ, 2008). The DOJ and FTC collaborate on antitrust laws enforcement.

The **Sherman Act of 1890** focuses on eliminating **monopolies,** which are healthcare organizations that control a market so that the consumer has no choice in their health care. It also targets **price fixing** among competitors; pricing fixing prohibits the consumer from paying a fair price because competitors establish a certain price (by either increasing or lowering prices) among themselves to stabilize the market. Healthcare facilities may also have an agreement on **market division**. This illegal action occurs when one or more health organizations decide which type of services will be offered at each organization. **Tying** refers to healthcare providers that will only sell a product to a consumer who will also buy a second product from them. **Boycotts** are also illegal according to this act. When healthcare providers have an agreement to not deal with anyone outside their group, that is considered interfering with the consumers' rights to choose. **Price information exchange** of services between providers can also be illegal (Miller, 2006). Healthcare providers are protected under the Act if it has been determined that hospitals have exclusive contracts with certain providers which excludes other providers from use of the hospital. This could be a violation of the Act. Violations of the Act are considered federal crimes.

The **Clayton Act of 1914** was passed to supplement the Sherman Act, as amended by the Robinson-Patman Act, which issues further restrictions on mergers and acquisitions. With the increasing development of hospital chains, this Act has focused on hospitals. There are no criminal violations of this Act, unlike the Sherman Act. Any organization considering a merger or acquisition above a certain size must notify both the Antitrust Division of DOJ and FTC. The Act also prohibits other business practices that, under certain circumstances, may harm competition. The Act also allows individuals to sue for three times their actual damages plus legal costs (DOJ, 2008).

The **Hart-Scott-Rodino Antitrust Improvement Act of 1976,** as an amendment to the Clayton Act, ensures those hospitals and other entities that entered mergers, acquisitions, and joint ventures must notify DOJ and FTC before any final decisions are made. This is a requirement for any hospitals with greater than $100 million in assets acquiring a hospital with more than $10 million in assets (Buchbinder & Shanks, 2007). The DOJ and FTC will make the final decision on these proposals. This ensures there will not be any type of monopoly within a certain geographic area.

INFORMED CONSENT

The concept of **informed consent** is based on the patient's right to make an informed decision regarding medical treatment. It is a legal requirement in all 50 states. It is more than a patient signing an informed consent form—it is the communication between the provider and patient regarding a specific medical treatment. The provider is responsible for discussing the following information with the patient: the diagnosis if it has been established, the nature of a proposed treatment or operation including the risks and benefits, any alternatives and the risks and benefits of the alternatives, and the risks and benefits of not agreeing to the procedure or treatment (American Medical Association, 2008). If a patient did not provide informed consent for a procedure or treatment, it is considered a case of negligence.

The first case of informed consent occurred in the late 1950s. Earlier consent cases were based on **battery**, which is the physically touching an individual without their permission that is considered harmful or offensive. The liability occurred as a result of the unpermitted touching. The patient did not consent to a procedure or treatment and therefore the provider was considered to commit battery (Miller, 2006). Most cases now revolve around whether a patient was provided adequate information prior to the procedure or treatment being implemented. The second component of informed consent is what information should be given to the patient that will constitute informed consent.

To determine what constitutes informed consent, there are two legal standards that are applied: the reasonable patient and reasonable physician standard. The **reasonable patient standard** focuses on the patient's information needs, including the risks and benefits that allow the patient to make a decision. The **reasonable physician standard** focuses on the standard information that would be given by any physician to a patient contemplating the same procedure or treatment. Most states utilize the reasonable patient standard (Miller, 2006).

PATIENT BILL OF RIGHTS

The **Patient Self-Determination Act of 1990** requires hospitals, nursing homes, home health providers, hospices, and managed care organizations that provide services to Medicare and Medicaid eligible patients to provide information on patient rights to patients upon admission. It virtually applies to every type of healthcare facility. The facility must provide adult patients with written information, under the state law, about making healthcare decisions. Based on the concept of informed consent, in 1972 the Board of Trustees of the American Hospital Association developed a Patient Bill of Rights. The **Patient Bill of Rights** states that the patient has the right to all information from this provider regarding any testing, diagnoses, and treatments. This information must be provided to the patient in terms that the patient will be able to understand (Rosner, 2004). Eligible health organizations will have the Patient Bill of Rights displayed.

PHYSICIAN-ASSISTED SUICIDE

The **Oregon Death with Dignity Act of 1994** legalized physician-assisted suicide, a type of euthanasia, by allowing an adult Oregon resident who is terminally ill to request a medication that will end his or her life. The person must have a disease that is considered incurable and will end the person's life within 6 months. An annual impact report on the Death With Dignity Act, analyzed data from 1997 to 2004, indicated that a total of 58 prescriptions were written by 49 physicians in 2002 with 67 prescriptions written in 2003, indicating the number of prescriptions written had increased each year. Of the 67 prescriptions written in 2003, 39 patients actually used the prescriptions. Nearly 94% of the patients requested lethal medications because they were afraid of losing their autonomy or ability to make decisions and act for them, 76% were afraid they would no longer enjoy life as they were dying, and 53% were afraid of losing control of their bodily functions (Sultz & Young, 2006). The state of Washington passed a similar law in December 2008 to legalize physician-assisted suicide. It will be interesting to see if there will be similar statistics regarding the usage of this law.

ADVANCE DIRECTIVES

Advance directives are written directions outlining your wishes if you are impaired and are unable to make a decision about your health care at that time.

These wishes must be legally carried out. Examples of advance directives are living wills, medical powers of attorney (POA), and do not resuscitate order (DNR).

A **living will** lists which types of medical treatments you will and will not accept, such as life-sustaining measures. A **medical POA** or **durable POA for health care** is a person that will represent you in case you are unable to make a medical decision. A DNR is a written directive that does not allow any life-saving measures if you suffer cardiac arrest. An advance directive is not needed for a DNR order. A doctor may place a DNR in your medical chart (Mayo Foundation for Medical Education and Research, 2009).

HEALTHCARE FRAUD

Increasing healthcare costs that have impacted public health insurance programs have emphasized the need to combat fraud and abuse of the healthcare system. The US government has estimated that fraud may account for 10% of healthcare expenditures. From 1995 to 2005, DOJ closed nearly 400 healthcare fraud cases worth $9.3 billion (Kesselheim & Studdert, 2008). The centerpiece for fraud recovery is the False Claims Act.

The **False Claims Act**, enacted in 1863, was originally passed to protect the federal government against defense contractors during the Civil War. The False Claims Act has been amended several times throughout the years; however, in the 1990s, the Act focused on healthcare fraud, most notably Medicare and Medicaid fraud. The **False Claims Act of 1995** imposed criminal penalties on anyone who tries to present fictitious claims for payment to the federal government. It is one of the most powerful government tools to combat civil fraud in health care (Memmott & Makwana, 2007). This act also provides financial incentives for whistle-blowers—allowing employees to blow the whistle about contractor fraud against the federal government. Private plaintiffs fulfilling this role are pursuant to the **qui tam** provisions of the Act, which means "he who sues" (Miller, 2006). The Deficit Reduction Act of 2005 introduced additional incentives for states to crack down on healthcare fraud by giving the states additional incentives under their own fraud law. What is controversial about this Act is that whistle-blowers may receive between 15% and 25% of proceeds in the case. As a result of the financial incentive program, the federal government has received $12 billion in returned funds (Carroll & Buchholtz, 2006). According to one report, in 2006, nearly 500 hospitals across the United States were the subject of Medicare fraud. The civil fines for each violation can be $5500 to $11,000. Many healthcare organizations may have hundreds of fines so their penalties can be huge (Degnan & Scoggin, 2007).

In December 2001, the federal government, as a result of an administrator employed by a private health insurer and an employer at a pharmaceutical company (the whistle-blowers), recovered $95 million from TAP, a pharmaceutical company that encouraged doctors to prescribe their product by providing the product free to doctors, who then billed Medicare for the cost of the product. In August 2001, several executives of a hospital chain, the physicians, and the auditors blew the whistle on Hospital Corporation of America, who submitted claims for unnecessary diagnostic services. The recovery was for nearly $72 million (Kesselheim & Studdert, 2008).

The Stark laws (named after Representative Pete Stark who authored the legislation), also known as the **Physician Self-Referral Laws** or the **Ethics in Patient Referral Act of 1989**, prohibits physicians, including dentists and chiropractors, from referring Medicare and Medicaid patients to other providers for **designated health services** in which they have a financial interest. These laws directly prohibit many referrals that may increase a provider or family members' financial interest. Designated health services include clinical laboratory services, outpatient prescription drug services, physical and occupational therapy, and imaging services such as magnetic resonance imaging (MRI), etc. The statute became effective on January 1, 1995, but the regulations interpreting the statute were not released until January 4, 2001 (Gosfield, 2003, 2008). Additional Stark amendments expanded the types of services a physician could not refer Medicare and Medicaid patients to if they or family member has a financial interest. These regulations protect the consumer by ensuring they will receive objective referrals for health services.

CONCLUSION

As both a healthcare manager and healthcare consumer, it is imperative that you are familiar with the different federal and state laws that impact the healthcare industry. It is also important that you understand the differences between civil and criminal law and the penalties that may be imposed for breaking those laws. Both federal and state laws have been enacted and policy has been implemented to protect both the healthcare provider and the healthcare consumer. New laws have been passed and older laws have been amended to reflect needed changes regarding health care to continue to protect its participants.

Despite these efforts, access to health care still remains a problem. US citizens continue to experience some of the poorest health outcomes in the industrialized world (Boat, Chao, & O'Neill, 2008). It is the responsibility of government, policy makers, clinicians, and researchers to become involved in progress of developing a systematic healthcare transformation in order to improve the health outcomes in this country. As discussed in Chapter 3, the goal of Healthy People 2010 is to improve the quality of life and to eliminate health disparities among different segments of the population. These goals must be supported by lawmakers to ensure that at

least a minimum standard is established to ensure that health justice is achieved (Braithwaite, 2008).

PREVIEW OF CHAPTER ELEVEN

As stated in this chapter, legal standards are the minimum and mandatory standard of action established for society's actions. Ethical standards are considered one level above legal standards and they are not required by law. Individuals have choices based on what is the "right thing to do." The concept of ethics is an integral component of health care. It is important to understand the impact ethics has on the different aspects of the healthcare industry. Ethical dilemmas in health care are often a conflict between personal and professional ethics. Chapter 11 will discuss ethical theories and different ethical dilemmas that impact both healthcare providers and healthcare consumers.

VOCABULARY

Alternative dispute resolution (ADR)

Americans with Disabilities Act of 1990

Antitrust law

Battery

Benefits Improvement Act of 2000

Boycotts

Children's Health Insurance Program (CHIP)

Civil law

Clayton Act of 1913

Common law

Consolidated Omnibus Budget Reconciliation Act of 1985

Contractual relationship to care for a designated population

Contractual right to admission

Corporation

Criminal law

Defensive medicine

Emergency Medical Treatment and Active Labor Act of 1986 (EMTALA)

Employee Retirement Income Security Act of 1974 (ERISA)

Employee wellness programs

Ethics in Patient Referral Act of 1989

Express contract

False Claims Act

Family Medical Leave Act of 1993

Federal Trade Commission

Federal Trade Commission Act

For-profit organizations

Genetic Information Nondiscrimination Act

Government owned

Hart-Scott-Rodino Antitrust Improvement Act of 1976

Health Insurance Portability and Accountability Act (HIPAA)

Hill-Burton Act of 1946

HIPAA National Standards to Protect Patients' Personal Medical Records of 2002

Implied contract

Informed consent

Intentional torts

Job lock

Joint ventures

Law, criminal and civil

Limited liability company

Limited partnerships

Medical malpractice

Mental Health Parity Act of 1996

Model Medical Accident Compensation Act

Monopolies

Negligence

Neo-no-fault insurance

Not-for-profit organizations

Oregon Death with Dignity Act of 1994

Patient Self-Determination Act of 1990

Patient Bill of Rights

Physician self-referral laws

Pregnancy Discrimination Act of 1978

Price fixing

Price information exchange

Professional corporation

Qui tam

Reasonable physician and patient standards

Rules and regulations

Sherman Antitrust Act

Sole proprietorship

Statutes

Tort

Tying

Unlimited liability

REFERENCES

American Medical Association. (2008). Retrieved November 10, 2009, from http://www.ama-assn.org/ama/pub/physician-resources/medical-ethics/code-medical-ethics/.

American Heritage Dictionary (p. 1060). (2000). Boston: Houghton Mifflin.

Anderson, R., Rice, T., & Kominski, G. (2007). *Changing the U.S. health care system*. San Francisco: Jossey-Bass.

Boat, T., Chao, S., & O'Neill, P. (2008). From waste to value in health care. *Journal of American Medical Association*, 299, 568–571.

Braithwaite, K. (2008). Health is a human right, right? *Journal of Public Health*, 98, S5–S7.

Buchbinder, S., & Shanks, N. (2007). *Introduction to health care management*. Sudbury, MA: Jones and Bartlett.

Carroll, A., & Bucholtz, A. (2006). *Business society: Ethics and stakeholder management*. Mason, OH: Thomson/Soutwestern.

Centers for Medicare and Medicaid Services. (2008). EMTALA overview. Retrieved September 1, 2008, from http://www.cms.hhs.gov/EMTALA.

Congressional Budget Office. (2008). Medicare, Medicaid, and SCHIP Benefits Improvement and Protection Act of 2000. Retrieved September 5, 2008, from http://www.cbo.gov/doc.cfm?index=3055&type=0.

Danzon, P. (1995). *Medical malpractice: Theory, evidence, and public policy*. Cambridge, MA: Harvard University Press.

Degnan, J., & Scoggin, S. (2007). *Medical defense and health law*. IADC Committee Newsletter, no. 9.

Department of Energy Office of Science. (2008). Genomic science program. Retrieved November 8, 2008, from http://www.ornl.gov/sci/techresources/Human_Genome/elsi/legislat.shmtl.

Department of Justice. (2008). Retrieved September 1, 2008, from http://www.doj.gov/atr/public/div_stats/211491.htm.

Department of Labor. (2008). Retrieved September 5, 2008, from http://www.dol.gov/ebsa/Regs/fedreg/final/2006009557.htm.

Emanuel, E. (2008). *Health care guaranteed*. New York: Public Affairs.

Equal Employment Opportunity Commission. (2008). Pregnancy discrimination. Retrieved September 3, 2008, from http://www.eeoc.gov/types/pregnancy.html.

Gosfield, A. (2003). *The stark truth about the STARK law: Part 1*. Retrieved September 1, 2008, from www.aafp.org/fpm.

Gosfield, A. (2008). Stark III: Refinement not revolution (part 2). Retrieved November 10, 2008, from http://www .aafp.org/fpm/20080400/25star.html.

Hickman, J., Gilligan, M., & Patton, G. (2008). FMLA and benefit obligations: New rights under an old mandate. *Benefits Law Journal, 21*, 3, 5–16.

Kesselheim, A., & Studdert, D. (2008). Whistleblower-initiated enforcement actions against health care fraud and abuse in the United States, 1996–2005. *Annals of Internal Medicine, 149*, 5, 342–349.

Lipton, S. (2005). EMTALA—Why don't we have all the answers? *Journal of Health Care Compliance*, March-April, 13–20.

Longenecker, J., Moore, C., Petty, L., & Palich, L. (2008). *Small business management* (14th ed.). Mason, OH: Thomson/Southwestern.

Longest, B., & Darr, K. (2008). *Managing health services organizations and systems*. Baltimore: Health Professions Press.

Mayo Foundation for Medical Education and Research. (2009). Living wills and advance directives for medical decisions. Retrieved September 5, 2009, from http://www.mayoclinic.com/health/living-wills/HA00014.

Memmott, S., & Makwana, K. (2007). Beware the whistleblower within—Recent False Claims Act settlements remind industry that almost anyone can be a whistleblower. *Journal of Health Care Compliance, 9*, 47–65.

Miller, R. (2006). *Problems in health care law* (9th ed.). Sudbury, MA: Jones and Bartlett.

Moran, A. (2008). Wellness programs: What's permitted. *Employee Relations Law Journal, 34*, 2, 111–116.

National Health Law Program. (2008). Retrieved November 10, 2009, from http://www.healthlaw.org/search/ download.74631#Hill-Burton.

National Human Genome Research Institute. (2009). Retrieved November 10, 2009 from http://www.genome.gov/About/.

Nelson III, L., Morrisey, M., & Kilgore, M. (2007). Damages caps in malpractice cases. *The Milbank Quarterly, 85*, 2, 259–286.

Noe, R., Hollenbeck, J., Gerhart, B., & Wright, P. (2009). *Fundamentals of human resource management* (3rd ed.). Boston: McGraw Hill.

Office of Technology Assessment. (1993). *Impact of legal reforms on medical malpractice cost*, (OTA-BP-H-19). Washington, DC: US Government Printing Office.

Ringholz, J. (2005). An outline of the basic requirements of EMTALA, as it relates to compliance. *Journal of Health Care Compliance*, January, 35–36.

Rosenbach, M. & Stone, A. (1990). Malpractice insurance costs and physician practice—1981–1986. *Health Affairs, 9*, 176–185.

Rosner, F. (2004). Informing the patient about a fatal disease: From paternalism to autonomy—The Jewish view. *Cancer Investigation, 22*, 6, 949–953.

Shi, L., & Singh, D. (2008). *Essentials of the U.S. health care delivery system*. Sudbury, MA: Jones and Bartlett.

Shone, P. (2005). Reduction in racial and ethnic disparities after enrollment in the State Children's Health Insurance Program. *Pediatrics, 115*, 6, 697–705.

Small Business Association. (2008). Retrieved November 10, 2009, from http://www.sba.gov/smallbusinessplanner/ start/chooseastructure/index.html.

Sultz, H., & Young, K. (2006). *Health care USA: Understanding its organization and delivery* (5th ed.). Sudbury, MA: Jones and Bartlett.

Waters, T., Budetti, P., Claxton, G., & Lundy, J. (2007). Impact of state tort reforms on physician malpractice payments. *Health Affairs, 26*, 2, 500–509.

NOTES

CROSSWORD PUZZLE

Instructions: Please complete the puzzle using the vocabulary words found in the chapter. There may be multiple-word answers. The numbers in the parenthesis indicate the number of words in the answers.

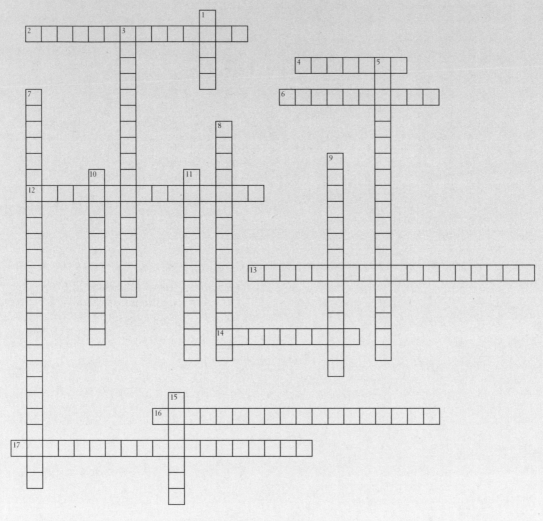

Created with EclipseCrossword © 1999–2009 Green Eclipse

STUDENT ACTIVITY 10-1

Across

2. This occurs when one or more organizations decide which services will be offered at each organization. (2 words)

4. Earlier cases were based on this concept that states that this occurs when a physician touches an individual without their permission. (1 word)

6. Organizations that are so large that they control a market, which does not allow consumers to choose. (1 word)

12. Patients' right to make an informed and education decision regarding their medical treatment. (2 words)

13. Improper or negligent treatment of a patient by a provider which results in injury, damage, or loss. (2 words)

14. As the judiciary system interprets previous legal decisions regarding a case, they are creating this. (2 words)

16. The simplest method of establishing a business. (2 words)

17. Also called the Patient Self-Determination Act of 1990. (4 words)

Down

1. This act was passed to promote patient information and confidentiality in a secure environment. (1 acronym)

3. Providers order more tests and provide more services than necessary to protect themselves from lawsuits. (2 words)

5. These are created by administrative agencies to interpret law. (3 words)

7. These laws prohibit physicians, including dentists and chiropractors, from referring patients for services where they have a financial interest. (4 words)

8. This is merely a mutual agreement between a patient and provider. (2 words)

9. This Act was passed in 1863 to protect the federal government against fraudulent defense contractors during the Civil War. (3 words)

10. A group of healthcare organizations decide amongst each other to collaborate with price raising, lowering, etc. (2 words)

11. This type of law's purpose is to protect the competition to ensure consumer choice in health care. (2 words)

15. This occurs when employees are afraid to change employment because they are afraid of losing their medical coverage. (2 words)

STUDENT ACTIVITY 10-2

IN YOUR OWN WORDS

Based on Chapter 10, please provide an explanation of the following concepts in your own words. DO NOT RECITE the text.

Advance directives: _____

_____

_____

Implied contracts: _____

_____

_____

Contractual right to admission: _____

_____

_____

Intentional torts: _____

_____

_____

Rules and regulations: _____

_____

_____

Common law: _____

_____

_____

Model Medical Accident Compensation Act: _____

_____

_____

Reasonable physician standard: _____

_____

_____

Tying: _____

_____

_____

Qui tam: _____

_____

_____

STUDENT ACTIVITY 10-3

REAL LIFE APPLICATIONS: CASE STUDY

A friend of the family is very upset because she feels that her grandmother was not properly treated when she was admitted to the emergency room a month ago. Her mother said that she felt that she was not given enough information about her medical condition in order to make a decision about her treatment. Also, she told your friend that she was transferred to another hospital when she went to the emergency room because she did not have health insurance. She actually did have health insurance but did not bring her insurance card so they sent her elsewhere because they could not verify it at the time.

Since her release, she has been treated by a physician that she likes. However, she feels as if her provider is sending her for unnecessary tests. She knows that you are studying health care and would like some advice on what to do next. She understands that you are not an attorney but would like to have a basic understanding of her situation.

ACTIVITY

(1) Identify any potential healthcare issues regarding her treatment in the emergency room and by her physician, (2) identify what laws, if any, have been violated, (3) what advice would you give her?, and (4) answer these questions using the information from the text.

RESPONSES

_____

_____

_____

_____

_____

_____

_____

_____

_____

_____

_____

_____

_____

_____

_____

_____

_____

STUDENT ACTIVITY 10-4

INTERNET EXERCISES

Write your answers in the space provided.

- Visit each of the Web sites listed here.
- Name the organization.
- Locate their mission statement on their Web site.
- Provide a brief overview of the activities of the organization.
- How do these organizations participate in the US healthcare system?

Web Sites

http://www.justice.gov

Organization Name: _____

Mission Statement:

_____

_____

_____

Overview of Activities:

_____

_____

_____

Importance of organization to US health care:

_____

_____

_____

http://www.genome.gov

Organization Name: _____

Mission Statement:

_____

_____

_____

Overview of Activities:

_____

_____

_____

Importance of organization to US health care:

_____
_____
_____

http://www.healthlaw.org

Organization Name: _____

Mission Statement:

_____
_____

Overview of Activities:

_____
_____
_____

Importance of organization to US health care:

_____
_____
_____

http://www.ccoc.qov

Organization Name: _____

Mission Statement:

_____
_____

Overview of Activities:

_____
_____
_____

Importance of organization to US health care:

_____
_____
_____

STUDENT ACTIVITY 10-4

http://www.healthcarecoach.com

Organization Name: _____

Mission Statement:

_____

_____

_____

Overview of Activities:

_____

_____

_____

Importance of organization to US health care:

_____

_____

_____

http://www.abanet.org

Organization Name: _____

Mission Statement:

_____

_____

_____

Overview of Activities:

_____

_____

_____

Importance of organization to US health care:

_____

_____

_____

Chapter 11

Ethics and Health Care

LEARNING OBJECTIVES

The student will be able to:

- Discuss the concept of ethics and its application to healthcare organizations.
- Define the four basic models of healthcare provider behavior.
- Define and discuss the four ethical models of a physician–patient relationship.
- Apply the concept of stakeholder management to the healthcare industry.
- Discuss the ethical dilemmas of organ transplants.
- Describe five different types of genetic testing.

DID YOU KNOW THAT?

- The concept of **bioethics** evolved as a result of the Nazi's human experimentation in the World War II prisoner camps.
- As of October 2008, there are 19,000 candidates waiting for organ donations—with only 9000 donors available.
- Xenotransplantation, which is transferring organs from one species to another, was first performed in 1984 when Baby Fae, a 5-pound infant, received the heart of a baboon.

- Euthanasia is from the Greek language meaning *letting die.*
- As the cost of US medical procedures has increased, **medical tourism** is becoming popular as more citizens travel overseas to have medical procedures performed because the procedures are less expensive overseas.

INTRODUCTION

As stated in Chapter 10, legal standards are the minimal standard of action established for individuals in a society. Ethical standards are considered one level above a legal action because individuals make a choice based on what is the "right thing to do," not what is required by law. There are many interpretations of the concept of ethics. Ethics has been interpreted as the moral foundation for standards of conduct (Taylor, 1975). The concept of **ethical standards** applies to actions that are hoped for and expected by individuals. Actions may be considered legal but not ethical. There are many definitions of ethics but, basically, **ethics** is concerned with what are right and wrong choices as perceived by society and its individuals.

The concept of ethics is tightly woven throughout the healthcare industry. It has been dated back to Hippocrates, the father of medicine, in the 4th century BC, and evolved into the Hippocratic Oath, which is the foundation for the ethical guidelines for patient treatment by physicians. In 1847, the American Medical Association (AMA) published a *Code of Medical Ethics* that provided guidelines for the physician–provider relationship, emphasizing the duty to treat a patient (AMA, 2008). To this day, physicians' actions have followed codes of ethics that demand the "duty to treat" (Wynia, 2007).

Applying the concept of ethics to the healthcare industry has created two areas of ethics: medical ethics and bioethics. **Medical ethics** focuses on the decisions healthcare providers make on the patient's medical treatment. Euthanasia or physician-assisted suicide would be an example of a medical ethic. **Advance directives** are orders that patients give to providers to ensure that, if they are terminally ill and incompetent to make a decision, certain measures will not be taken to prolong that patient's life. If advance directives are not provided, the ethical decision of when to withdraw treatment may be placed on the family and provider. These issues are legally defined, although there are ethical ramifications surrounding these decisions.

This chapter will focus primarily on **bioethics**, which emerged as a field in World War II when Nazis in Germany used prisoners in war camps as medical experiments, illustrated the rights of human subjects in medical research. This field of study is concerned with the ethical implications of certain biologic and medical procedures and technologies, such as cloning; **alternative reproductive methods**, such as in vitro fertilization; organ transplants; genetic engineering; and care of the terminally ill, which will be discussed in this chapter (History of Bioethics, 2009). Additionally, the rapid advances in medicine in these areas raised questions about the influence of technology on the field of medicine (Coleman, Bouesseau, & Reis, 2008).

It is important to understand the impact of ethics in different aspects of providing health care. Ethical dilemmas in health care are situations that test a provider's belief and what the provider should do professionally. Ethical dilemmas are often a conflict between personal and professional ethics. A **healthcare ethical dilemma** is a problem, situation, or opportunity that requires an individual, such as a healthcare provider, or an organization, such as a managed care practice, to choose an action that could be unethical. This chapter will discuss ethical theories, codes of healthcare conduct, informed consent, confidentiality, special populations, research ethics, ethics in public health, end-of-life decisions, genetic testing and profiling, and biomedical ethics, which focuses on technology use and health care.

HEALTHCARE STAKEHOLDER MANAGEMENT MODEL

A **stakeholder** is an individual or group that has an interest in an organization or activity. This term should not be confused with a "shareholder," who actually has a financial interest in an organization because they own part of the organization. The concept of **stakeholder management** focuses on the relationship between organizations and all of their constituents, including shareholders, and how management recognizes the different expectations of each group. For example, a customer stakeholder would have a large interest in an organization where they purchase a product or a service. For some organizations, the government is an important stakeholder because the government regulates the organization's activities. Managing the interests of all of the stakeholders is a challenge for management, particularly in the healthcare industry. The pressure that stakeholders may impose on a manager can impact their ethical decision-making process (Carroll & Buchholtz, 2008).

The basic stakeholder relationship in the healthcare industry is the relationship between the physician and the patient. However, Oddo (2001) has proposed that there are several other stakeholders that play a role in their relationship. The patient will have relationships that impact their interaction with the physician. The physician also has relationships with other stakeholders who have expectations of the physician. For example, the patient will have family and friends and the health insurance company or the government that is paying for the health procedure. The family and friends have expectations that the physician will cure their friend or family member. They have an emotional relationship. The health insurance company's relationship with the patient is professional. They will reimburse standardized treatment procedures.

The physician's stakeholder relationships are more complex. They may be a part of a managed care facility or have admitting privileges at a hospital so they have the relationship with that entity and the entity might have expectations of how they will treat the patient. Physicians are also impacted by health insurance companies who want them to treat the patient according to standardized diagnostic procedures. Drug companies also have an interest in the physician because they want the provider to use their products. All of these stakeholders have expectations on the simple relationship between the patient and provider. When these stakeholders place undue pressure on this relationship, the decision-making process of the provider may not always place the patient first although, as stated previously, the provider is ethically bound to treat the patient.

PHARMACEUTICAL MARKETING TO PHYSICIANS

There have been many cases regarding how drug companies market their products to physicians. Over the past two decades, this relationship has received more scrutiny. The drug companies provide free samples and information to physicians because the companies want the provider to use their products. Wazana (2000) reviewed several studies published over a 13-year period and estimated that physicians met with drug sales reps four times per month and residents accepted at least six gifts per year. According to a *New England Journal of Medicine* article, Campbell (2007) reports that physicians surveyed regarding this issue indicated that nearly 80% receive free drug samples, nearly 85% receive free meals, 35% receive reimbursement from drug companies for travel to medical conferences, and 28% receive consulting fees for enrolling patients in drug trials. Although providers deny that these "perks" influence their decisions in choosing drugs, federal legislation, **Physician Payment Sunshine Act**, is being debated in Congress that would require drug companies with annual revenues of $100 million or more to disclose the amount of money or other benefits given to physicians. Two states, Vermont and Minnesota, have made this type of reporting mandatory. In 2002, the **Pharmaceutical Research and Manufacturers of America** (PhRMA) implemented a new code of conduct governing physician–industry relationships (PhRMA, 2009). The code discourages gifts to physicians and other monetary rewards, emphasizing the relationship should focus on enhancing the quality of treatment of the patient. It emphasizes ethical marketing to the physicians. Eli Lilly, a large drug company, announced in September 2008 that it would publicly report all payments to physicians for any speaking and consulting services (Peng, 2008). These initiatives are increasing the transparency of the relationship between the provider and the companies, thereby providing

more accountability of the use of certain prescriptions by providers. This type of relationship can test the ethical relationship between the provider and patient.

According to Beauchamp and Childress (2001) and Gillon (1994), the role of ethics in the healthcare industry is based on five basic values that all healthcare providers should observe:

- **Respect for autonomy**: decision making may be different and healthcare providers must respect their patients' decisions even if they differ from their own.
- **Beneficence**: the healthcare provider should have the patient's best interests when making a decision.
- **Nonmalfeasance**: the healthcare provider will cause no harm when taking action.
- **Justice**: healthcare providers will make fair decisions.
- **Dignity**: patients should be treated with respect and dignity.

Each of these principles will be discussed in depth because these concepts are important to understanding the role of ethics in the healthcare industry. **Autonomy**, which is defined as self-rule, is an important concept to healthcare because it is applied to **informed consent**, which requires a provider to obtain the approval of a patient who has been provided adequate information to make a decision regarding intervention. As discussed in Chapter 10 regarding healthcare law, informed consent is a legal requirement for medical intervention. As part of the autonomy concept, it is also important that the provider respect the decision of their patient even if the patient's decisions do not agree with the provider's recommendation. A friend who has been diagnosed with a very advanced stage of cancer was told by her provider that she could enroll her in an experimental program that would give her 2 to 3 months to live. The intervention is very potent with severe side effects. My friend decided to try a homeopathic medicine to attack her disease. Her doctor was not in agreement with her choice but she respected her patient's decision. She told her that if she needed pain medication, she could come see her and she would help her. This situation is an excellent example of autonomy in medicine.

Beneficence in the healthcare industry means that the best interest of the patient should always be the first priority of the healthcare provider and healthcare organizations and **nonmalfeasance** further states that healthcare providers must not take any actions to harm the patient. As discussed in the paragraph on autonomy, this concept appears to be very easy to understand; however, there may be an interpretation between the provider and the patient as to what is best for the patient. For example, Jehovah's Witnesses, a religious sect, do not believe in blood transfusions and will not give consent during an operation for a transfusion to occur, despite the procedure's ability to possibly save a life (Miller, 2006). The provider has been trained to believe in beneficence and malfeasance. However, from the provider's point of view, if they respect the wishes of the patient and family, they will be potentially harming their patient.

Justice or fairness in the healthcare industry emphasizes that patients should be treated equally and that health care should be accessible to all. Justice should be applied to the way healthcare services are distributed, which means that healthcare services are available to all individuals. Unfortunately, in the United States, the healthcare system does not provide accessibility to all of its citizens. Access to health care is often determined by the ability to pay either out of pocket or by an employer- or government-sponsored program. In countries with universal healthcare coverage, justice in the healthcare industry is more prevalent. With over 45 million uninsured and 25 million underinsured in the United States, can one say that justice has not prevailed in the health care industry (Centers for Disease Control and Prevention, 2008).

ETHICS AND THE DOCTOR–PATIENT RELATIONSHIP

In Chapter 10 there was a discussion regarding the legal relationships between the provider and patient. This chapter examines the ethical relationship between the two parties.

The foundation of health care is the relationship between the patient and physician. In 2000 and 2001, the **American College of Physicians and Harvard Pilgrim Health Care Ethics Program** developed a statement of ethics for managed care. The following is a summary of the statements:

- Clinicians, healthcare plans, insurance companies, and patients should be honest in their relationship with each other.

- These parties should recognize the importance of the clinician and patient relationship and its ethical obligations.
- Clinicians should maintain accurate patient records.
- All parties should contribute to developing healthcare policies.
- The clinician's primary duty is the care of the patient.
- Clinician has the responsibility to practice effective and efficient medicine.
- Clinicians should recognize that all individuals, regardless of their position, should have health care.
- Healthcare plans and their insurers should openly explain their policies regarding reimbursement of types of health care.
- Patients have a responsibility to understand their health insurance.
- Health plans should not ask clinicians to compromise their ethical standards of care.
- Clinicians should enter agreements with healthcare plans that support ethical standards.
- Confidentiality of patient information should be protected.
- Clinicians should disclose conflicts of interest to their patients.
- Information provided to patients should be clearly understood by the patient (Povar et al., 2004).

This statement was developed as a result of the continued economic and policy changes in the healthcare industry. It provided guidelines to healthcare practitioners, healthcare organizations, and the healthcare insurance industry about ethical actions in the changing healthcare environment.

It is important to further discuss the relationship between the practitioner and the patient. There are several different models that can be applied to this relationship. Veatch (1972) identified four models that apply to the doctor–patient relationship: engineering model, priestly model, contractual model, and collegial model. The **engineering model** focuses on the patient and their power to make decisions about their health care. The provider gives the patient all of the necessary information to make a decision. The provider empowers the patient with knowledge to make a decision. The **priestly model** assumes the doctor will make the best decisions for the patient's health. The patient assumes a very passive role, giving the provider great power in the decision-making process. This is a very traditional relationship that often would occur between the elderly and physicians because they were taught to revere the medical world. The **contractual model**, based on a legal foundation, assumes there is an agreement between the two parties, assuming mutual goals. It is a relationship between the two parties with equal power. The patient understands the legal ramifications of the relationship. The **collegial model** assumes trust between the patient and doctor and that decision making is an equal effort (Veatch, 1972). These models are dependent on what type of relationship a patient expects with their practitioner. In any case, in each model, ethics plays a role in the relationship. Although the provider may play different roles in each of these models, the underlying foundation is assuming that the doctor's actions are ethical, representing the best interest of the patient.

ETHICS AND PUBLIC HEALTH

In contrast to the bioethicist view of the relationship between physician and patient, ethical analysis has expanded to public health. There are several ethics in public health that focus on the design and implementation of measures to monitor and improve the community's health (Coleman et al., 2008). Issues in public health include: inaccessibility to health care for certain populations, response to bioterrorism, research in developing countries, health promotion and its infringement on individual's lifestyle choices, and public health's response to emergencies. The concept of **paternalism** and public health is the concern that individual freedom will be restricted for the sake of public health activities because the government infringes on individual choices for the sake of protecting the community (Ascension Health, 2008).

The **Nuffield Council on Bioethics**, based on Great Britain, has proposed a stewardship model that outlines the principles public health policy makers should utilize globally. This model addresses the issues of paternalism in public health. The **stewardship model** states that public health officials should achieve the stated health outcomes for the population while minimizing restrictions on people's freedom of choice. As stated in Chapter 8, the focus of public health is to reduce the population's health risks from other people's actions such as drunken driving, smoking in public places, environmental conditions, inaccessibility to

health care, and maintaining safe working environments. While promoting a healthy lifestyle, according to the Nuffield Council on Bioethics, it is also important that public health programs do not force people into programs without their consent or introduce interventions that may invade people's privacy. The Council also introduces the concept of an intervention ladder that establishes a ranking of the type of public health intervention introduced, which may minimize people's choices. As the intervention moves up the ladder, the higher the justification is required for the action (Nuffield Council on Bioethics, 2007).

Childress, Faden, and Gaare (2002) specify five justifications for public health interventions that infringe on individual choices. The criteria are: (1) effectiveness, (2) need, (3) proportionality, (4) minimal infringement, and (5) public education. **Effectiveness** is essential to demonstrating that the public health efforts were successful and, therefore, it was necessary to limit individual freedom of choice. The **need for a public health intervention** must be demonstrated to limit individual freedom. If the **proportionality of the public health intervention** outweighs freedom of choice, then the intervention must be warranted. If the public health intervention satisfies effectiveness, need, and proportionality, the least restrictive intervention or **minimal infringement** on individual freedoms should be considered first. Lastly, public health must provide **public education** to explain their interventions and why the infringement on individual choices is warranted. For example, bioterrorism is now a viable threat. If it has been determined that a public health threat exists as a result of some biological weapons, then mandatory blood tests, possible quarantines, and other measures that would infringe on individual freedom of choice must be implemented (Buchanan, 2008).

Another ethical public health issue is the duty of practitioners to treat individuals during a public health crisis. If there is a natural disaster, what is the **duty to treat** during a time of crisis? During Hurricane Katrina, several healthcare professionals volunteered to stay behind in a local hospital. Unfortunately, several patients in the hospital died and the providers were accused of murdering their patients. As a result of this incident, many professionals are now wary of volunteering during a crisis. From their perspective, they commit to an ethical reaction and they may be rewarded with a criminal liability. There are civil liability protections that differ from state to state, such as Good Samaritan laws. Physicians practicing in free clinics are protected by federal law. Federal lawmakers should pass legislation that protects these healthcare professionals during public health emergencies (Wynia, 2007).

ETHICS AND RESEARCH

Conducting research involving human subjects requires the assessment of the risks and benefits to the human subjects, which must be explained clearly to them before the consent to participate in the research is given. The principles of ethical research are outlined in **Institutional Review Boards** (IRBs). An IRB is a group that has been formally designated to review and monitor biomedical research involving human subjects. An IRB has the authority to approve, require modifications in (to secure approval), or disapprove research. This group review serves an important role in the protection of the rights and welfare of human research subjects (Food and Drug Administration [FDA], 2009). Any organization that performs research should develop an IRB for their organization. The ethical component of an IRB is to protect the participants of the study. The IRBs require the researchers to maximize the benefits and minimize the risks to the participant and explain these assessments clearly. It is important that the IRB does not approve a study that imposes significant risks on the subjects.

Assuming the study clears the IRB's assessment of risks and benefits, it is important the subject understands the study and its impact on them. Informed consent, as discussed in Chapter 10 as it relates to treatment, is one of the basic ethical protections for human subject research. It is designed to protect human subjects and increase autonomy. Informed consent protects human subjects because it allows the individual to consider personal issues before participating in medical research. Informed consent increases autonomy because it provides the individual with the opportunity to make a choice to exercise control over their lives (Mehlman & Berg, 2008). Research informed consent requires the disclosure of appropriate information to assist the individual in project participation. Both the Department of Health and Human Services (HHS) and FDA have outlined common rule regulations that comprise the elements of informed consent.

Common rule elements include: a written statement that includes the purpose and duration of the study, the procedures and if they are experimental, any foreseen risks and potential benefits, and any alternative

procedures that may benefit the subject (FDA, 2009; Korenman, 2009). Additional requirements are needed for children, pregnant women, people with disabilities, mentally disabled people, prisoners, etc. It is clear that the IRB must provide guidelines for parents that have children participate in research and for those subjects that may be mentally disabled who could be unduly influenced (Mehlman & Berg, 2008).

HEALTHCARE CODES OF ETHICS

As a result of many public ethical crises that have occurred, particularly in the business world, many organizations have developed codes of ethics, which are guidelines for industry participants' actions. Codes of ethics provide a standard for operation so that all participants understand that if they do not adhere to this code, there may be negative consequences. The healthcare industry is no different. Physicians have been guided by many healthcare codes of ethics. The statement of ethics discussed previously in this chapter is a type of code of ethics; AMA created a code of ethics for physicians in 1847. This code was revised and adopted in 2001. Each healthcare professional has a code of conduct. The American Nurses Association (ANA) established a code for nurses in 1985, which was revised in 1995 and most recently in 2001 (ANA, 2009). Healthcare executives have a code of ethics that was established in 1941 that discusses the relationship with their stakeholders. The American College of Healthcare Executives (ACHE) represents 30,000 executives internationally who participate in the healthcare system (ACHE, 2008). They also offer ethical policy statements on relevant issues such as creating an ethical culture for employees. They also offer an ethics self-assessment tool that enables employees to target potential areas of ethical weakness. Many hospitals have established a code of ethics, which may help providers when they are dealing with medical situations, such as organ donations.

Interestingly, the **Advanced Medical Technology Association** (AdvaMed), an industry association that represents medical products, has also developed a code of ethics that addresses interactions with healthcare professionals who are potential customers of their products. Their ethical issues are similar to the pharmaceutical industry because they want physicians to use their medical devices and encourage the use by providing physicians with incentives such as gifts or paying for healthcare providers' travel or medical conferences (AdvaMed, 2008).

BIOETHICAL ISSUES

Designer or Donor Babies

Alternative reproductive methods are methods of conception that parents use to have children, such as in vitro fertilization, which means that the embryo is fertilized in a clinic using the sperm from the father. **Preimplantation genetic diagnosis** (PGD) is when the embryo is tested for tissue compatibility with their siblings prior to being transplanted into the mother. If one of the siblings becomes ill, the "designer baby" can save the existing sibling's life by providing bone marrow transplants. If it has been determined that the embryo is not compatible, it could be destroyed. This procedure is considered very controversial because many people consider the embryo early human life. Secondly, are the physicians and parents "playing God" by determining whether the embryo should be saved? Does this type of control dehumanize **procreation** or creation of life? Another question is what kind of impact occurs on the child who will eventually be aware that s/he was created to save a sibling (Dayal & Zarek, 2008).

Cloning

All human beings possess **stem cells**, which are "starter" cells for the development of body tissue that have yet to be formed into specialized tissues for certain parts of the body (Sullivan, 2006). The term **cloning** applies to any procedure that creates a genetic replica of a cell or organism. There are two major types of cloning: **reproductive cloning**, which creates cloned babies, and **therapeutic** or **research cloning**, which uses the same process but the focus is replicating sources for stem cells to replaced damaged tissues. The most famous reproductive clone was Dolly, the sheep that was cloned in 1996 from an adult cell (Baylis, 2002). Several countries have banned cloning for reproductive purposes but have been more lenient in therapeutic cloning. There are several ethical issues regarding cloning. People feel that cloning humans is unnatural and "playing God" rather than allowing procreating to progress naturally. People are highly focused on the reproductive cloning issues rather than the potential research success of cloning that could result in effective treatment of many diseases. However, therapeutic cloning also is considered unethical because it is destroying embryos to obtain healthy stem cells for research.

Research has focused on stem cells that could replace damaged body tissues from spinal injuries or cure diseases such as Parkinson disease. These stem cells could be derived from surplus human embryos that are stored at in vitro fertilization clinics and were not used for fertility procedures. The ethical issue, similar to the designer baby issues, is that, in order to use the stem cells, they would be destroying human embryos for research purposes because embryos are considered human life by many people. The issue in both cases also is what should happen to the excess embryos that are stored in clinics? Studies have indicated there may be an estimated 400,000 embryos stored in US clinics (The Coalition of Americans for Research Ethics, 2008) that may eventually be destroyed. Could these embryos be used to develop therapies and cures for disease?

Genetic Testing

Genetic testing is carried out on populations based on age, gender, or other risk factors to determine if they are at risk for a serious genetic disease or if they have a carrier gene that they may pass on to their children. Genetic tests may be analyzed from bodily tissue, including blood, cells from your mouth, saliva, hair, skin, tumors, or fluid surrounding the fetus during pregnancy (National Human Genome Research Institute [NHGRI], 2009). The specimen is analyzed by a laboratory. There are several different types of tests:

- **Diagnostic testing** is used to identify the disease when a person is exhibiting symptoms.
- **Predictive and asymptomatic** (no symptoms) tests are used to identify any gene changes that may increase the likelihood of a person developing a disease.
- **Carrier testing** is used to identify individuals who carry a gene that is linked to a disease. The individual may exhibit no symptoms but may pass the gene to offspring who may develop the disease or carry the gene themselves.
- **Prenatal testing** is offered to identify fetuses with potential diseases or conditions.
- Newborn screening is performed during the first 1 to 2 days of life to determine if the child has a disease that could impact its development.
- **Pharmacogenomic testing** is performed to assess how medicines react to an individual's genetic makeup.
- **Research genetic testing** focuses on how genes impact disease development.

The **Human Genome Project**, a long-term government-funded project completed in 2003, identified all of the 20,000 to 25,000 genes found in human DNA. They catalogued these genes which has made it easier to quickly determine the genes an individual possesses. As a result of genetics research, several genes have been identified as markers of prediction of disease in families such as breast cancer, colon cancer, cystic fibrosis, and Down syndrome in fetuses (Oak Ridge National Laboratory, 2009).

Although this information gained from genetic testing is important to individuals and their families, there are several ethical issues regarding genetic testing. If employers were aware of this information, would they use it to discriminate against employees? Would parents decide against having a child because of a result of a genetic test? How accurate are the genetic tests? There are no regulations regarding genetic tests so individuals and families may make decisions based on faulty laboratory tests. It is important that genetic testing is provided in conjunction with genetic counseling to ensure that individuals understand the results. Recently, private companies have developed home kits for genetic testing. This type of information without discussion with a genetic counselor or physician may have repercussions because an individual may make decisions based on lack of comprehension.

Euthanasia: Treating the Terminally Ill

End-of-life issues of a patient can be an ethical challenge. Healthcare providers may find this concept difficult to understand because they have been trained to save lives. The term **euthanasia** is the term most often associated with end-of-life issues. This Greek word for *letting die* may seem unethical because you are allowing an individual to die. Letting a patient die may be morally justifiable if it has been determined that any medical intervention is completely futile. Although euthanasia is illegal in all states except Oregon and most recently Washington (physician-assisted suicide), it is important to examine end-of-life issues because many of us will face them ourselves or with a loved one. There is confusion regarding the difference between euthanasia and physician-assisted suicide. **Physician-assisted suicide** refers to the physician providing the means for death, most often with a prescription. The patient, not the physician, will ultimately administer the lethal medication. Euthanasia generally means that the physician would act directly, for instance by giving a lethal injection, to end the patient's life.

There are two major types of euthanasia: voluntary and nonvoluntary. **Voluntary euthanasia** is assisting a patient with ending his or life at the patient's request. **Nonvoluntary euthanasia** means ending the life of an incompetent patient usually at the request of a family member. The two most famous nonvoluntary euthanasia cases are Karen Quinlan and Terri Shiavo. In 1975, the New Jersey Supreme Court granted Ms. Quinlan's father the right to remove his daughter's respirator which resulted in her death 10 years later. She had remained in a coma or persistent vegetative state for 10 years. Because she was not able to make the decision herself, the judge granted the father the right to limit any medical interventions to continue her life. Terri Shiavo suffered a heart attack in 1990 and remained in a coma on a feeding tube until 2005, when the Florida Supreme Court allowed the husband of Terri Schiavo to remove her feeding tube despite her parent's protests (Euthanasia.com, 2008).

Voluntary euthanasia is only legal in the United States in the state of Oregon and Washington. As of this writing, worldwide, it is only legal in Belgium (2002) and the Netherlands (2001). The **Oregon Death with Dignity Act**, which was discussed in Chapter 10, allows physicians to prescribe lethal medications to assist terminally ill patients to die on their own terms if it has been determined that the patient only has 6 months to live (Sultz & Young, 2006). This has been a controversial piece of legislation that has generated more commentary throughout the country and worldwide. Healthcare providers who support euthanasia feel that (1) it is an opportunity to relieve the pain a patient is experiencing at the end of their life; (2) it is an example of autonomy in a person's life by allowing them to choose when they are dying; and (3) it allows an opportunity to be released from a life that no longer has quality. Healthcare providers who believe that euthanasia is unethical feel that (1) it devalues the concept of life, (2) it may merely be an opportunity to contain medical costs for both the families and health insurance companies and, most importantly, and (3) a provider should not be directly involved in killing a patient (Sullivan, 2005). The opponents of euthanasia also feel that a physician cannot, with medical certainty, tell a patient that they will die within 6 months. The patient's emotional state and response to medication may alter that prognosis.

Dr. Jack Kevorkian and Dr. Phillip Nitschke

It is important to mention two physicians who have strongly supported euthanasia throughout the years. US physician, Dr. Jack Kevorkian or Dr. Death, had provided assisted suicide services to at least 45 ill patients. In 1989, he developed a suicide machine that allowed patients to administer a lethal injection of medication to themselves. In 1997, the US Supreme Court ruled that individuals who want to kill themselves, but are physically unable to do so, have no constitutional right to end their lives. Dr. Kevorkian was sentenced to 10–25 years in prison that same year. He was paroled in 2007 because he was in failing health (Soylent Communications, 2008).

Australian physician, Dr. Phillip Nitschke, travels internationally presenting "how-to-commit suicide" clinics. Several years ago, he created a concoction from household ingredients which he calls the "Peaceful Pill." He believes that if there is a right to life, there is also a right to die and that individuals should have the right to choose to end life. He does not restrict this right to just the terminally ill. He also believes that the depressed, the elderly, and the grieving should have the right to end their lives (Exit International, 2009).

Transplantation

Transplantation is the general procedure of implanting a functional organ from one person to another. This procedure can include blood transfusions or complicated procedures such as heart and lung transplants and bone marrow transplants. Organ transplants are becoming a more common approach to the treatment of diseased organs, making organ donations important to saving lives. Many patients have a significant chance for long-term survival because of impressive gains in the field (Burrows, 2004; Woloschak, 2003). Organs can be harvested from a living or dead person. As a result, the waiting list for organs has increase from 35,000 to 85,000 while the number of organ donors has remained stagnant (Berman, 2005). There are two major ethical and legal issues associated with organ transplants between humans including (1) the decision-making process for who receives the organ and (2) financial remuneration from selling organs, which has resulted in a black market for buying organs. It is important to note that since 1984, as a result of the passage of the

National Organ Transplant Act, it is illegal in the United States to buy and sell organs, which has resulted in 6500 Americans dying annually because lack of available organs. By 1990, many countries and the World Health Organization issued similar bans. The Ethics Committee of the Transplantation Society issued a policy statement further supporting the ban on illegally buying and selling organs (Friedman & Friedman, 2006). As of January 2007, nearly 9500 patients were awaiting an organ transplant (Berman, 2005; Bramstedt & Xu, 2007; Burrows, 2004). It is projected that by 2010, there will be 100,000 patients waiting for an organ with the average wait time nearly a decade (Xue, Ma, & Louis, 2001).

Who Should Receive the Organ?

According to the **United Network for Organ Sharing** (UNOS), there were 18,660 organ waiting list candidates, with 9941 donors available—a nearly 2 to 1 ratio (UNOS, 2009). There are ethical questions when making the decision as to who receives an organ. In the United States, there is an organ waiting list. Should the sickest recipient waiting on the organ list receive the organ or should the patient who may live longer receive the organ? Under the current UNOS, patients awaiting a transplant are assigned a priority based on medical need. If a patient is waiting for a heart transplant, the patient who is on life support or is in intensive care has first priority. Kidneys are allocated based on a point system maintained by UNOS. Liver transplants also include guidelines on alcohol abuse, which often destroys livers. UNOS guidelines require 6 months of sobriety prior to a transplant. Should the alcoholic receive a liver transplant at all? Some organ transplant centers will not provide any liver transplants to any alcoholics (Giuliano, 1997).

A recent trend over the last decade is transplanting organs in the elderly. The number of people over the age of 65 who have received organ transplants has tripled between 1996 and 2005. The ethical dilemma for a surgeon is whether to transplant an organ in an older patient rather than trying to save the life of a younger patient. Studies have indicated that survival rates for elderly lung recipients are acceptable—73.6% 3-year survival rate compared to 74.2% for younger patients (Davis, 2008). However, does the surgeon opt to shorten the life of a younger patient in order to give an additional 3 years of life to an elderly patient who already has lived a full life?

Consent for Organ Donations

As stated in the previous paragraph, organ donations may also occur when a person dies. Depending on the state of residence, individuals may enroll in a program that gives permission for organ harvest when they die, alleviating the pressure on families of having to make that decision to harvest the organs. However, in some states, permission is required by the family which places pressure on them. Some families feel it is unethical to donate their family member's body for science because of religious or personal philosophical reasons. In the United States, proximately 40% to 60% of US families consent to organ harvesting. A 2005 study indicated that the media had a huge influence on the family's decision to give consent to organ donations. Because the media has sensationalized the illegal buying and selling of organs and the unscrupulous behavior of physicians who are selling body parts for greed have influenced their decisions (Morgan et al., 2005).

In other parts of the world, countries use **presumed consent**, which means that if a parent does not actively oppose the transplantation, the procedure automatically occurs. In the United States, the consent must be actively received from the family first. As a result of presumed consent, those countries receive significantly more donations (Burrows, 2004). Is it an ethical policy to assume the family will consent to organ donations? Oftentimes, a family is frozen with grief and cannot make a coherent decision.

Organ Transplants from Family Member

Often, organ transplants may occur between two family members because it has been determined that the compatibility is very high, which would result in less risk for an organ to be rejected. An ethical issue with this situation is the pressure a family member feels from other family members to agree to give one of their organs to another member. Most parents would gladly donate organs to their sick offspring. What about siblings who don't like each other? Should they feel compelled to give an organ? Are they being pressured by other family members to go into surgery? The donors are also at risk. Any time surgery is performed there is a risk to the individual. Should physicians provide a "medical excuse" to the potential family donor as a way to rationalize their decision not to give their organ to a family member? The family member should not be coerced or forced to have the surgery.

Financial Payoff for Organ Donations

Living donor organ transplantation is the only field in medicine in which two individuals are ultimately involved—the person donating the organ and the person receiving the organ. Because of the success of organ transplantation, more treatments are focusing on this alternative. As stated previously, the statistics indicate that the need for organ donations is far outstripping the number of donors. Because of the ongoing need for organs, creative financial incentives are becoming more common, such as offering to pay for funeral expenses if a family would consent to donating an organ from their deceased family member (which is offered in Pennsylvania). In Wisconsin, they offer a $10,000 tax credit for families that consent to organ donations from deceased family members (Burrows, 2004).

Also, as a result of the increasing need for organs, a black market, which is an illegal form of commerce, has developed for the buying and selling of organs. **Organs Watch**, established in 1999 at the University of California at Berkeley, has monitored organ transplants in 12 countries worldwide. They have witnessed Israeli patients who travel to Turkey to receive kidneys sold by Romanians and European and North American patients receiving kidneys purchased from Manila whose operations were set up by an independent liver broker, Liver4You. Despite these practices, no surgeons have been investigated. The procurement of body parts from poor people may be considered illegal in most countries in the world and certainly unethical, but nothing has been done because many of the organ recipients need these organs to live and those individuals that sell the organs are making an informed choice (Scheper-Hughes, 2003).

As a result of the inequity between the supply and demand of organs, the concept of medical tourism or "medical value travel" has evolved. US organ transplants can cost $100,000, but are considerably less expensive overseas. IndUShealth and Global Health Administrators, Inc., have collaborated with insurance companies to arrange for US residents to obtain medical treatment in India. United Group Programs offers living and deceased organ donor transplants from foreign countries such as Thailand (Bramstedt & Xu, 2007). In 2006, The Blue Ridge Paper Products, Inc., and American company, integrated a medical tourism component as part of their employee benefit package. Employees were offered incentives including a $10,000 bonus if they had surgery in India because it was more cost-effective (Burkett, 2007). Although these programs are cost-effective, concerns about follow-up care or complications may determine the effectiveness of these medical value plans. Are these programs ethical? Are insurance companies focusing on cost rather than safety of the patient? Is the patient fully aware of the risk of these types of options?

Xenotransplantation

Another type of transplantation is **xenotransplantation**, which is the transfer of organs from one species to another. This has evolved as a result of the shortage of human organs available for donation. The first xenotransplantation was the transfer of a baboon heart into a 5-pound infant in 1984. Baby Fae survived 3 weeks before the baboon heart was rejected (Ascension Health, 2008). Since that time, several other xenotransplants have occurred using pig livers and hearts. Although xenotransplantation is promising, the ethical dilemma is that we are killing animals for these procedures, which are considered experimental. Is there a difference between killing animals for food and killing them for organ transplants? Although we may be ultimately saving lives, for some individuals, xenotransplantation is not ethical. Another issue is the contraction of animal disease to humans. If xenotransplantation is to be successful, it is important that the animals be screened for any diseases humans may contract such as rabies and viruses.

CONCLUSION

There are several ethical issues discussed in this chapter involving the healthcare industry and its stakeholders. There are two components of ethics in health care: medical ethics, which focus on the treatment of the patient, and bioethics, which focus on technology and how it is utilized in health care. The most important stakeholder in healthcare is the patient. The most important relationship with this stakeholder is their healthcare provider. Their relationship is impacted by the other stakeholders in the industry, including the government who regulates healthcare provider activities, the insurance companies who interact with both provider and patient, and healthcare facilities, such as hospitals or managed care facilities, where the physician has a relationship. All of these stakeholders can influence how a healthcare provider interacts with the patient because they have an interest in the outcome. For that reason, many organizations that represent these stakeholders have developed codes of ethics so individuals are provided guidance for ethical behavior. Codes of ethics for the physicians and other healthcare providers, nurses, pharmaceutical companies, and medical equipment companies were discussed that emphasize how these stakeholders should interact with both the healthcare providers and patients.

Another major area of ethics is the treatment of patients who are dying. Euthanasia, including physician-assisted suicide, illegal in all states but Oregon and most recently, Washington, has been a controversial patient issue for years. There are supporters of euthanasia because they feel it is the individual's right to choose when they want to end their life and they should have assistance from a physician, if needed. Opponents feel it is unethical because it is the responsibility of a physician to save a life, or not to take a life. This issue is tied into advance directives which a patient gives to the provider requesting that certain treatments be administered or not. If the patient is incompetent, advanced directives provide guidance on how the provider should treat the patient at the end of their life.

Another area of ethical discussion is organ transplantation. There are not enough organ donors in the United States, thereby creating a long waiting list. With limited supply, the ethical dilemma of organ transplants is how to determine who should receive an organ. For example, the famous New York Yankee baseball player, Mickey Mantle, a long time alcoholic, received a liver transplant. He needed a liver transplant as a result of his alcoholism. There was a public outcry because people felt that he received the liver because he was famous. Although the doctors explained that was not the case, people were upset because they felt that his addiction caused the liver failure. Why should he receive a liver that he damaged? As a result of designer or donor babies, children must be included in the transplant discussion. Should parents have another child specifically to save another child's life? The child who was designated as the donor baby may have emotional issues because they will eventually be aware that they were created specifically for their sibling's transplant needs.

When Dolly the sheep was cloned in 1995, she created an international furor. There are diametrically opposing views on cloning. Opponents feel that cloning takes the natural procreation process and turns it into a scientific experiment. Supporters feel that the scientific community has provided an opportunity to recreate a specimen, at will, with the desired genes.

And, finally, it is necessary to address the ethical foundation of our healthcare system. With over 45 million uninsured citizens in the United States, is it unethical that there is no universal healthcare system? The United States is the only industrialized nation, with the exception of South Africa, that has no universal healthcare coverage. Other nations have stated that health care is a right, not a privilege. Is it unethical for the United States to have a system that does not provide for all citizens? This text cannot provide answers to ethical situations because ethics is viewed differently by each individual. This chapter can only provide questions for the reader so they can assess their ethical viewpoint as it relates to the healthcare industry.

PREVIEW OF CHAPTER TWELVE

Mental disorders are common in the United States. They are the leading cause of disability in the United States and Canada for people ages 15 to 44. Consumers of mental health services have an average life expectancy of 25 years less than the general public. Despite these issues, access to mental health services has been limited. The causes of mental health disorders have often been less defined and less understood compared to traditional medical problems. As a result, they are often not diagnosed accurately. Also, insurance companies are hesitant to cover mental health services because the treatment is also less defined. Chapter 12 will discuss the history of the US mental health system, mental healthcare law, insurance issues, populations at risk, and an analysis and recommendations to improve US mental health care.

VOCABULARY

Advance directives

Alternative reproductive methods

American College of Physicians and Harvard Pilgrim Health Care Ethics Program

Autonomy

Beneficence

Bioethics

Cloning

Collegial model

Common rule

Contractual model

Dignity

Effectiveness

Engineering model

Ethical standards

Ethics

Euthanasia

Genetic testing

Healthcare ethical dilemma

Human Genome Project

Institutional Review Boards

Justice

Medical ethics

Medical tourism

Minimal infringement

Nonmalfeasance

Nonvoluntary euthanasia

Nuffield Council on Bioethics

Oregon Death with Dignity Act

Organs Watch paternalism preimplantation genetic diagnosis

Pharmaceutical Research and Manufacturers of America

Physician-assisted suicide

Physician Payment Sunshine Act

Presumed consent

Priestly model

Public education

Reproductive cloning

Research cloning

Respect for autonomy

Stakeholder

REFERENCES

Advanced Medical Technology Association. (2008). Retrieved November 10, 2009, from http://www.advamed.org/MemberPortal/About/code/.

American College of Healthcare Executives. (2008). Retrieved November 10, 2009, from http://www.advamed.org/MemberPortal/About/code/.

American Medical Association. (2008). Retrieved November 10, 2009, from http://www.ama-assn.org/ama/pub/physician-resources/medical-ethics.shtml.

American Nurses Association. (2009). NursingWorld. Retrieved November 10, 2009, from http://www.nursingworld.org/MainMenuCategories/EthicsStandards.aspx.

Ascension Health. (2008). Retrieved November 9, 2008, from http://www.ascensionhealth.org/ethics/public/cases/case4.asp.

Baylis, F. (2002). Human cloning: Three mistakes and an alternative. *Journal of Medicine and Philosophy*, 27, 3, 319–337.

Beauchamp, T., & Childress, J. (2001). *Principles of biomedical ethics* (5th ed.). Oxford: Oxford University Press.

Berman, R. (2005). Lethal legislation. *Robert Kennedy School Review*, 6, 13–18.

Bramstedt, K., & Xu, J. (2007). Checklist: Passport, plane ticket, organ transplant. *American Journal of Transplantation*, 7, 1698–1701.

Buchanan, D. (2008). Autonomy, paternalism and justice: Ethical priorities in public health. *American Journal of Public Health*, 98, 15–21.

Burkett, L. (2007). Medical tourism. Concerns, benefits, and the American legal perspective. *The Journal of Legal Medicine*, 28, 223–245.

Burrows, L. (2004). Selling organs for transplantation. *The Mount Sinai Journal of Medicine*, 71, 4, 251–254.

Campbell, E. (2007). Doctors and drug companies—Scrutinizing influential relationships. *New England Journal of Medicine*, 357, 18, 1796–1796.

Carroll, A., & Bucholtz, A. (2006). *Business society: Ethics and stakeholder management*. Mason, OH: Thomson/Southwestern.

Centers for Disease Control and Prevention. (2008). Retrieved November 9, 2009, from http://www.cdc.gov/Features/Uninsured/.

Childress, J., Faden, R., & Gaare, R. (2002). Public health ethics: Mapping the terrain. *Journal of Law Medical Ethics*, 30, 170–178.

The Coalition of Americans for Research Ethics. (2008). Retrieved November 8, 2008, from http://www.stemcellresearch.org.

Coleman, C., Bouesseau, M., & Reis, A. (2008). The contribution of ethics to public health. *Bullletin of the World Health Organization*, 86, 8, 578–589.

Davis, R. (2008). *More elderly patients are having transplantation surgery*. Retrieved November 8, 2009, from http://www.usatoday.com/news/health/2008-02-04-transplant_N.htm.

Dayal, M., & Zarek, S. (2008). Preimplantation genetic diagnosis. Retrieved November 10, 2009, from http://emedicine.medscape.com/article/273415-overview.

Exit International. (2009). Retrieved November 9, 2009, from http://www.exitinternational.net.

Food and Drug Administration. (2009). Information sheet guidances guidance for institutional review boards, clinical investigators, and sponsors. Retrieved November 4, 2009, from http://www.fda.gov/oc/ohrt/irbs/facts.html#IRBOrg.

Friedman, E., & Friedman, A. (2006). Payment for donor kidneys: Pros and cons. *International Society of Nephrology*, January, 960–962.

Gillon, R. (1994). Principles of medical ethics. *British Medical Journal*, *309*, 184.

Giuliano, K. (1997). Organ transplants: Tackling the tough ethical questions. *Nursing*, *27*, 34–40.

History of Bioethics. (2009). Retrieved November 10, 2009, from http://science.jrank.org/pages/8456/Bioethics-History-Bioethics.html.

Korenman, S. G. (2009). Teaching the responsible conduct of research in humans. Retrieved November 4, 2009, from http://ori.hhs.gov/education/products/ucla/chapter2/page04b.htm.

Mehlman, M., & Berg, J. (2008). Human subjects protections in biomedical enhancement research: Assessing risk and benefit and obtaining informed consent. *Journal of Law, Medicine & Ethics*, Fall, 546–559.

Miller, R. (2006). *Problems in health care law* (9th ed.). Sudbury, MA: Jones and Bartlett.

Morgan, S., Harrison, T., Long, S., Afiffi, W., Stephenson, M., & Reichert, T. (2005). Family discussions about organ donations: How the media influences opinions about organ donations. *Clinical Transplant, 19*, 674–682.

National Human Genome Research Institute. (2009). Retrieved November 10, 2009, from http://www.genome.gov/10002335.

Nuffield Council on Bioethics Report. (2007). *Public health: Ethical issues guide to the report*. Retrieved November 4, 2009, from http://www.nuffieldbioethics.org/fileLibrary/pdf/Public_Health_-_short_guide.pdf.

Oak Ridge National Laboratory. (2009). Retrieved November 9, 2009, from http://www.ornl.gov/sci/techresources/Human_Genome/home.shtml.

Oddo, A. (2001). Health care ethics: A patient-centered decision model. *Journal of Business Ethics*, *29*, 126.

Peng, T. (2008). Opening the books. Retrieved October 29, 2008, from www.newsweek.com/id/160894?from=rss?nav=slate.

Pharmaceutical Research and Manufacturers of America. (2008). Retrieved November 8, 2009, from http://www.phrma.org/about_phrma/.

Povar, C., Blumen, H., Daniel, J., Daub, S., Evans, L., Holm, R., et al. (2004). Ethics in practice: Managed care and the changing health care environment. *American College of Physicians*, *4*, 2, 131–136.

Scheper-Hughes, N. (2003). Keeping an eye on the global traffic in human organs. *Lancet*, *361*, 1645–1648.

Soylent Communications. (2008). Jack Kevorkian. Retrieved November 9, 2008, from http://www.nndb.com/people/272/000023203/.

Sullivan, D. (2005). Euthanasia versus letting die: Christian decision-making in terminal patients. *Ethics and Medicine*, *21*, 2, 109–118.

Sullivan, D. (2006). Stem cells 101—An audio/MP3 version. Retrieved November 2, 2008, from http://www.bioethics.com/?page_id=533.

Sultz, H., & Young, K. (2006). *Health care USA: Understanding its organization and delivery* (5th ed.). Sudbury, MA: Jones and Bartlett.

Taylor, P. (1975). *Principles of ethics: An introduction to ethics* (2nd ed.). Encino, CA: Dickinson.

United Network for Organ Sharing. (2009). Retrieved November 2, 2009, from http://www.unos.org.

Veatch, R. (1972). Medical ethics: Professional or universal. *Harvard Theological Review, 65,* 531–559.

Wazana, A. (2000). Physicians and the pharmaceutical industry: Is a gift ever just a gift? *Journal of American Medical Association*, *283,* 373–380.

Woloschak, G. (2003). Transplantation: Biomedical and ethical concerns raised by the cloning stem cell debate.

Zygon, 8, 599–704.

Wynia, M. (2007). Ethics and public health emergencies: Encouraging responsibility. *The American Journal of Bioethics*, *7,* 1–4.

Xue, J., Ma, J., & Louis, T. (2001). Forecast of the number of patients with end-stage renal disease in the United States to the year 2010. *Journal of American Sociological Nephrology*, *12,* 2753–2758.

STUDENT ACTIVITY 11-1

CROSSWORD PUZZLE

Instructions: Please complete the puzzle using the vocabulary words found in the chapter. There may be multiple-word answers. The numbers in the parenthesis indicate the number of words in the answers.

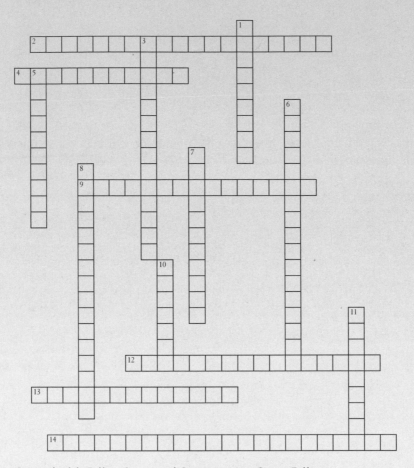

Created with EclipseCrossword © 1999–2009 Green Eclipse

STUDENT ACTIVITY 11-1

Across

2. This procedure transfers organs from one species to another. (1 word)

4. The healthcare provider should have the best interest of the patient when making a decision. (1 word)

9. General procedure of transferring an organ from one person to another. (1 word)

12. This model focuses on the provider giving the patient all of the information to make a decision. (2 words)

13. The provider will make the best decisions for the patient's health. (2 words)

14. Ending the life of a patient usually at the request of a family member. (3 words)

Down

1. Starter cells for the development of body tissue. (2 words)

3. The healthcare provider will cause no harm to the patient when taking action. (2 words)

5. Greek phrase for "letting die." (1 word)

6. This type of test is used to identify a disease when a person exhibits symptoms. (2 words)

7. An individual or group that has an interest in an organization or activity. (1 word)

8. Public health officials should protect the health of the population while minimizing restrictions on people's freedom of choice. (2 words)

10. Any type of procedure that recreates a cell or organism. (1 word)

11. This field of study applies ethics to the healthcare industry. (1 word)

STUDENT ACTIVITY 11-2

IN YOUR OWN WORDS

Based on Chapter 11, please provide an explanation of the following concepts in your own words. DO NOT RECITE the text.

Paternalism: _____

_____

_____

Medical tourism: _____

_____

_____

Therapeutic cloning: _____

_____

_____

Stem cell: _____

_____

_____

Transplantation: _____

_____

_____

Xenotransplantation: _____

_____

_____

Presumed consent: _____

_____

_____

Autonomy: _____

_____

_____

Stewardship model: _____

_____

_____

Institutional Review Boards: _____

_____

_____

REAL LIFE APPLICATIONS: CASE STUDY

A friend from high school who you had not seen for 5 years moved into your neighborhood. Although you were close friends in high school, you had lost touch but were very happy to welcome her and her family into the neighborhood. You were pleased because she has children that were the same age as your children. She was also pregnant with her third child. You invite her over to the house so the children can play with each other and catch up. She told you that her eldest child was very ill and required a bone marrow transplant. There were no matching donors on the national list. She and her husband decided to have a baby that could be used to save her other child. She asked what you thought of her actions. You could not respond because you were unclear of the actual process and ethical ramifications of the situation. Before making any statements that could hurt your friend, you decide to do some research on the topic and talk to your spouse about it.

ACTIVITY

(1) Explain this type of procedure and what the procedure entails, (2) identify any ethical issues associated with this type of procedure, and (3) provide an opinion on this procedure—would you do it or not and why?

RESPONSES

_____

_____

_____

_____

_____

_____

_____

_____

_____

_____

_____

_____

_____

_____

STUDENT ACTIVITY 11-4

INTERNET EXERCISES

Write your answers in the space provided.

- Visit each of the Web sites listed here.
- Name the organization.
- Locate their mission statement on their Web site.
- Provide a brief overview of the activities of the organization.
- How do these organizations participate in the US healthcare system?

Web Sites

http://www.nursingworld.org

Organization Name: _____

Mission Statement:

_____

_____

_____

Overview of Activities:

_____

_____

_____

Importance of organization to US health care:

_____

_____

_____

http://www.thehastingscenter.org

Organization Name: _____

Mission Statement:

_____

_____

_____

Overview of Activities:

_____

_____

_____

STUDENT ACTIVITY 11-4

Importance of organization to US health care:

_____
_____
_____

http://www.phRMA.org

Organization Name: _____

Mission Statement:

_____
_____
_____

Overview of Activities:

_____
_____
_____

Importance of organization to US health care:

_____
_____
_____

http://www.procon.org

Organization Name: _____

Mission Statement:

_____
_____
_____

Overview of Activities:

_____
_____
_____

Importance of organization to US health care:

_____
_____
_____

STUDENT ACTIVITY 11-4

http://www.ornl.org

Organization Name: _____

Mission Statement:

_____

_____

_____

Overview of Activities:

_____

_____

_____

Importance of organization to US health care:

_____

_____

_____

http://www.stemcells.nih.gov

Organization Name: _____

Mission Statement:

_____

_____

_____

Overview of Activities:

_____

_____

_____

Importance of organization to US health care:

_____

_____

_____

Mental Health Issues

LEARNING OBJECTIVES

The student will be able to:

- List the six types of mental health professionals and their roles in mental health care.

- List and define at least 10 mental health disorders as defined by the American Psychiatric Association's *Diagnostic and Statistical Manual of Mental Disorders*.

- Discuss at least five liability issues surrounding mental health professionals.

- Define mental health behavioral companies and discuss their relationship to mental health care.

- Discuss mental health issues in high-risk populations.

- Define and discuss why posttraumatic stress disorder (PTSD) occurs.

- Evaluate the importance of the National Institute for Mental Health and the American Psychological Association (APA) to mental health care.

DID YOU KNOW THAT?

- Surveys indicate that one in four Americans suffer from a mental disorder in any one year.

- The life expectancy rate for the mentally disabled is 25 years less than that of the general public.

- Half of all lifetime mental health illnesses begin by age 14; three quarters occur by age 24.

- The annual economic, indirect cost of mental illness is estimated to be $79 billion.

- Over 50% of students with a mental disorder age 14 and older dropout of high school—the highest drop out rate of any disability group.

INTRODUCTION

Mental disorders are common in the United States. Mental disorders are the leading cause of disability in the United States and Canada for ages 15 to 44 and many suffer from more than one mental disorder at the same time (Kochanek, Murphy, & Anderson, 2004). Consumers of mental health services, on an average, have a life expectancy of 25 years less than the general public (Everett, Mahler, Biblin, Ganguli, & Mauer, 2008). This premature mortality of the people with mental disabilities has several national organizations focusing on the healthcare needs of this population. The recipients of mental health services are a small subpopulation of those who are actually afflicted with a mental health problem. Access to mental health services has been limited because of myths associated with mental health problems and the treatment of mental health illnesses (Sultz & Young, 2006). Although mental health is a disease that requires medical care, its characteristics set it apart from traditional medical care.

David Satcher, US Surgeon General, released a landmark report in 1999 on mental health illness, *Mental Health: A Report of the Surgeon General*. The Surgeon General's report on mental health defines **mental disorders** as conditions that alter thinking processes, moods, or behavior that results in dysfunction or stress. It can be psychological or biological in nature. The most common conditions include **phobias,** which are excessive fear of objects or activities; substance abuse; and affective disorders, which are emotional states such as depression. Severe mental illness would include schizophrenia, major depression, and psychosis. Obsessive–compulsive disorders (OCD), mental retardation, Alzheimer's disease, and dementia are also considered mentally disabled conditions. According to the report, mental health ranks second to heart disease as a limitation on health and productivity (US Public Health Service, 1999). People who have mental disorders often exhibit feelings of anxiety, or may have hallucinations or feelings of sadness or fear that can limit normal functioning in their daily life. Because the cause or etiology of mental health disorders are less defined and less understood compared to traditional medical problems, interventions are less developed than other areas of medicine (Anderson, Rice, & Kominski, 2007). This chapter will provide a discussion on the following topics: the history of the US mental healthcare system, a background of healthcare professionals, mental healthcare law, insurance coverage for mental health, barriers to mental health care, the populations at risk for mental disorders, the types of mental health disorders as classified by the American Psychiatric Association's *Diagnostic and Statistical Manual of Mental Disorders* (DSM), liability issues associated with mental health care, an analysis of the mental healthcare system, and guidelines and recommendations to improve US mental health care.

HISTORY OF US MENTAL HEALTH CARE

Over the past three centuries, the mental health system has consisted of a patchwork of services that has become very fragmented (Regier et al., 1993). Initially, mentally ill individuals were relegated to care by their families. State governments built insane asylums, later known as hospitals. In the mid-18th century, the state of Pennsylvania opened a hospital in Philadelphia where the mentally ill were housed in the basement. During this period, Virginia was the first state to build an asylum in its capital city of Williamsburg. If the mentally ill were not cared for by their families or sent to an asylum, they were found in jails or almshouse. It was not until the 19th century that the mentally ill were treated with sensitivity. This **moral treatment** approach was used in Europe earlier with success. Mental health patients in hospitals were treated while participating in work and educational activities. The first mental health reformers in the United States were Dorothea Dix and Horace Mann who crusaded for this moral movement by convincing the public that some mentally ill patients can be treated in a controlled environment outside the confines of an asylum. Asylums should be focused on housing those mentally ill with chronic conditions that were untreatable. During this period, more states built more asylums, which became overcrowded. It is important to note that the local governments were responsible for funding the care of the asylum residents, which resulted in deteriorating conditions and exposure of the patients to inhumane treatment. State Care Acts were passed that mandated state funding for treatment between 1894 and World War I. Asylums were renamed mental hospitals. Psychiatric units were also opened in general hospitals to promote mental health as part of general health care (http://www.mentalhealth.samhsa.gov).

After World War I, many war veterans returned home with mental disorders, or what is now known as PTSD, because of their war experiences. It was not until the 1930s that prescriptions became available. However, other controversial treatments were used, such as electrotherapy. Brain surgery or lobotomies became a method to treat the mentally ill. World War II further focused the government on mental health issues and the National Institute of Mental Health was created. Government funding was awarded for mental health training and research. The Department of Veteran Affairs (VA) established psychiatric hospitals and clinics. During this period, most health care focused on inpatient services. The VA also developed mental health disorder categories in order to better treat their war veterans. By the mid-1950s, over 500,000 mental health patients were being treated in government mental health hospitals. In 1952, the American Psychiatric Association published their first DSM, which was coordinated with the World Health Organization's (WHO) International Classification of Disease (American Psychiatric Association, 2009) to encourage acceptance of mental health disorders.

Finally, the first psychoactive medication was developed which allowed outpatient treatment of mentally disabled patients. In 1955, the US Commission on Mental Health was established. They investigated the quality of mental hospitals and allocated funding for outpatient facilities. As more psychotropic medications were developed, Congress provided more funding allocations for community-based services. Medicaid, Medicare, Supplemental Security income (SSI), Social Security, and Disability insurance became accessible for mental health care (Grob, 1983, 1994; Sultz & Young, 2006).

During the 1960s and 1970s, community mental health centers were developed and supported by the federal government. Most of the funding focused on the less severe mentally ill who could live normally with outpatient services. In the late 1970s, President Carter appointed a Presidential Committee on Mental Health, which had limited success; however, Medicaid payments for outpatient mental health services were increased. Patients with severe mental illness became eligible for SSI funding. Unfortunately, budget cuts reduced SSI benefits for the mentally ill. By 1990, most mental health services were offered as outpatient services. Over the past 15 years, increased funding has increased the quality of mental health services, yet access to mental health services still remains limited for many reasons (Grob, 1994; Sultz & Young, 2006).

BACKGROUND OF MENTAL HEALTH SERVICES

Mental Health Professionals

Mental health services are provided by psychiatrists, psychologists, social workers, nurses, counselors, and therapists (see Chapter 6). Social workers will receive training in counseling, normally a master's degree, and can provide support for an individual with a mental health disability. Family and vocational counselors may also be involved in the treatment plan as well as recreational therapists. Mental health can be such a complex condition that impacts different aspects of the life of a mentally ill person that often many different mental health professionals are there for support and treatment. Most of these mental health professionals provide outpatient or ambulatory care for the mentally ill. Inpatient care may be offered in the psychiatric units of a hospital, mental hospitals, or substance abuse facilities (Pointer, Williams, Isaacs, & Knickman, 2007).

Mental health problems impact not only the individual but family members and friends as well. As a result of the vast impact of mental health disabilities, behavioral services are provided by psychiatrists, psychologists, social workers, nurses, counselors, and therapists (Shi & Singh, 2008). **Psychiatrists** are specialty physicians who can prescribe medication and admit patients to hospitals. Psychologists, who also participate in the treatment of mental health, cannot prescribe drugs but provide different types of therapy. Social workers focus on mental health counseling. Nurses may also specialize in psychiatric care. There may be additional counselors and therapists who participate in the treatment of the mentally disabled.

However, there are liability issues that mental health professionals may face. A recent study (Woody, 2008) indicated that there were seven reasons mental health professionals are at high risk for liability and complaints:

- When mental health professionals provide services to both children and their families, they are at risk for more complaints from their patients regarding care. Families may be wary when a mental health professional provides services to their children. A recent study has indicated that 70% of complaints are a result of child mental health services.

- Because of the increased government regulations of the licensing of practitioners, professionals no longer have a say in establishing standards for care.

- The litigious US society has included the mental health profession in their complaints.

- Patients have become more distrustful of their providers and are not always willing to adhere to treatment guidelines. If they are not cured, they blame the provider.

- Managed care has imposed restrictions on the number of sessions that have increased the liability of providers.

- Because of the high cost of health care, more patients are abandoning their healthcare treatment, which has reduced revenues. As a result, practitioners have developed practices to cut costs, which may result in more errors.

■ Mental health practitioners are ignoring their professional liability issues and do not hire professionals to resolve their problems. As a result, many practitioners are ill prepared to defend their actions and are found liable.

Mental Health Commitment Law

Commitment laws are laws that enable family members, law enforcement, or healthcare professionals to commit a person to a facility or a treatment program. **Commitment may be voluntary**, which occurs when people commit themselves willingly to receive care. If a person voluntarily commits for treatment, they can leave of their own free will. **Involuntary commitment** occurs when people are being forced to receive treatment or are committed to a facility against their wishes. A hearing must be held to prove the person is dangerous to themselves or others or is suffering from a mental disorder. If they are committed, they are not free to leave (Pointer et al., 2007). An involuntary commitment may occur as an outpatient mental health treatment plan. This type of involuntary commitment is normally a court-ordered program for mental health services.

Insurance Coverage for Mental Health

Mental health services are provided by distinct components of the healthcare system. There are specialty healthcare providers, as explained previously, such as psychiatrists and psychologists. However, the primary care provider (e.g., family physicians, internists, etc.) is often the initial contact for the mentally ill and may often serve as the provider for their problems. An important component of their care is the social service sector, such as social service workers and counselors, who provide assistance to both the individual and the family. Finally, there is a growing sector of nonprofit groups and organizations for the mentally ill that provide education and support. These components are known as the **de facto mental health service system** (Fig. 12-1) (US Public Health Service, 1999). Funding for mental health services are provided by both private insurance and public funding such as Medicare and Medicaid. However, as managed care has become the major model of providing health care, annual or lifetime limits on mental health care have been incorporated in managed care plans. As a result of cost concerns of

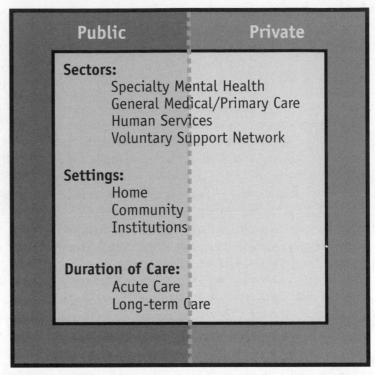

Figure 12-1 The mental health service system. (Source: US Public Health Service. [1999]. *Mental Health: A Report of the Surgeon General*. Retrieved November 5, 2009, from http://mentalhealth. samhsa.gov/features/surgeongeneralreport/chapter2/sec7.asp.)

mental health care, managed care organizations contracted with external vendors that focused on mental health care. These external vendors became known as managed care behavioral organizations.

Barriers to Mental Health Services

There is still a stigma that is attached to being mentally disabled. Individuals may be embarrassed to admit they may have a mental health problem and ignore it or they do not understand what is happening to them. Families can be embarrassed by a member that is mentally disabled. Another major barrier that still remains regarding mental health is the inadequacy of insurance coverage. A patient's primary care provider may also be uncomfortable with dealing with a patient that may have a mental health disorder.

Who are the Mentally Ill?

According to the newest revision of the DSM, diagnoses are based on 17 general categories:

■ Disorders diagnosed in infancy, childhood, or adolescence, which include mental retardation, autism, behavioral, and attention disorders

- Delirium, dementia, amnesia, and other cognitive disorders, which focus on memory deficits

- Mental disorders caused by a general medical condition

- Substance-related disorders related to drug use and abuse including alcohol and tobacco

- Schizophrenia and other psychotic disorders, a prevalent mental health disorder, focuses on hallucinations, delusions, multiple personalities, or other types of similar behavior

- Mood disorders such as manic/depressive disorders and behavior as a result of alcohol use

- Anxiety disorders, such as panic attacks and phobias, and PTSD, which is a condition that often occurs post-war experience or as a result of a life-changing event

- Somatoform disorders cannot be explained by substance abuse or medical condition but the disorder is present in an individual

- **Factitious disorders**, which are characterized by physical or psychological symptoms, are actually developed by patients to pretend they are ill

- **Dissociative disorders** focus on a disruption of an individual's memory, identity, or environmental awareness

- Sexual and gender disorders that focus on any type of sexual dysfunctions, which include fantasies and obsessions

- Eating disorders that focus on disturbances in overeating or undereating, which can be life threatening

- Sleep disorders that focus on abnormal sleep patterns

- **Impulse control disorders**, which could include gambling addiction or a pyromaniac who has an obsession with fire

- Adjustment disorders that focus on an individual's reaction to stress; this category is not as severe as category 7

- Personality disorders that are long term, such as paranoia and OCD

- Other conditions that are related to abuse or neglect and noncompliance with treatments and occupational issues (American Psychiatric Association, 2009; Sultz & Young, 2006)

Based on these categories, the prevalence of these types of disorders within a 12-month and lifetime prevalence were analyzed. The top two specific categories of 12-month prevalence of mental health disorders were anxiety disorders (19%) and substance abuse disorders (11%). The top two specific categories of lifetime prevalence of mental health and substance abuse disorders were anxiety disorders (29%) and substance abuse or dependence (27%) (Kessler & Uston, 2004).

SPECIAL POPULATIONS

Children and Adolescents

According to the **National Institute of Mental Health** (NIMH), 1 in 10 children suffer from a mental health disorder that requires treatment. Fewer than one in five will receive appropriate treatment. They can be diagnosed with the following:

- Attention deficit hyperactivity disorder (ADHD), attention deficit disorder (ADD)

- Autism spectrum disorders (pervasive developmental disorders)

- Bipolar disorder

- Borderline personality disorder

- Depression

- Eating disorders

- Schizophrenia

In some instances, these disorders can follow them throughout their life. It is particularly difficult to assess teen mental disorders because of their stage in life. Many teens are worried about peer pressure, family issues, schoolwork and activities, and making decisions about going to college or not. It is important that there is open communication with both children and teens either with their parents, counselors, or friends to ensure that, if there is a mental disorder, it will be addressed. Suicide is a major concern among children and adolescents, being the fifth leading cause of death among ages 5 to 14 years of age (Agency for Healthcare Research and Quality, 2009; NIMH, 2009)

Treatment for Children and Adolescents

According to the APA, it is important that parents recognize problems in their children so that they can be treated appropriately. The most common mental disorders are depression, ADHD, and conduct disorders. Although there is limited research on mental disorders in children, it is estimated that 1 in 10 children may suffer from persistent feelings of sadness, which can lead to depression. In some instances, children may not be able to verbalize their emotions so it is important to notice any behavioral changes such as poor school performance, loss of interest in hobbies, angry outbursts, anxiety, alcohol or drug abuse, and irrational behavior (Children and Adolescents, 2009).

ADHD symptoms include impulsiveness, inability to focus, and hyperactivity. This type of behavior can impair normal functioning for a child in school and socially. It is more common in males than females. It develops before the age of 7. As a parent, a child that has ADHD may trouble listening, may not be able to finish their schoolwork, may be excessively active, can be easily distracted, may talk incessantly, may have trouble in groups, and may have learning disabilities. Approximately 70 to 80% of children diagnosed with this disorder respond to medication.

Conduct disorder means that children consistently ignore their social norms. It is one of most frequently diagnosed disorders in teens. Many of these symptoms may be confused with a child that is considered "trouble." Symptoms such as stealing, lying, skipping school, starting fights, setting fires, cruelty to animals, destroying property, etc., can be indicative of a mental health disorder. Therefore, it is important to monitor these patterns of behavior over a period of 3 to 6 months. Treatment for conduct disorders involves either group or individual therapy.

The following is a list of medications that are being used for the treatment of children. This is a summary of the recommendations made by NIMH (NIMH, 2009).

Antidepressant and Antianxiety Medicine

These types of medications are prescribed almost as frequently as stimulant medications among children and adolescents. They are used for depression, a disorder recognized only in the last 20 years as a problem for children, and for anxiety disorders, including OCD.

Antipsychotic Medications

These medications are used to treat children with schizophrenia, bipolar disorder, autism, Tourette syndrome, and severe conduct disorders. Some of the older **antipsychotic medications** have specific indications and dose guidelines for children. Some of the newer medications, which have fewer side effects, are also being used effectively for children.

Mood Stabilizing Medications

These medications are used to treat bipolar disorder (manic-depressive illness). However, because there is very limited data on the safety and efficacy of most

mood stabilizers in youth, treatment of children and adolescents is based mainly on experience with adults.

Elderly and Mental Health

As the US population ages and continues to live longer, mental health disorders will become more prevalent in the elderly. As we age, we will experience loss of family members and friends, which is a major trigger of depression and possibly suicide. Unfortunately, many elderly are not treated for mental illness for several reasons. Often the elderly are being treated for other traditional illnesses, so the focus is treating those illnesses. Also, as we age, society assumes that we lose our memory and some of our faculties as part of the normal aging process, which is not an inevitable fact, so primary care providers and family members do not attribute these symptoms to dementia or Alzheimer's disease, both mental disorders. It is also more difficult to see a specialist because of lack of transportation. The elderly are focused on seeing their primary care provider for their main ailments, so both the patient and the provider may ignore the symptoms. Also, the primary care provider may not be comfortable addressing mental health issues. If the primary care provider refers the elderly patient to a psychologist, a recent APA survey indicated that fewer than 30% of psychologists have had graduate coursework in **geropsychology**, which deals with mental health issues in the elderly, and that 70% would be interested in attending programs in geropsychology (American Psychiatric Association, 2009). The APA has provided guidelines, called **Guideline 20**, for psychologists for older adults. Finally, the family of an elderly person may not want to acknowledge the problems because they may be afraid of hurting their feelings. Alzheimer's disease and other dementias are difficult for a family member to acknowledge because of knowing the end result of these diseases. It is important that the primary care provider, the family, and the patient work together to assess the elderly patient's mental status. Research estimates that over 60% of elderly patients do not receive treatment for mental health disorders (Kessler et al., 2006).

COMMON TYPES OF MENTAL DISORDERS IN THE ELDERLY

Depression and Dementia

Depression may strike more than 10% of the elderly population. It can imitate dementia because its victims withdraw, cannot focus, and appear confused at times. **Dementias**, which have symptoms of memory loss and confusion, are often considered a part of growing old—but they are not an inevitable part of the aging process. Only 15% of the elderly population suffers from dementia. Of that percentage, over 60% suffer from Alzheimer's disease, for which there is no cure as of this writing. Approximately 40% of dementias can be caused by conditions such as high blood pressure or a stroke or other diseases such as Parkinson and Huntington diseases, which are disorders that, in their advanced stages, can cause dementia (American Psychiatric Association, 2009).

Alzheimer's Disease

This disease causes the death of brain cells that control memory. The longer the person has **Alzheimer's disease**, the greater the memory loss as more cells die. One million people 65 years or older have severe Alzheimer's disease with approximately 2 million in the moderate stages of the disease (American Psychiatric Association, 2009).

Pseudo (False) Dementias

Pseudo dementias may develop as a result of medications, drug interactions, poor diet, or heart and gland diseases. These dementias may occur accidentally because of these conditions. Many elderly have multiple prescriptions so it is important to note any potential interactions that could result in dementia. Also, if the elderly person does not eat well and has poor nutrition, this habit could also cause dementia as well. It is important that family members or providers monitor the dietary habits of the elderly patient. Fortunately, because of the causes, most of these pseudo dementias are reversible if treated.

MENTAL HEALTH AND CULTURE, RACE, AND ETHNICITY

Mental health disorders occur across race and culture; however, according to NIMH, diverse communities are often underserved. Suicide is a particular issue among Native Americans. Minority cultures have fewer outpatient visits and less use of mental health specialists. African Americans are admitted to inpatient care at a higher rate than whites yet may not receive follow-up care. It is important to note that culture plays an important role on how diverse communities access health services. Any new immigrants to the United States may have language barriers. Asian Americans find that mental health services are stigmatizing and are therefore uncomfortable to access (Anderson et al., 2007).

US research has been based predominantly on White- and European-based populations and does not attempt to understand the importance of cultural beliefs in accessing mental health services. For example, African Americans can be distrustful of the medical system which is a reason they may not want follow-up care. They may also decide that they will seek spiritual guidance for help. The level of religious commitment is higher among African Americans who use prayer for stress relief. Also, community participation is important to them and so African Americans may turn to their community for assistance. As a result, there may be higher rates of disability resulting from mental disorders because of their lack of access to mental health care (American Indians and Native Alaskans may also have cultural beliefs that impact their access to mental health care). Unfortunately, substance abuse is prevalent in both cultures, which can impact mental health. Both cultures believe in both the modern medical care system and traditional healing techniques, which they will rely on first. Therefore, there may still be mistrust in the mental healthcare system. As a result, there may be less treatment for mental health disorders in both populations (US Public Health Service, 2009).

It is important to recognize the differences in cultural beliefs and adapt the system to recognize these value systems. Language barriers may also be a reason why minority cultures do not access the system. Hiring mental health counselors and providers that are from the same culture would be a first step in encouraging more culturally diverse individuals to use the system.

Women and Mental Health

Depression affects women significantly more than men—nearly twice as often as men. They tend to experience it earlier, longer, and more severely. Women many experience depression as a result of biologic and social reasons. **Premenstrual dysphoric disorder**, a severe disorder that relates depression and anxiety to menstruation, impacts between 3 and 5% of women. Women may also feel depressed as a result of infertility, miscarriage, and menopause. Married women suffer depression more than married men. The more children a woman has, the more likely they may suffer from depression.

Women who have been victims of sexual abuse or domestic violence may also suffer from depression.

As the baby boomer generation ages, there will be unique psychologic needs for older women (Smith, 2007). By the year 2030, as stated in previous chapters, 20% of the population will be 65 years or older. Per decade above 65 years of age, the proportion of women increases. Older women comprise the large majority of nursing home residents. Unfortunately, women in nursing homes do not often receive mental health care. Throughout their lives, women have been traditional caregivers. Women may provide up to 13 hours of care a day for more than 20 years for both physical and emotional illnesses (Bradley, 2003). As a result of this role, many elderly women experience more depression and anxiety. Unfortunately, research indicates that healthcare providers do not provide appropriate mental health care to a large majority of older females (Qualls, Segal, Norman, Niederehe, & Gallagher-Thomson, 2002).

The Homeless and Mental Health

There are approximately 3.5 million people in the United States who are homeless. The majority live in urban areas, over 20% live in suburban areas, and nearly 10% live in rural areas. Los Angeles has the largest homeless population in the United States. Approximately two thirds of the homeless population is single men, and 20% are women. Approximately 15% are parents with children. The majority of the homeless are between 25 and 44 years of age although this population is aging. Nearly 25% of the homeless are veterans. The homeless statistics may increase as a result of the recent housing crisis and downturn in the economy. The health status of the homeless is overall poor because of lack of housing. They are exposed to more disease and do not have adequate access to health care, thus their health status deteriorates over time. Mental health and substance abuse problems are common in the homeless population. Nearly 90% of the homeless population has experienced at least one mental health or substance abuse problem in their life—over 50% have a mental health problem. One third of homeless adults suffer from types of personality disorders. As a result of their lack of stability, it is difficult to provide adequate mental health care; however, recent statistics indicate that in the previous year, nearly 75% used some type of health services although less than 20% have used outpatient medical services (Pointer et al., 2007).

MENTAL HEALTH ISSUES AND DISASTERS, TRAUMA, AND LOSS

Disasters can impact communities and their citizens. Natural disasters can be natural, such as hurricanes, earthquakes, floods, and tornadoes, or manmade events such as the September 11, 2001, terrorist attacks or the wars in Iraq and Afghanistan. Many losses occur after any of these events such as the loss of family and loved ones, pets, neighbors, colleagues, and the community infrastructure such as schools, churches, and homes. These disasters may be short or long term. These events may impact individuals emotionally. They may experience fear and anxiety because of the uncertainty in their lives. According to the International Society for Traumatic Stress Studies (ISTSS), individuals may experience feels of shock, disbelief, grief, anger, guilt, helplessness, and emotional numbness. They may have difficulty with cognitive thinking and may experience physical reactions such as fatigue and illness (ISTSS, 2009). They may also have difficulty interacting with others. As with any mental health condition, it is important to reach out for assistance before the condition controls an individual's life.

Mental Health Impact of September 11, 2001, and Hurricane Katrina, August 2005

September 11, 2001

Terrorist attacks are different than natural disasters such as hurricanes, earthquakes, avalanches, or tornados because these attacks are deliberately aimed at harming populations. An evaluation of the federal emergency mental health program indicated that over 1 million New Yorkers received one or more face-to-face counseling or public education services as a result of the September 11 terrorist attacks (Neria et al., 2007). Interestingly, the emotional impact of the terrorist attacks was felt nationwide. The federal emergency preparedness model of the **Federal Emergency Management Agency** (FEMA) and the **Substance Abuse and Mental Health Services Administration** (SAMSHA), which is outlined in the chapter on public health, is helpful to victims with short-term mental health issues as a result of different types of disasters (Felton, 2004). The **American Psychological Association**

Task Force on Promoting Resilience in Response to Terrorism has produced fact sheets that are intended to provide information to psychologists assisting those target populations impacted by terrorist events (APA, 2009) However, those inflicted with long-term mental health issues as a result of these types of events are often not treated. The assumption is that the traditional healthcare system will treat those long-term mentally ill. However, as discussed previously, individuals who have long-term mental health issues feel stigmatized about seeking mental health services. Those individuals who have experienced traumatic events often feel uncomfortable because they feel that they should have recovered from the events without help.

Hurricane Katrina

Hurricane Katrina devastated nearly 90,000 square miles that were declared a natural disaster area. At least 1 million individuals, including 370,000 school-aged children, were displaced. Many were evacuated to throughout 46 states (Cook, 2006). Parents were very anxious because their homes were destroyed and had to start a new life elsewhere, which was not their choice. The Centers for Disease Control and Prevention (CDC) surveyed Hurricane Katrina survivors in October 2005 and found that 50% needed mental health services and 33% needed an intervention, with only 2% actually receiving assistance (Weisler, Barbee, & Townsend, 2006). Mental health providers reported grief, anxiety, and fear. This experience was magnified for survivors who had previous history of trauma and who suffered from mental health disorders. Long-term mental health care is needed for the survivors of Hurricane Katrina. It is critical that mental health issues be included in the health care of those impacted by events such as terrorist and natural disasters. Mental health issues do not only impact the survivors but also the providers of care to those survivors.

MENTAL HEALTH AND VETERANS

With nearly 155 hospitals serving nearly 8 million war veterans and current servicemen, the VA operates the largest healthcare system and is the largest single employer of psychologists in the country. In 1989, the National Center for Posttraumatic Stress Disorder was created within the VA to address the needs of the military-related PTSD (National Center for PTSD, 2009). Approximately 19% of veterans experience PTSD, a mental disorder that results from traumatic events in individuals' lives such as war, terrorism,

violence, and accidents. A 2004 survey study (Hoge et al., 2004) of 1709 Marines and soldiers deployed to Iraq and Afghanistan indicated that as many as 17% of these war veterans demonstrated symptoms of PTSD and depression. Of those individuals who met the criteria of a mental disorder, approximately 40% indicated they were interested in receiving help and only 25% indicated they have received help in the past year. Their reasons for not seeking help were because of the fear of being stigmatized for seeking these types of service. The Army, which has a longtime policy of requiring the commanding officer to be notified if a soldier voluntarily seeks counseling, is seeking to suspend this rule (Zoroya, 2009). This fear of stigmatization is similar in the general population. There are new military healthcare models to ensure that mental health services are being offered confidentially to allay these fears.

PRIVATE AND PUBLIC FUNDING FOR MENTAL HEALTH

Private insurance coverage for the mental health conditions and substance abuse or behavioral care is less generous than the coverage for traditional medical care. Many small companies do not offer mental health coverage. Employers routinely impose higher employee copayments and may limit outpatient visit reimbursement. The Mental Health Parity Act of 1996, enacted in 1998, provided the mental health field with more equity with health insurance coverage to ensure mental health services were being reimbursed on an equal level of traditional medical care.

Medicare and Medicaid are a large source of mental health funding, particularly for those individuals with serious mental disabilities who often cannot work. Medicaid is the single largest payer for state-financed mental health care (Shi & Singh, 2008). Medicare does impose a 50% copayment rate for outpatient services other than initial diagnoses and drug management. The normal copayment rate is 20% for traditional medical care (Anderson et al., 2007).

MANAGED BEHAVIORAL HEALTH CARE

Managed behavioral healthcare organizations (MBHOs), also known as behavioral healthcare carve outs, are specialized managed care organizations that focus on mental health services. MBHOs dominate private mental health coverage. Research has indicated that the MBHOs have reduced mental health treatment costs (Zuvekas, Rupp, & Norquist, 2008). The National Committee for Quality Assurance (NCQA) Managed Behavioral Health Accreditation Program provides information to employers, health plans, and consumers regarding quality MBHO programs. As the MBHO programs grew in the 1980s, there was a need for an accreditation program to set objective criteria for quality care. Currently, there are 300 MBHOs that serve 120 million US citizens. The NCQA program is designed to:

- Develop accountability measures for quality of care
- Provide employers and consumers with MBHO information
- Develop quality improvement MBHO programs
- Encourage coordination of behavioral care with medical care treatment

As of December 2008, there are 35 fully accredited MBHO programs by the NCQA (NCQA, 2008).

NATIONAL INSTITUTE FOR MENTAL HEALTH STRATEGIC PLAN

As the lead federal government agency on mental health, NIMH developed a long-term or strategic plan for mental health care in the United States. Revised in 2008, they identified four core areas of focus, which include:

- Research in mental health illness: to promote research in the behavioral sciences on the causes of mental health disorders
- Prevention and treatment: chart mental health illnesses over time to determine how to develop effective interventions
- Development of new interventions: develop interventions that incorporate the diverse needs and circumstances of the mentally ill
- Public health application to mental health interventions: provide funding that focuses on community-based mental health prevention (NIMH, 2008)

These strategic objectives will be the focus of NIHM over the next 5 years.

The Virginia Tech Massacre: A Case Study of the Mental Health System

On April 16, 2007, a senior Virginia Tech student, Seung Hui Cho—who had been diagnosed with and treated for severe anxiety disorders in middle school until his junior year of high school, had been accused of stalking two female students at Virginia Tech, had been declared mentally ill by a Virginia special justice, and was asked to seek counseling by at least one Virginia Tech professor—killed 32 people, students and professors. It was the worst school massacre in US history.

The Virginia Tech Review Panel was charged by Virginia Governor Kaine to review the mental health history of Cho. According to the Panel's findings, even as a young boy, Cho was extremely shy and often refused to speak. He was uncomfortable in his school surroundings and was often bullied. As a result of testing, he did receive counseling throughout middle and high school until he was 18 years of age. He had responded well to the counseling and did not want to continue the counseling so his parents allowed him to stop. When he decided to go to Virginia Tech, the school did not know of his mental health issues because of personal privacy issues. The **Family Educational Rights and Privacy Act of 1974** (FERPA) and the Americans with Disabilities Act (ADA) generally allow for special education records to be transferred to a higher education facility. However, the law prohibits a university from making an inquiry preadmission about an applicant's disability status. After a student's admission, they may make inquiries on a confidential basis. Cho could have made his disability known to the University but chose not to. Unfortunately, Virginia law allowed Cho to purchase a handgun without detection by the National Instant Criminal Background Check System (NCIS) (Virginia Tech Review Panel, 2007). As a result of this tragic event, a more stringent federal law was passed that strengthened the NCIS. The state mental health laws were also reviewed and recommendations were made to develop communication protocols to share mental health information between the University and mental health providers/facilities.

RECENT MENTAL HEALTHCARE EFFORTS

New Freedom Commission on Mental Health

In 2002, President George W. Bush established the **New Freedom Commission on Mental Health** that was charged with implementing an analytical study on the US mental health service system and developing recommendations to improve the public mental health system that could be implemented at the federal, state, and local levels. This was the first study performed since 1978 when President Jimmy Carter's Mental Health Commission's report.

In 2003, the Commission issued a final report that contained nearly 20 recommendations that focused primarily on mental illness recovery including a comprehensive approach to mental health care, including the screening of mental illness for children and other high-risk populations (APA, 2003).

The Mental Health Parity and Addiction Equity Act of 2008

This Act, included in the Emergency Economic Stabilization Act and signed into law on October 3, 2008, attempts to correct the inequities between general medical benefits and mental health and substance use disorders. The law requires that mental health benefit deductibles, covered hospital days, copayments, and mental health visits are equal to traditional medical care reimbursement (Lehmann, 2008). This law was passed because employer surveys indicated that nearly 90% of their healthcare plans limited the benefits compared to traditional healthcare benefits. This Act applies to employers with 51 or more members of a group health plan. This Act also includes those with self-insurance health plans who were previously exempt as a result of the Employee Retirement Income Security Act (ERISA). Unfortunately, the Act does not mandate mental health benefits be included in all healthcare plans; however, if mental health benefits are offered, they must be equitable to traditional healthcare benefits. This Act is effective as of January 2010 (Luongo, 2008).

ALTERNATIVE APPROACHES TO MENTAL HEALTH CARE

Alternative approaches to mental health care emphasize the relationships between the body, mind, and spirituality (Center for Mental Health Services, 2009). Established in 1992, the National Center for Complementary and Alternative Medicine at the National Institutes of Health evaluates different types of alternative therapies and treatments and whether to integrate them into traditional medicine culture. The following techniques are outlined in a fact sheet from the National Mental Health Information Center. The following is a discussion of the different types of treatment:

- **Self-help organizations:** Many mentally ill individuals often seek comfort in self-help organizations. They find solace with others who have experienced similar conditions. Many of them are nonprofit and are free of charge. They also provide education and support to the caregivers for those individuals who are mentally. Often, these organizations are anonymous because of the stigma attached to mental disorders.

- **Nutrition:** Some research has demonstrated that certain types of diets may assist with certain mental disorders. Eliminating wheat and milk products may alleviate the severity of symptoms of children with autism.

- **Pastoral counseling:** Mental health counselors have recognized that incorporating spiritual guidance with traditional medical care may alleviate mental disorder symptoms.

- **Animal-assisted therapies:** Animals are often used to increase socialization skills and encourage communication among the mentally ill. Integrating animals into individual's lives may alleviate some symptoms of the mental ill.

- **Art therapy:** Art activities such as drawing, painting, and sculpting may help people express their emotions and may help treat disorders such as depression. There are certificates in art therapy for this purpose.

- **Dance therapy:** Moving a body to music may help with those individuals recovering from physical abuse because the movement may help develop a sense of ease with their bodies.

- **Music therapy:** Research supports that music elevates a person's emotional moods. It has been used to treat depression, stress, and grief.

Culturally Based Healing Arts

Oriental and Native American medicine believe that wellness is a state of balance between the physical, spiritual, and emotional needs of an individual and that illness results as a result of an imbalance (Center for Mental Health Services, 2009). Their remedies focus on natural medicine, nutrition, exercise, and prayers to regain the balance.

Acupuncture is the Chinese practice of the insertion of needles in specific points of the body to balance the system. Acupuncture has been used to treat stress and anxiety, depression, ADHD in children, and physical ailments. Acupuncture is often used in conjunction with chiropractic medicine.

Ayurveda medicine incorporates diet, meditation, herbal medicine, and nutrition to treat depression and to release stress.

Yoga is an Indian system that uses breathing techniques, stretching, and meditation to balance the body. Yoga is offered at many athletic clubs and gyms and has become a popular mainstream form of exercise. It has been used for depression and anxiety.

Native American practices include ceremonial dances and baptismal rituals as part of Indian health. These dances and rituals are used to treat depression, stress, and substance abuse.

Relaxation and Stress Reduction Techniques

Biofeedback is a technique that focuses on learning to control heart rate and body temperature. This technique may be used in conjunction with medication to treat depression and schizophrenia. Biofeedback may used to control issues with stress and hyperventilation.

Visualization is when a patient creates a mental image of wellness and recovery. This may be used by traditional healthcare providers to treat substance abuse, panic disorders, and stress.

Massage therapy manipulates the body and its muscles and is used to release tension. It has been used to treat depression and stress.

Technology-based Applications

Technology aided development of electronic tools that can be used from home and increase access to isolated geographic areas.

Telemedicine is when providers and patients are connected using the Internet for communication for consultation. Those who are mentally ill living in rural areas, for example, have an opportunity to have access to providers.

Telephone counseling is an important part of mental health care. As stated previously, because of the stigma attached to receiving mental health services, individuals prefer to talk to a counselor on the telephone because they do not have to face anyone and do not have to tell anyone where they are going if they have an appointment in an office. Counselors receive training for telephone counseling. Like telemedicine, telephone counseling provides an opportunity for outreach for individuals who live in isolated locations.

The Internet, including email services (**electronic communication**), has provided an opportunity to increase an individual's exposure to knowledge regarding their condition. Consumer groups and medical Web sites can be accessed anonymously.

Radio psychiatry has been used in the United States for over 30 years. Radio psychologists and psychiatrists provide advice, information, and referrals to consumers. Both the APA and the American Psychiatric Association have issued guidelines for radio show programs that focus on mental health.

CONCLUSION

Mental health issues impact millions of US citizens. Mental health disabilities limit the life expectancy of individuals by 25 years. Treatment of mental health disorders have been traditionally underfunded because of attitude of the traditional healthcare system, confusion by health insurance companies, and fear by individuals who are mentally ill that they will be discriminated against because of their conditions. In 1999, Surgeon General David Satcher's report on mental health brought awareness to the issues with the US mental healthcare system. The Mental Health Parity Act of 1996 was an attempt to establish a fair system of treatment between mental health disorders and traditional healthcare conditions by mandating annual and lifetime limits to be equal between mental health care and traditional health care. President Bush's Freedom Commission on Mental Health focused on an analysis of the mental health system and recommendations to improve mental health care. The recent Mental Health Parity Act of 2008 further emphasized the need to ensure that mental health conditions in the United States are treated fairly by mandating that copayments, deductibles, hospital stays, and mental health visits were covered.

In a January 2008 *Nation's Review* commentary, state government has been applauded for mandating mental health parity. Although parity laws vary in their comprehensiveness, 30 states have passed mental health parity laws. Connecticut, Maryland, Minnesota, and Vermont have developed comprehensive parity laws. Connecticut and Vermont cover all of the mental illnesses identified in the DSM, which were identified previously in the chapter (Johnson, 2008). In a 2002 article, Wang, Demler, and Kessler performed a quantitative analysis of the US mental health system. Using data from the National Comorbidity Survey, results indicated that less than one in six people who had a serious mental health illness received care that was minimally adequate (Wang, Demler, & Kessler, 2002). The study also indicated that nearly 9 million mentally ill individuals received inadequate treatment on an annual basis. These statistics indicate that there is a dire need for the government to reassess the US mental healthcare system and to allocate funds to develop effective programs for the homeless, elderly, children, and other high-risk populations.

PREVIEW OF CHAPTER THIRTEEN

There have been many critics of the US healthcare system because of its cost and because it does not provide universal coverage to all of its citizens. The number of uninsured and underinsured continues to rise. This chapter will provide an overview of the US healthcare system, an international comparison of this system to other developed countries, and a discussion of whether universal coverage can be implemented here in the United States. There will also be a discussion of healthcare trends in the United States, including the impact of information technology on healthcare services.

VOCABULARY

Acupuncture

Alternative approaches to mental health care

Alzheimer's disease

American Psychiatric Association

American Psychological Association Task Force on Promoting Resilience in Response to Terrorism

Animal-assisted therapies

Antipsychotic medications

Art therapy

Attention deficit hyperactivity disorder (ADHD)

Ayurveda

Biofeedback

Conduct disorder

Dance therapy

De facto mental health service system

Dementia

Diagnostic and Statistical Manual of Mental Disorders

Dissociative disorders

Electronic Communication

Factitious disorders

Family Educational Rights and Privacy Act of 1974 (FERPA)

Federal Emergency Management Agency

Geropsychology

Guidelines 20

Hurricane Katrina

Impulse control disorders

Involuntary commitment

Managed behavioral healthcare organizations

Massage therapy

Mental disorders

Mental Health Parity Act of 1996

Mental Health Parity and Addiction Equity Act

Mood stabilizing medications

Moral treatment

Music therapy

National Center for Posttraumatic Stress Disorder

National Institute of Mental Health

Native American Practice

New Freedom Commission on Mental Health

Phobias

Posttraumatic stress disorder

Premenstrual dysphoric disorder

Pseudo dementias

Psychiatrists

Radio psychiatry

Substance Abuse and Mental Health Services Administration

Telemedicine

Telephone counseling

Visualization

Vocabulary

Voluntary commitment

Yoga

REFERENCES

Agency for Healthcare Research and Quality. (2009). Retrieved December 7, 2008, from http://www.ahrq.gov/research/feb02/0202RA8.htm.

American Psychiatric Association. (2009). Retreived November 9, 2009, from http://www.psych.org/MainMenu/Research/DSMIV.aspx.

American Psychological Association. (2003 July 22). Office of Public Affairs. American Psychological Association applauds final report of President's New Freedom Commission on Mental Health. *American Psychological Association Press Release*. Retrieved December 19, 2008, from http://www.apa.org/releases/mentalhealth_rpt.html.

American Psychological Association. (2004). Guidelines for psychological practice with older adults. *American Psychologist*, *59*, 4, 236–260.

American Psychological Association. (2009). Fostering resilience in response to terrorism: Fact sheets for psychologists. Retrieved November 9, 2009, from http://www.apa.org/psychologists/resilience.html.

Anderson, R., Rice, T., & Kominski, G. (2007). *Changing the U.S. Healthcare System* (pp. 439–479). San Francisco, CA: Jossey-Bass.

Bradley, P. (2003). Family caregiver assessment: Essential for effective home health care. *Journal of Gerontological Nursing*, *29*, 29–36.

Center for Mental Health Services. (2009). Alternative approaches to mental health care. Retrieved January 24, 2009, from http://mentalhealth.samhsa.gov/publications/allpubs/ken98-0044/default.asp.

Children and Adolescents with Mental, Emotional and Behavioral Disorders. (2009). Retrieved November 10, 2009, from http://mentalhealth.samhsa.gov/publications/allpubs/CA-0006/default.asp.

Cook, G. (2006). Schooling Katrina's kids. *American School Board Journal*, *193*, 18–26.

Everett, A., Mahler, J., Biblin, J., Ganguli, R., & Mauer, B. (2008). Improving the health of mental health consumers. *International Journal of Mental Health*, *37*, 2, 8–48.

Felton, C. (2004). Lessons learned since September 11 2001 concerning the mental health impact of terrorism, appropriate response strategies and future preparedness. *Psychiatry*, *67*, 2, 147–153.

Grob, G. (1983). *Mental illness and American society: 1875–1940*. Princeton, NJ: Princeton University Press.

Grob, G. (1994). *The mad among us: A history of the care of America's mentally ill*. New York: Free Press.

Hoge, C., Castro, C., Messer, S., McGurk, D., Cotting, D., & Koffman, R. (2004). Combat duty in Iraq and Afghanistan, mental health problems and barriers to care. *New England Journal of Medicine*, *351*, 1, 13–22.

International Society for Traumatic Stress Studies. (2009). Mass diasters, trauma, and loss. Retrieved January 4, 2009, from http://www.istss.org/resources/disaster_trauma_and_loss.cfm.

Johnson, T. (2008). Parity can reduce costs, improve access. *The Nation's Health*, December/January, 23.

Kessler, R. C., Chiu, W. T., Colpe, L., Demler, O., Merikangas, K. R., Walters, E. E., et al. (2006). The prevalence and correlates of serious mental illness (SMI) in the National Comorbidity Survey Replication (NCS-R). In Manderscheid, R. W., & Berry, J. T. (Eds.). *Mental health, United States, 2004* (DDHA Publication No. SMA-06-4195). Rockville, MD: Center for Mental Health Services.

Kessler, R. C., & Ustun, T. B. (2004). The World Mental Health (WMH) survey initiative version of the World Health Organization (WHO) composite international diagnostic interview (CIDI). *International Journal of Methods in Psychiatric Research*, *13*, 93–121.

Kochanek, K., Murphy, S., & Anderson, R. (2004). Deaths: Final data for 2002. *National Vital Statistics Reports*, *53*, 5, 1–115.

Lehmann, R. (2008). Bailout sweet-tart: Mental health parity. *Best's Review*, *109*, 7, 12.

Luongo, T. (2008). The Mental Health Parity and Addiction Equity Act of 2008: Equal footing for those suffering from mental health and addition disorders. Retrieved January 22, 2009, from http://www.hrtutor.com/en/news_rss/articles/2008/12-02-Mental-Health-Parity-and-Addiction-Equity-Act-of-2008.aspx.

National Center for Posttraumatic Stress Disorder. (2009). Retrieved December 22, 2008, from http://www.ptsd.va.gov/about/mission/history_of_the_national_center_for_ptsd.asp.

National Committee for Quality Assurance. (2008). Report card for managed behavioral healthcare organizations. Retrieved December 19, 2008, from http://hprc.ncqa.org/mbho/Results.asp.

National Institute of Mental Health. (2009). Child and adolescent mental health. Retrieved November 5, 2009, from http://www.nimh.nih.gov/health/topics/child-and-adolescent-mental-health/index.shtml.

National Institute of Mental Health. (2008). The National Institute of Mental Health strategic plan. Retrieved December 19, 2008, from http://www.nimh.nih.gov/about/strategic-planning-reports/index.shtml.

Neria, Y., Gross, R., Litz, B., Maguen, S., Insel, B., Seirmarco, G., et al. (2007). Prevalence and psychological correlates of complicated grief among bereaved adults 2.5–3.5 years after September 11 attacks. *Journal of Traumatic Stress*, *20*, 3, 251–262.

Pointer, D., Williams, S., Isaacs, S., & Knickman, J. (2007). *Introduction to U.S. health care*. Hoboken, NJ: Wiley Publishing.

Qualls, S., Segal, D., Norman, D., Niederehe, G., & Gallagher-Thomson, D. (2002). Psychologists in practice with older adults: Current patterns, sources of training, and need for continuing education. *Professional Psychology: Research and Practice*, *33*, 435–442.

Regier, D., Narrow, W., Rae, D., Manderscheid, R., Locke, B., & Goodwin, F. (1993). The de facto US mental and addictive disorders service system. Epidemiologic catchment area prospective 1-year prevalence rates of disorders and services. *Archives of General Psychiatry*, *50*, 85–94.

Shi, L., & Singh, D. (2008). *Essentials of the U.S. health care delivery system*. Sudbury, MA: Jones and Bartlett.

Smith, H. (2007). Psychological service needs of older women. *Psychological Services*, *4*, 277–286.

Sultz, H., & Young, K. (2006). *Health care USA: Understanding its organization and delivery* (5th ed.). Sudbury, MA: Jones and Bartlett.

US Public Health Service. (1999). Mental Health: A Report of the Surgeon General. Retrieved November 5, 2009, from http://mentalhealth.samhsa.gov/features/surgeongeneralreport/chapter2/sec7.asp.

Virginia Tech Review Panel. (2007). *Mass shootings at Virginia Tech: Report of the Review Panel presented to Governor Kaine, Commonwealth of Virginia*. Retrieved December 22, 2008, from http://www.governor.virginia.gov/TempContent/techPanelReport.cfm.

Wang, P., Demler, O., & Kessler, R. (2002). Adequacy for treatment for serious mental illness in the United States. *American Journal of Public Health*, *92*, 92–98.

Weisler, R., Barbee, J., & Townsend, M. (2006). Mental health and recovery in the Gulf Coast after Hurricanes Katrina and Rita. *Journal of the American Medical Association*, *296*, 585–588.

Woody, R. (2008). Obtaining legal counsel for child and family mental health practice. *The American Journal of Family Therapy*, *36*, 323–331.

Zoroya, G. (2009). Army aims to get more GIs help. *USA Today*, January 12, 2009.

Zuvekas, S., Rupp, A., & Norquist, G. (2008). The impacts of mental health parity and managed care in one large employer group: A reexamination. *Health Affairs*, *24*, 1668–1671.

CROSSWORD PUZZLE

Instructions: Please complete the puzzle using the vocabulary words found in the chapter. There may be multiple-word answers. The number in the parenthesis indicates the number of words in the answers.

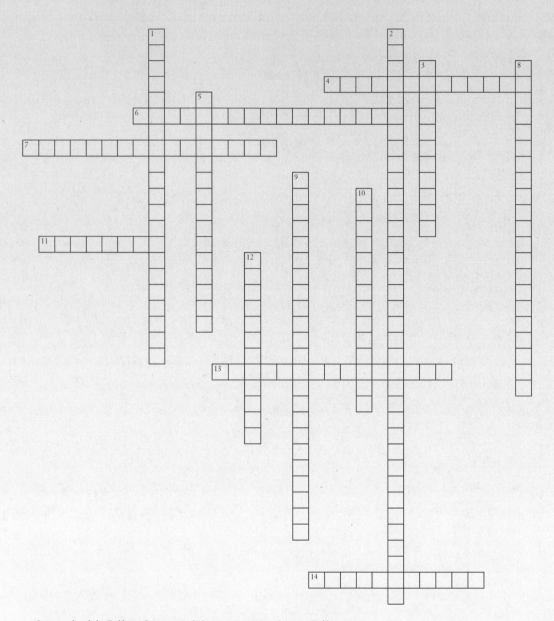

Created with EclipseCrossword © 1999–2009 Green Eclipse

STUDENT ACTIVITY 12-1

Across

4. The patient creates a mental image of wellness and recovery. (1 word)

6. This condition causes brain cells that control memory to die. (2 words)

7. This 2005 natural disaster devastated nearly 90,000 square miles in the southern part of the United States. (2 words)

11. This type of medicine focuses on diet, meditation, and herbal medicine to treat depression. (1 word)

13. These disorders develop as a result of poor diet, medication, or drug interactions. (2 words)

14. This Chinese practice inserts needles in specific points of the body to balance the system. (1 word)

Down

1. This act was passed in 1996 to ensure that there was equity in providing both mental health and traditional healthcare benefits in health insurance plans. (4 words)

2. These are managed care organizations that focus on mental health care. (4 words)

3. This type of technique focuses on learning to control heart rate and respiration. (1 word)

5. Conditions that alter thinking, moods, or thought processes that impact daily living. (2 words)

8. This type of therapy may bring dogs to the mentally ill to encourage communication. (3 words)

9. Gambling addiction or obsession of fire are examples of these disorders. (3 words)

10. The mentally ill were treated sensitively in Europe in the 19th century with success using this type of treatment. (2 words)

12. This type of therapy elevates people's moods and may be used to treat depression. (2 words)

STUDENT ACTIVITY 12-2

IN YOUR OWN WORDS

Based on Chapter 12, please provide a definition of the following vocabulary words in your own words. DO NOT RECITE the text definition.

Posttraumatic stress disorder:

_____

_____

_____

Mental disorders:

_____

_____

_____

Moral treatment approach:

_____

_____

_____

Factitious disorders:

_____

_____

_____

Dissociative disorders:

_____

_____

_____

Attention deficit hyperactivity disorder:

_____

_____

_____

Psychiatrists:

_____

_____

_____

New Freedom Commission on Mental Health:

_____

_____

_____

The Family Educational Rights and Privacy Act:

_____

_____

_____

Ayurveda:

_____

_____

_____

STUDENT ACTIVITY 12-3

REAL LIFE APPLICATIONS: CASE STUDY

You have been concerned about your grandmother recently. She has become forgetful. Yesterday, she left the stove on when she went out to the grocery store. Your grandfather has been chronically ill for years and she is his main caregiver. She regularly visits her primary care provider who has told her that it is nothing more than old age. You decide to research mental health issues and the elderly and have found very interesting statistics about the elderly and mental health, particularly women.

ACTIVITY

(1) Provide three statistics about mental health issues in the elderly, (2) discuss four reasons why mental health issues are not addressed with the elderly, and (3) discuss three reasons why elderly women may be at higher risk for mental disorders.

RESPONSES

_____

_____

_____

_____

_____

_____

_____

_____

_____

_____

_____

_____

_____

_____

_____

_____

_____

_____

STUDENT ACTIVITY 12-4

INTERNET EXERCISES

Write your answers in the space provided.

- Visit each of the Web sites listed here.
- Name the organization.
- Locate their mission statement on their Web site.
- Provide a brief overview of the activities of the organization.
- How do these organizations participate in the US healthcare system?

Web Sites

http://www.apa.gov

Organization Name:

_____

Mission Statement:

_____

_____

_____

Overview of Activities:

_____

_____

_____

Importance of organization to US health care:

_____

_____

_____

http://www.samhsa.gov

Organization Name:

_____

Mission Statement:

_____

_____

Overview of Activities:

_____

_____

_____

STUDENT ACTIVITY 12-4

Importance of organization to US health care:

_____

_____

_____

http://www.istss.org

Organization Name:

_____

Mission Statement:

_____

_____

_____

Overview of Activities:

_____

_____

_____

Importance of organization to US health care:

_____

_____

_____

http://www.psych.org

Organization Name:

_____

Mission Statement:

_____

_____

_____

Overview of Activities:

_____

_____

_____

Importance of organization to US health care:

_____

_____

_____

STUDENT ACTIVITY 12-4

http://www.nimh.nih.gov

Organization Name:

_____

Mission Statement:

_____

_____

_____

Overview of Activities:

_____

_____

_____

Importance of organization to US health care:

_____

_____

_____

http:// www.aaom.org

Organization Name:

_____

Mission Statement:

_____

_____

_____

Overview of Activities:

_____

_____

_____

Importance of organization to US health care:

_____

_____

_____

Analysis of the US Healthcare System

LEARNING OBJECTIVES

The student will be able to:

- Discuss the cost efficiency of e-prescribing.

- Describe the universal healthcare systems of Massachusetts and San Francisco, California.

- Describe the major components of the healthcare delivery systems of Japan, France, and Switzerland.

- Discuss the Green House project and its potential importance to long-term care.

- Assess the pros and cons of a pay-for-performance (P4P) healthcare system.

- Evaluate the differences between the types of universal health coverage programs.

DID YOU KNOW THAT?

- More than 7000 medication-related deaths occur each year as a result of incompatible drug interactions and drug allergies. These deaths are caused by illegible handwritten prescriptions and because the healthcare provider is unaware of patient allergies.

- In April 2006, the state of Massachusetts passed legislation to implement a type of universal healthcare coverage for their residents.

- Robotic hands used in surgery are so sensitive that they can easily peel a grape or thread a needle.

- Second only to the United States, Switzerland spends the largest portion of its gross domestic product on health care.

- California operates the largest P4P healthcare program in the United States.

INTRODUCTION

As discussed in the previous 12 chapters of this text, it is apparent that the US healthcare system is very complex. The US healthcare system has long been recognized as providing state-of-the-art health care. It has also been recognized as the most expensive healthcare system in the world and the price tag is expected to increase. Despite offering two large public programs—Medicare and Medicaid for the elderly, indigent, and disabled—current statistics indicate that nearly 47 million individuals are uninsured. This number is expected to increase because of the recession. Experts indicate that there needs to be a healthcare reform policy to rectify some of these major issues to improve the US healthcare system.

This chapter will provide an international comparison between the US healthcare system and the healthcare systems of other countries and discuss whether universal healthcare coverage should be implemented in the United States. This chapter will also discuss US healthcare trends that may positively impact the healthcare system, including the increased use of technology in prescribing medicine and providing health care, complementary and alternative medicine use, a nursing home model, P4P health care, and a discussion of the newly implemented universal healthcare coverage programs in Massachusetts and San Francisco, California.

HIGHLIGHTS OF THE US HEALTHCARE SYSTEM

The US healthcare system is a complicated system that is comprised of both public and private resources. Health care is available to those individuals who have health insurance or are entitled to health care through a public program. I think of the healthcare system as several concentric circles that surround the most important circle—the healthcare consumers and providers. Immediately surrounding this relationship is the circle that contains healthcare insurance companies and government programs, healthcare facilities, pharmaceutical companies, and laboratories that all provide services to the consumer to ensure that they receive quality health care and support the provider to ensure that they are able to provide quality health care. The next circle consists of peripheral stakeholders that do not immediately impact that main relationship but are still important to the industry: professional associations, research organizations, and medical and training facilities.

GOVERNMENT'S ROLE

The federal government plays an important role in the healthcare system; it provides funding and policy that are implemented at the state and local government levels. Federal healthcare regulations are implemented at the state and local levels and are enforced at these levels. Primarily, funding is distributed from the federal government to the state government, which consequently allocates funding to their local health departments. Local health departments provide the majority of services for their constituents. More local health departments are working with physicians to increase their ability to provide services such as immunizations, education, and prevention to local organizations such as schools.

PUBLIC HEALTH

For the past 7 years, public health has received increased publicity because of the terrorist attacks in 2001, the anthrax attacks against the postal service, the natural disaster of Hurricane Katrina, and, most recently, the flooding in the Midwest. Funding has increased for public health activities because of these events and the concept of bioterrorism is now a topic of conversation. Because public health is now considered an integral component in battling terrorism and, consequently, a matter of national security, federal funding has dramatically increased. Since 2002, the federal budget for public health activities at all government levels has increased by $2 billion with continued funding expected (Turncock, 2007). However, in order to continue to receive increased funding levels, it is important that public health markets itself to both the policy makers and the public so they understand the increased importance of public health's role in national security.

OUTPATIENT SERVICES

The healthcare industry has recognized that outpatient services are a cost-effective method of providing quality health care. This type of service is the preferred method of receiving health care by the consumer. In 2004, there were over 900 million visits to doctor's offices, which is the traditional method of ambulatory care (Shi & Singh, 2008). However, as medicine has evolved and more procedures can be performed on an outpatient basis such as surgeries, different types of outpatient care have evolved. As discussed previously, there are more outpatient surgical centers, imaging centers, urgent/emergent care centers, and other services that used to be offered on an inpatient basis and there will continue to be an increase in outpatient services being offered. The implementation of the patient's electronic health record (EHR) nationwide will be the impetus for the development of more electronic healthcare services being offered.

HEALTHCARE PERSONNEL

Healthcare personnel represent one of the largest labor forces in the United States. There are more than 200 occupations and professions among the 13 million healthcare workers (Sultz & Young, 2006). The healthcare industry will continue to evolve as the following trends in the United States change: demographics, disease and public health patterns, cost and efficiency issues, insurance issues, technological influences, and economic factors. More occupations and professions will develop as a result of these trends. The major trend to impact the future of the US healthcare industry will be the growth of its aging population. The **Bureau of Labor Statistics (BLS)** predicts that half of the next decade's fastest growing jobs will be in the healthcare industry (BLS, 2009). In December 2008, the US economy was in a recession where millions of its citizens lost their jobs. The loss of these jobs most likely included the loss of health insurance coverage supplied by employers. The number of uninsured and underinsured will continue to rise and healthcare facilities may need to provide more charitable care, reducing the profits of their organizations. Government programs that provide healthcare benefits will be maximized and overloaded because this economic trend will place a huge burden on the healthcare industry. Healthcare personnel may be overworked because of the state of the economy. As healthcare costs continue to increase, cost-cutting measures will be the focus while continuing to provide quality health care.

HEALTHCARE EXPENDITURES

As healthcare expenditures continue to increase, the major focus of the healthcare industry is cost control, in both the public and private sectors. For years, healthcare costs were unchecked. The concept of retrospective reimbursement methods (when a provider submitted a bill for healthcare services to a health insurance company and was automatically reimbursed) gave healthcare insurers no incentive to control costs in health care. This type of reimbursement method contributed to expensive health care for both the healthcare insurance companies and the individual who was paying out-of-pocket for services. As a result, the establishment of prospective reimbursement system for Medicare (reimbursement is based on care criteria for certain conditions, regardless of providers' costs) became an incentive for providers to manage how they were providing services.

MANAGED CARE

The managed care model for healthcare delivery was developed for the primary purpose of containing healthcare costs. By administering both the healthcare services and the reimbursement of these services, and therefore eliminating a third-party health insurer, the industry felt that this model would be very cost-effective. The consumer's (or patient) and the physician's concerns were the same—worry about providing quality care while focusing predominantly on cost. The consumer was also worried about loss of freedom of choice of their primary care provider. The physician was worried about loss of income.

As managed care evolved, managed care organizations (MCOs) were developed, which allowed more choice for both the consumer and the physician. Eventually, there were models such as preferred provider organizations (PPOs) and point-of-service plans (POPs) that allowed a consumer to more freely choose their provider; however, there was a financial disincentive to use a provider outside the network of the MCO. The provider was also able to see non-MCO patients, which increased their income, but also received a financial deterrent because any MCO patient was given health care at a discounted rate.

INFORMATION TECHNOLOGY

The healthcare industry has lagged behind in utilizing information technology as a form of communicating important data across healthcare systems nationally. Even so, there have been specific applications of information technology, such as e-prescribing, telemedicine, e health, and specific applied technology (i.e., Intellifinger, Docketscanner, the Phreesia Pad, Accuson P210, and the PiccoloXpress), that are excellent advances in medicine. Healthcare organizations have recognized the importance of information technology and have hired chief information officers and chief technology officers to manage their data. However, the healthcare industry must embrace the need to implement an electronic patient record across all of its health systems. This will enable patients to be treated effectively and efficiently anywhere in the nation. Having the ability to access patients' health records would assist in reducing medical errors.

HEALTHCARE LAW

As both a healthcare manager and healthcare consumer, it is imperative that you are familiar with the different federal and state laws that impact the healthcare industry. It is also important that you understand the differences between civil and criminal law and the penalties that may be imposed. Both federal and state laws have been enacted and policy has been implemented to protect both the healthcare provider and the healthcare consumer. New laws have been passed and older laws have been amended to reflect needed changes regarding health care to continue to protect its participants.

Despite these efforts, access to health care still remains a problem. US citizens continue to experience some of the poorest health outcomes in the industrialized world. It is the responsibility of the government and policy makers, clinicians, and researchers to become involved in progress of developing a systematic healthcare transformation in order to improve the health outcomes in this country. As discussed in Chapter 4, the goal of Healthy People 2010 is to improve the quality of life and to eliminate health disparities among different segments of the population. These goals must be supported by lawmakers to ensure that at least a minimum standard is established to ensure that health justice is achieved (Department of Health and Human Services [HHS], 2000).

HEALTHCARE ETHICS

There are several ethical issues involving the healthcare industry and its stakeholders. There are two components of ethics in health care: medical ethics, which focus on the treatment of the patient, and bioethics, which focus on technology and how it is utilized in health care. The most important stakeholder in health care is the patient. The most important relationship with this stakeholder is the physician. Their relationship is impacted by the other stakeholders in the industry including the government that regulates healthcare provider activities, the insurance companies that interacts with both provider and patient, and healthcare facilities, such as hospitals or managed care facilities, where the physician has a relationship. All of these stakeholders can influence how a physician interacts with the patient because they have an interest in the outcome. For that reason, many organizations that represent these stakeholders have developed codes of ethics so individuals are provided guidance for ethical behavior. Codes of ethics for the physicians, nurses, pharmaceutical companies, and medical equipment companies emphasize how these stakeholders should interact with both the healthcare providers and patients.

It is also necessary to discuss ethics as it relates to our healthcare system. With 47 million uninsured citizens in the United States, is it unethical that there is no universal healthcare system? The United States is the only industrialized nation, with the exception of South Africa, that has no universal healthcare coverage. Other nations have stated that health care is a right not a privilege. Is it unethical for the United States to have a system that does not provide health care for all citizens? This text cannot provide answers to ethical situations because ethics is viewed differently by individuals. This textbook can only provide questions for the reader so they can assess their ethical viewpoint as it relates to the healthcare industry.

MENTAL HEALTH

A difficult issue for the healthcare system is mental health illness. Mental health issues impact millions of US citizens. Mental health disabilities limit the life expectancy of individuals by 25 years. The treatments for mental health disorders have been traditionally underfunded because of the attitude of the traditional healthcare system, confusion by health insurance companies, and fear by individuals who are mentally ill that they will be discriminated against because of their conditions. In 1999, Surgeon General David Satcher's report on mental health brought awareness to the issues of the US mental healthcare system. The Mental Health Parity Act of 1996 was an attempt to establish a fair system of treatment between mental health disorders and traditional healthcare conditions by mandating annual and lifetime limits to be equal between mental health care and traditional health care. President Bush's Freedom Commission on Mental Health focused on an analysis of the mental health system and recommendations to improve mental health care. The recent Mental Health Parity Act of 2008 further emphasized the need to ensure that mental health conditions in the United States are treated fairly by mandating that copayments, deductibles, hospital stays, and mental health visits be covered.

TRENDS IN HEALTH CARE
Complementary and Alternative Medicine

Complementary and alternative medicine (CAM) is a group of diverse medical care practices that are not considered part of traditional medicine. Examples of CAM include acupuncture, chiropractic manipulation, diet therapies, meditation, natural products (e.g., flaxseed and fish oil), yoga, and massage. Complementary medicine is used in conjunction with traditional medicine, and alternative medicine is used in place of traditional medicine. In 2007, approximately 38% of adults used CAM. CAM use is more predominant in females and those individuals with higher education and income. The National Center for Health's 2007 statistics indicate that back pain was the most common reason people used CAM (National Center for Complementary and Alternative Medicine, 2009). However, as more people lose their health insurance because of unemployment, there will most likely be a rise in CAM use because it is less costly. US consumers spend an average of $34 billion on CAM. A 2005 study analyzed the cost-effectiveness of CAM therapies. Results indicated that the following were cost-effective compared to the usual traditional care for the following conditions: acupuncture of migraine headaches, manual therapy for neck pain, spa therapy for Parkinson disease, complementary relaxation therapy for patients with cardiac issues, and complementary pre- and postoperative nutritional supplements for lower gastrointestinal surgery (Herman, Craig, & Caspi, 2005). It is anticipated that more CAM therapies, particularly alternative medicine therapies, will be used because of the rising cost of health care and the increasing number of uninsured.

Nursing Home Trends

In 2001, the Robert Wood Johnson Foundation funded a pilot project developed by Dr. Bill Thomas, the **Green House Project**, which is a unique type of nursing home that focuses on creating a residence that provides services but also focuses on the concept of being a home to the residents not an institution where they receive care. It alters the size of the facility, the physical environment, and delivery of services (Fine, 2009).

The home is managed by a team of workers who share the care of the residents, including the cooking and housekeeping. The daily staff members are certified nursing assistants (CNAs). All mandated professional personnel, such as physicians, nurses, social workers, and dieticians, form visiting clinical support teams that assess the **elders** and supervise their care (Kane, Lum, Cutler, Degenholtz, & Yu, 2007).

The residents can eat their meals when they choose. The word "patient" is not used; all residents are called "elders." The Green House is designed for 6 to 10 elders. Each resident has a private room and private bathroom. The elder rooms have lots of sunlight and are located near the kitchen and dining areas. There are patios and gardens for elders and staff to enjoy.

Although these new types of nursing homes look like a residential home, they adhere to all long-term housing requirements. It looks like other homes in their designated neighborhood (Fine, 2009).

Residents can also have their own pets, which are not allowed in traditional nursing homes. According to a recent study performed by the University of Minnesota, the residents of the Green House are able to perform their activities of daily living longer and are less depressed than residents of traditional nursing homes and are able to be self-sufficient longer than residents from traditional nursing homes. The staff also enjoy working at the Green House. There is less staff turnover (Kane et al., 2007).

The first Green House was constructed in Tupelo, Mississippi. There are now 18 homes nationwide. Dr. Thomas eventually partnered with NCB Capital Impact, which is a not-for-profit organization that provides financial assistance to underserved communities. The NCB Capital Impact has a loan program that provides financial assistance up to $125,000 to support engineering, architectural, and other expenses for a selected Green House site. The borrower must contribute 25% of the loan amount (NCB Capital Impact, 2009).

Pay-for-Performance Health Care

Pay-for-performance (P4P) or **value-based purchasing** (VBP) are terms that describe healthcare payment systems that reward healthcare providers for their efficiency, which is defined as providing higher quality care for less cost. From a healthcare consumer's perspective, these stakeholders should hold healthcare providers accountable for both the cost and high quality of their care. Since most health care in the United States has been historically provided by employers, in VBP, employers should select healthcare plans based on demonstrated performance of quality and cost-effective health care (Agency for Healthcare Research and Quality [AHRQ], 2009). For the past decade, the Centers for Medicare and Medicaid Services (CMS) has been collaborating with the National Quality Forum, The Joint Commission, the National Committee for Quality Assurance, AHRQ, and the American Medical Association to implement initiatives to assess P4P systems nationwide. Despite national recommendations and successful programs that have been implemented nationwide, these efforts remain experimental because of lack of empirical evidence (Damberg, Raube, Teleki, & dela Cruz, 2009).

For example, California's **Integrated Healthcare Association's** (IHA) P4P program, started in 2003, has operated the largest experimental program nationally. The program targets 225 medical groups representing 35,000 physicians that contracted with the 7 largest health maintenance organizations (HMOs) and P4Ps in the state, which have 6.2 million enrollees. The IHA scored physician care based on the healthcare effectiveness data and information measures and paid performance-based payments. Results indicated that 25 of the physician organizations felt that the P4P positively impacted behavior by focusing on quality accountability, 21 physician groups hired more staff to capture data to demonstrate their results, and 29 of the groups modified incentives to increase physician quality activities (Damberg et al., 2009). However, despite these positive results, there were no major breakthrough improvements in quality. Questions regarding the amount and type of incentives need to be reevaluated. Also, the type of quality indicators may also need to be reevaluated. The concept of P4P is a valid concept for health care. As more experimental programs are evaluated, lessons that were learned from the first round of experimental programs must be taken into account. Although, despite these efforts, employers seldom use this type of information when selecting benefits for their workers. A recent telephone interview of 609 employers in 41 markets, which represented 78% of US urban population, indicated that premium rates and geographic coverage motivated their decisions. Despite these issues, *Futurescan: Healthcare Trends and Implications* 2006–2011 survey indicates that P4P may be more commonplace (Rosenthal et al., 2007).

Electronic Prescribing

E-prescribing developed as a result of the Medicare Prescription Drug, Improvement and Modernization Act. Part D, which authorized a drug prescription program for enrollees, also supported a voluntary electronic prescription program for providers. It also called for the adoption of technical standards to develop a system that would support e-prescribing. This electronic system would enable physicians to check the ingredients of the drugs which would enable an increased use of generic drugs because they could automatically compare the drug ingredients to brand name prescription drugs (Friedman, Schueth, & Bell, 2009). E-prescribing is not only more efficient, it enhances patient safety. More than 7000 medication-related deaths occur each year as a result of incompatible drug interactions and drug allergies. These deaths are because of illegible handwritten prescriptions and because the healthcare provider is unaware of patient allergies. E-prescriptions are immediately notified about patient-specific drug allergies and potential drug interactions (Brunetti & Jay, 2009).

A recent study of Massachusetts physicians who e-prescribed indicated that being able to provide more generic drugs could save both the consumer and health insurance companies, which could result in a savings of $845,000 per 100,000 patients annually (Fischer et al., 2008). In January 2009, Medicare and some private healthcare plans began paying a bonus to physicians who e-prescribe to their Medicare patients. Medicare will also penalize physicians who do not e-prescribe by 2012 by reducing their reimbursement rates by 1% (CMS, 2009). E-prescribing use will continue to increase because of the Medicare mandate and because more health insurance companies recognize the cost savings in e-prescribing. In April 2009, CVS Caremark and Horizon Blue Cross Blue Shield of New Jersey announced that, since 2004, both companies had processed 5.5 million electronic prescriptions. This was one of the largest single-payer e-prescribing initiatives in the country (Alexander & Frederick, 2009).

Telemedicine

Telemedicine refers to the use of information technology to enable healthcare providers to communicate with rural care providers regarding patient care or to communicate directly with patients regarding treatment. The basic form of telemedicine is a telephone consultation. Telemedicine is most frequently used in pathology and radiology because images can be transmitted to a distant location where a specialist will read the results. Telemedicine is becoming more common because it increases healthcare access to remote locations such as rural areas. It also is a cost-effective mode of treatment. Currently, more than 1.5 million Americans have access to a telephonic medical consultation and significant growth is projected as more Americans utilize cell phones. It is also possible that employers and health plans recognize the potential to improve access to medical care while reducing medical costs (Gingrich, Boxer, & Brooks, 2008). An example of telemedicine can be found at http://www.SwiftMD.com, which provides electronic consulting by experienced board-certified physicians who are trained in emergency medicine and who are also trained in telemedicine. Enrollees pay a low monthly fee ($18) and a fee for a consult (currently $55) from one of the physicians. However, telemedicine may not be appropriate for emergency conditions or conditions that require seeing a specialist. But for routine medical care, it may be a cost-effective method. This type of consumer-centric approach may become more popular.

Robotic Surgery

Robots were first introduced as a surgical tool in 1987. **Robotic surgery** is a type of minimally invasive surgery (MIS) that it is less invasive than traditional surgery—there are smaller incisions, which reduces the risk of infection, shortens hospital stays, and reduces recuperation times. Surgeons manipulate robotic arms to perform surgeries normally performed by human hands. Surgeons have to be trained in robotic surgery and use a machine that will reduce the possibility of errors caused by tremors in the surgeons' hands.

As robotic surgery became more popular, National Aeronautic and Space Administration (NASA) developed the concept of **telesurgery**, which combines virtual reality, robots, and medicine. The US Army also became involved in robotic surgery because they were interested in bringing surgery to the soldiers who were fighting and needed surgery immediately. They hoped robotic surgery would reduce war mortality rates. It is important to note that there are also other tools that can be used for MIS. Studies have indicated that some procedures such as an appendectomy show very little difference if performed by the traditional method or the robotic method. However, robotic surgeries performed on the prostate have shown significant positive outcomes (Guidarelli, 2006; Loisance, 2007).

The robotic system that has dominated the current market is the **da Vinci Surgical System**, which was developed by Intuitive Surgical of Sunnyvale, California. It is used in areas of cardiac, urologic, gynecologic, and general surgery. This tool was used for 1500 cases in the year 2000, but use increased to 20,000 cases in 2004. The initial investment for a da Vinci system is $1.5 million, with an annual upkeep of $100,000 (Intuitive Surgical, Inc., 2009). Despite the initial cost, experts feel that the actual procedure is cost-effective because recuperation time is far less for the patients. Medical students will also have an opportunity to be trained in a fellowship once their initial training has been completed. Indications are that robotic surgery will continue to evolve as a surgical tool. As with any technological advances, the

costs should decrease and the tool will become more advanced and more efficient.

INTERNATIONAL HEALTHCARE SYSTEMS

For years, there has been a movement toward healthcare reform in the United States because many feel that because the United States is so powerful and wealthy, compared to the rest of the world, we should not have nearly 50 million uninsured citizens. However, universal healthcare coverage may not be the answer. It, too, has problems.

There is continued controversy over the expense of the US healthcare system. If we spend so much of our gross domestic product on health care, why are there geographic disparities on who receives it? This results in lower health indicators of the United States, such as life expectancy and infant mortality rates, compared to the rest of the world. Although the United States can provide state-of-the-art health care, we are reminded of the Institute of Medicine report that estimates 44,000–90,000 annual deaths are a result of medical errors (Kohn, Corrigan, & Donaldson, 1999). As with any large system, there are system errors that were just outlined. The United States is not the only country with a healthcare system that has problems. Using the Organisation for Economic Co-operation and Development (OECD) data from Chapter 2, I have selected Japan, France, and Switzerland as having outranked the United States in healthcare indicators. These analyses will demonstrate that although these countries offer a type of universal healthcare coverage, they also have problems.

UNIVERSAL HEALTHCARE CONCEPTS

Countries with national healthcare programs provide universal access to health care to all citizens. They have a **single-payer system** which means the government pays for the healthcare services. There are three models for structuring a universal or national healthcare system: national health insurance, national health system, and socialized health insurance. **National health insurance**, as in Canada, is funded by the government through general taxes although the delivery of care is by private providers. In a **national health system**, as in Great Britain, taxes support the system but the government also manages the infrastructure for healthcare delivery. In a **socialized health insurance system**, as in Germany, the government mandates financial contributions by both the employer and employee with private providers delivering health care. Sickness funds, which are not-for-profit insurance companies, collect the contributions and pay the healthcare providers (Shi & Singh, 2008). The US healthcare system is employer–employee based and government funded. The US system provides 100% coverage of people older than 65 years of age with the Medicare program, and 82% coverage for people younger than 65 years of age through employer-based insurance, Medicaid, Indian Health Services, Veterans' Administration (TRICARE), and the federal government employee program. In Chapter 2, the US health status was compared to several countries that participate in the OECD. The following OECD countries that had better health status indicators than the United States will be discussed: Japan, France, and Switzerland.

Japan

Similar to Germany's socialized health insurance system, Japan's healthcare system centers on mandatory employment-based insurance. Health spending is 8% of their gross domestic product. Japan has universal coverage which is comprehensive, including dental and prescription drug coverage. Average annual spending per person is $2358, which breaks down as $1927 from government funds, $71 from private insurance, and $360 out of pocket by consumers. With the graying of their population, approximately 90% of Japan's healthcare costs are the result of the elderly utilization of the healthcare system. It is anticipated that Japan will triple government spending on health care in the next 20 years (NPR News, 2008; OECD, 2009).

There is compulsory employer–employee financed national health insurance and a government-paid program for people older than 70 years of age, the indigent, and small businesses. Most large employers, who have 700 or more employees, have their own health programs similar to large US companies that have self-insured programs. The employers and employees are each required to pay 4% of the salary to a nonprofit, community-based insurance plan. There are copayments of 30% for any outpatient care and 20% for hospitalization with a cap on out-of pocket costs. This system is characterized by long hospital stays and frequent provider visits (NPR News, 2008; OECD, 2009).

Similar to Switzerland, Japan's insurance companies cannot deny a claim, which is unlike the United States. The government sets fees for doctors through negotiation and sets hospital rates (NPR News, 2008), which is

similar to the United States for Medicare and Medicaid and managed care organizations. In 2003, a recent policy development was the use of a reimbursement system for inpatient care called diagnosis–procedure combination (DPC) (Shi & Singh, 2008). Hospitals receive daily fees for conditions and treatment regardless of the actual actions by the hospital. This new policy development is very similar to the US diagnosis-related groups that are established rates of care based on similar chronic conditions. Both the Japanese and US reimbursement systems are prospective reimbursements that provides incentives for more efficient care to the consumer. Like the United States, Japan is very focused on the integration of technology in health care.

France

France's healthcare system has many characteristics of a socialized health insurance program similar to Germany and Japan. Many healthcare experts feel that France's system should be examined when retooling the US healthcare system. Health spending is 11.1% of their gross domestic product, which is the third most expensive in the world. They have universal coverage for approximately 99% of French citizens. France has several health insurance funds heavily regulated by the government. The largest fund, the General National Insurance Scheme, covers approximately 85% of French residents. Average annual spending per person is $3374, which breaks down as $2693 from government, $448 from private insurance, and $233 from the consumer out of pocket (NPR News, 2008; OECD, 2009).

Payroll taxes provide the largest source of funding. Employers pay 13.1% of employees' salary to the national health insurance program. Employees only pay 0.75% of their salary to the program. Income taxes provide care to the indigent, disabled, unemployed, and retired. There is also a 5.25% general social contribution tax on income and taxes from alcohol, tobacco, and pharmaceutical company revenues. Nearly 90% of citizens have a supplemental insurance policy from private-for-profit insurers that they purchase from their employer. Often, the employer pays for the supplemental policy (NPR News, 2008; OECD, 2009; Tanner, 2008).

Private health insurers are central to the French system because of the supplemental insurance policies that most citizens purchase. More than 118 insurance companies offer some form of health insurance coverage. The national system pays 100% of costs for 30 chronic conditions including cancer and diabetes (NPR News, 2008; OECD, 2009). Unlike the United States, the government makes it very difficult for insurance companies to deny any coverage because of preexisting conditions. Citizens who are very ill receive increased care and coverage, which is unlike the US system where individuals may go financially bankrupt because of their cost sharing during a chronic disease.

All physicians in France participate in the nation's public health insurance (like Medicaid). The average American physician earns more than five times the average US wage while the average French physician makes only about two times the earnings of the average French wage. However, in France, medical schools, although extremely competitive to enter, are tuition free. Therefore, French physicians enter their careers with minimal debt. Unlike US physicians who pay high malpractice premiums, they pay much lower malpractice insurance premiums because their society is much less likely to sue a physician. French physicians have less administrative expenses because the government has created a standardized efficient system for physician billing and patient reimbursement using electronic funds. It is interesting to note that the French government allows physicians to charge more than the government's reimbursement schedule although physicians employed by hospitals are not allowed to set their own fees. Most physicians do not overcharge because of the intense competition in their field (Dutton, 2007). The government has also attempted to limit the use of prescription drugs by focusing on less expensive, generic-type drugs. Because physicians prescribe a tremendous amount of drugs on an annual basis, the French government recently developed a list of drugs that would not be reimbursed by the government. However, a recent study indicated that 90% of asthmatics did not receive the appropriate medication. Citizens may purchase drugs not on the reimbursable list for which they will have to pay (OECD, 2009).

Critics of France's healthcare system say that it is rigid and does not react well to healthcare crises. For example, 15,000 elderly died in the summer of 2003 as a result of a heat wave because the system did not adequately address this emergency. In 2004, during a flu epidemic, there was a shortage of hospitals beds for those afflicted (Tanner, 2008).

The United States is focusing on increasing the use of electronic systems by e-prescribing and electronic health and medical records for patients. Like the United States, French employers are less willing to hire employees because of their responsibility to the healthcare system.

France's healthcare system is experiencing a billion-dollar deficit that is largely responsible for France's overall budget deficit. The French government is examining a healthcare system based on taxes, fees, and income levels. Consumers have had no restrictions on physician selection; they may visit several physicians before they find a physician they prefer. This type of **medical nomadism** drives up healthcare costs. In response to this issue, in 2005, the government established a **coordinated care pathway** which is similar to the US managed care system (NPR News, 2008; Tanner, 2008). Individuals are recommended to choose a preferred doctor and follow the doctor's pathway for their care. At this point, this is not a mandate; this is a choice for the citizens. Despite these problems, according to a 2004 survey, the French had the highest level of satisfaction with their healthcare system worldwide (Tanner, 2008).

Switzerland

Switzerland's healthcare system is unique because all residents are required to purchase health insurance, so, in a sense, it is a country with universal healthcare coverage. Health spending is 11.6% of their gross domestic product. They are second to the United States in percentage of gross domestic product. They have universal coverage with individuals buying insurance directly from private insurance providers. The Swiss system is similar to the "managed competition" healthcare plan proposed by the Clintons in the early 1990s (Shafrin, 2008). Swiss law requires all citizens to purchase a health insurance package. Insurers cannot reject an applicant based on their health status. Healthier consumers pay higher premiums to subsidize the costs for the less healthy. Nonsmokers pay less costly premiums than smokers. Insurers compete on price.

Unlike the other countries discussed in this chapter, few Swiss employers provide insurance or contribute to insurance so individuals bear the full cost of insurance plans. They pay twice the amount of out-of-pocket expenses than the United States. Average annual spending per person is $4177, which breaks down as $2493 from the government, $408 from private insurance, and $1276 from consumer out-of-pocket expenses (Rovner, 2008).

The government subsidizes the indigent. Their health-care insurance industry is private but regulated by the government. Their citizens pay more for health insurance in Europe than other countries. Government controls prescription drug prices, of which consumers pay 10% (Rovner, 2008). Like the United States and Japan, Switzerland has focused on health technology. Unlike the United States, Switzerland has strong regulations for nonphysician healthcare professionals such as nurse practitioners, etc., which results in more expensive provider care. The government also sets rates for all providers and hospitals. Insurance companies may not make a profit on a basic insurance plan, which is very comprehensive, but can make a profit on supplemental insurance policies that cover dental, alternative medicine, or private or semiprivate hospital rooms. Consumers, however, can adjust their premium up or down by choosing a larger or smaller annual deductible, or by joining an HMO-type plan. Switzerland ranks second only to the United States in ability of patients to choose their provider (Rovner, 2008; Shafrin, 2008; Tanner, 2008;).

LOCAL GOVERNMENT HEALTHCARE REFORM

Massachusetts Universal Healthcare Program

In April 2006, the state of Massachusetts passed legislation to implement a type of universal healthcare coverage for their residents. The legislation mandated that all adult residents obtain health insurance coverage by July 1, 2007. The cost would be based on the income of the individual. For those residents who did not register, a financial penalty of up to 50% of the health insurance plan cost would be assessed. By July 1, 2007, employers with 11 or more employees were required to provide health insurance coverage or pay a **fair share** contribution of $295 annually per employee. Employers were also required to offer a Section 125 Cafeteria Plan that permits employees to purchase health care using pretax funds. A specially designed health coverage option was available for residents 19–36 years of age (Brown, 2008).

As part of the healthcare reform, the state established a clearinghouse system, the **Commonwealth Health Insurance Connector**, which facilitated the buying, selling, and administration of affordable, quality, private insurance coverage for employers with 50 or fewer employees. A major component of this reform was the provision of government-funded subsidies to low income individuals to assist with the purchase of health insurance. Plans offered through the Commonwealth Care have no deductibles and are offered by Medicaid managed care organizations (Commonwealth Health Insurance Connector, 2009).

Any resident could purchase coverage through the clearinghouse or a nonresident could purchase insurance if their employer designated the nonresident as part of their group plan. Insurance purchased through this clearinghouse could be transferred within the state, during periods of unemployment, part-time employment, or self-employment (Haisimaier & Owcharenko, 2006). As a result of this program, an estimated 440,000 individuals have health insurance coverage. However, a major problem resulting from this new program is a lack of primary care physicians. Many uninsured that now have insurance require the services of a primary care physician. There are now huge waiting lists to obtain appointments for an initial visit. This problem is reflective of the geographic maldistribution of primary care physicians in the United States—there are more specialists than there are primary care physicians. The state has passed incentive legislation, such as loan forgiveness for their medical training, to encourage primary physicians to practice in Massachusetts (Brown, 2008). Despite this issue, this program is being examined by other states as a way to provide more health insurance coverage for those who are underinsured.

Healthy San Francisco Program

In April 2007, the city's **Healthy San Francisco (HSF) Program** was established and it made comprehensive health care available to the 73,000 uninsured residents between 18 and 65 years of age. Employers with 100 employees or more are also required to spend $1.76 per work hour per employee on health benefits. Employees with 20–99 employees are required to spend $1.17 per hour. It is not an insurance program, but a restructuring of the county's program for the uninsured (Department of Public Health, San Francisco, 2009). This type of managed care program provides inpatient and outpatient care, prescription coverage, lab services, and treatments for mental health and substance abuse. Any resident is eligible to apply for the program regardless of income status, preexisting conditions, or immigration status. Those eligible must choose a primary care provider home among the 14 clinics and they are provided with an identification card and a handbook explaining the services. Small fees are charged based on income. Recent data indicated that 70% of enrollees have incomes 100% at or below the federal poverty levels. As of May 2009, there are 41,000 enrollees in the program (Katz, 2008).

The administrators evaluated the cost of this program compared to a private health insurance programs' (Blue Cross and Kaiser Permanente) premium costs for an uninsured person. If an uninsured had to pay a premium to either of the Blue Cross or Kaiser Permanente programs, they would pay a monthly premium of $388 and $618, respectively. The HSF premium was $280 (Department of Public Health, San Francisco, 2009), so there is a substantial cost savings.

Both the Massachusetts and San Francisco programs focus on the uninsured in their geographic areas and attempt to provide affordable and quality medical care to all individuals, regardless of income.

LESSONS TO BE LEARNED FROM OTHER HEALTHCARE SYSTEMS

Japan, France, and Switzerland have types of universal health insurance programs, but their systems all have flaws. Although Japan ranks at the top in the OECD country rankings for infant mortality rates and life expectancy, there are issues with their system. Like the United States, employer insurance provides a large percentage of their health care. Like the United States, the elderly use the healthcare system more than any other demographic and, as a result of this, Japan's healthcare spending is expected to triple over the next several years. In the United States, Medicare spending is out of control. **A huge advantage to the Japanese system, unlike the United States, is that health insurance companies cannot deny a claim, which means that more Japanese will receive appropriate health care. That may be a possibility for the US healthcare system.**

France, which has been applauded for a quality healthcare system, also has its problems. Similar to the United States, employers pay a portion of an employee's health insurance premium. However, unlike the United States, employers are mandated to pay a percentage of the employee's salary to a national health insurance program, not to a private health insurance plan. In France, the taxes on tobacco, alcohol, and pharmaceutical company revenues are used for health care. Using alcohol and tobacco taxes for health care may be a possibility in the United States. Similar to the United States, private health insurance companies participate in their healthcare industry because 90% of citizens purchase supplemental insurance. Their role in the United States could be altered for this goal. **However, unlike the United States, the more sick a citizen/resident becomes, the more coverage they receive from the government. That is a feature that may be pursued in this country.**

There are 30 chronic conditions for which the French government will pay the coverage, such as cancer and diabetes. In the United States, some citizens become bankrupt if they have chronic conditions because they cannot pay for the out-of-pocket expenses. France's healthcare providers all participate in public health insurance, which is similar to Medicare and Medicaid. Unlike the United States, physicians voluntarily enroll in the program. The French providers earn much less than US providers but medical school tuition is free.

As with the US system, France is experiencing an overall budget deficit for health care. Their government is now examining the possibility of developing a new system that is based on increased taxes, fees, and the income of individuals. There is a continual outcry regarding raising individual's personal taxes for a universal healthcare program in the United States. **However, increased taxes on certain consumer purchases may be an option in the United States.** Like the United States, France is developing a managed care–type program that will encourage citizens to select a provider who will become the gatekeeper for their care. Managed care contained costs in the United States during the 1990s and has become commonplace in the US healthcare system.

Switzerland has an expensive healthcare system. The program is similar to the new healthcare system in Massachusetts because they both require all of their residents to purchase healthcare insurance. Like Japan, Swiss insurers cannot reject any applicant based on their health status. They also cannot make any profit on the basic insurance package but can make a profit on the supplemental insurance packages that most citizens buy. **This type of system could be introduced in the United States because it restricts insurance plans from charging exorbitant prices but it allows them to make a profit on supplemental policies.** The government supports the indigent like the United States does with its Medicaid program.

CONCLUSION

The US healthcare system continues to evolve. Technology will continue to have a huge impact on health care. Consumers have more information to make healthcare decisions because of information technology. Healthcare providers have more opportunities to utilize technology in their delivery such as robotic surgery, e-prescribing, and clinical decision support systems that will assist them with diagnoses. The Green House Project is an exciting initiative that may transform how long-term care will be implemented. As our population becomes grayer, more citizens will want to live as independently as possible for a longer period of time and the Green House Project is an excellent template for achieving this goal. All of these initiatives are exciting for the healthcare consumer. The implementation of an EHR, which will enable providers to share information about a patient's health history, will provide the consumer with the opportunity to obtain more cost-effective and efficient health care. The Veteran's Administration hospitals use the EHR system. Duke University Health System also uses an EHR system across North Carolina (Ritzenthaler, 2009). There are hospitals, physician practices, and other healthcare organizations that utilize EHR systems across the country. Even though implementing the system nationally will be extremely expensive—costs have been estimated in the billions—it will eventually be a cost-saving measure for the United States.

These analyses indicate that all countries have problems with their healthcare systems. Establishing a universal healthcare system in the United States may not be the answer. There are aspects of each of these programs that could be integrated in the US system. There were surprisingly many similarities. The major differences were the control the government placed on pharmaceutical prices and the health insurers. They limited their profitability in order to increase healthcare access to their citizens. The main difference between these three countries and the United States are the citizens' willingness to pay more so all citizens can receive health care. That collectivistic attitude is not prevailing here in the United States; that would be difficult to change. Finally, if a universal federal healthcare coverage program is not politically feasible, perhaps more states will develop initiatives to ensure a portion of the 47 million uninsured will be provided health care. Both Massachusetts and San Francisco have implemented types of universal healthcare coverage programs. They are both too new to fully assess the success of the programs, but they need to be monitored by the federal government. Other states may be able to learn some valuable lessons from these local governments.

VOCABULARY

Bureau of Labor Statistics

Commonwealth Health Insurance Connector

Coordinated care pathway

da Vinci Surgical System

Elders

Electronic prescribing (e-prescribing)

Green House Project

Healthy San Francisco Program

Integrated Healthcare Association

Medical nomadism

National health insurance

National health system

Pay-for-performance/value-based purchasing (P4P/VBP)

Robotic surgery

Single-payer system

Socialized health insurance system

Telesurgery

REFERENCES

Agency for Healthcare Research and Quality. (2009). Theory and reality of value-based purchasing: Lessons from the pioneers. Retrieved June 1, 2009, from http://www.ahrq.gov/qual/meyerrpt.htm.

Alexander, A., & Frederick, J. (April 20, 2009). CVS Caremark, Blue Cross of NJ hit milestone in e-prescribing adoption. Retrieved November 10, 2009, from http://www.drugstorenews.com.

Brown, K. (2008). Mass health care reform reveals doctor shortages. Retrieved June 2, 2009, from http://www.npr.org/templates/story/story.php?storyId=97620520.

Brunetti, L., & Jay, R. (2009). Using technology for more effective pharmacy benefit management. *Benefits & Compensation Digest*, *46*, 16–21.

Bureau of Labor Statistics. (2009). Retrieved November 10, 2009, from http://www.bls.gov/oco/cg/cgs035.htm#outlook.

Centers for Medicare and Medicaid Services. (2009). Retrieved June 2, 2009, from http://www.cms.hhs.gov/partnerships/downloads/11399.pdf.?counter=1343.

Commonwealth Health Insurance Connector Authority. (2009). Retrieved June 3, 2009, from http://www.mahealth-connector.org.

Damburg, C., Raube, K., Teleki, S., & de la Cruz, E. (2009). Taking stock of pay-for performance: A candid assessment from the front lines. *Health Affairs*, *28*, 2, 517–525.

Department of Health and Human Services. (2000). Healthy People 2010. Retrieved November 10, 2009, from http://www.healthypeople.gov/Publications.

Department of Public Health, San Francisco. (2009). Retrieved June 2, 2009, from http://www.healthysanfrancisco.org/about_us/Reports.aspx.

Dutton, P. V. (2007). France's model healthcare system. Retrieved June 2, 2009, from http://www.boston.com/news/globe/editorial_opinion/oped/articles/2007/08/11/frances_model_healthcare_system/.

Fine, S. (2009). Where to live as we age. *Parade Magazine*, May 31, 8–9.

Fischer, M., Vogeli, C., Stedman, M., Ferris, T., Brookhart, M., & Weissman, J. (2008). Effect of electronic prescribing with formulary decision support on medication use and cost. *Archives of Internal Medicine*, *168*, 2433–2439.

Friedman, M., Schueth, A., & Bell, D. (2009). Interoperable electronic prescribing in the U.S.: A progress report. *Health Affairs*, *28*, 2, 393–403.

Gingrich, N., Boxer, R., & Brooks, B. (2008). Telephone medical consults answer the call for accessible, affordable and convenient health care. Retrieved November 6, 2009, from http://www.healthtransformation.net/galleries/default-file/teladoc.pdf.

Guidarelli, M. (2006). Robotic surgery. *The Next Generation: An Introduction to Medicine*, 2. Retrieved June 2, 2009, from http://www.nextgenmd.org/vol2–5/robotic_surgery.html.

Haisimaier, E., & Owcharenko, N. (2006). The Massachusetts approach: A new way to restructure state health insurance markets and public programs. *Health Affairs*, *25*, 6, 1580–1590.

Herman, P., Craig, B., & Caspi, O. (2005). Is complementary and alternative medicine (CAM) cost effective? A systematic review. *BMC Complementary and Alternative Medicine*, *5*, 11, 5–11.

Intuitive Surgical, Inc. (2009). da Vinci surgery. Retrieved June 2, 2009, from http://www.davincisurgery.com.

Kane, R., Lum, T., Cutler, L., Degenholtz, H., & Yu, T. (2007). Resident outcomes in small-house nursing homes: A longitudinal evaluation of the initial Green House program. *Journal of Geriatrics Society*, *55*, 6, 832–839.

Katz, M. (2008). Golden Gate to health care for all? San Francisco's new universal-access program. *New England Journal of Medicine*, *258*, 4, 327–329.

Kohn, L. T., Corrigan, J. M., & Donaldson, M. S. (1999). *To err is human: Building a safer health system*. Washington, DC: National Academy Press.

Loisance, A. (2007). Robotic surgery and telesurgery: Basic principles and description of a novel concept. *Journal de Chirugie*, *3*, 3, 211–214.

National Center for Complementary and Alternative Medicine. (2009). Retrieved November 10, 2009, from http://nccam.nih.gov/about/.

NCB Capital Impact. (2009). Retreived November 10, 2009, from http://www.ncbcapitalimpact.org/default .aspx?id=146&terms=Green+House.

NPR News. (2008). Compare international medical bills. Retrieved June 2, 2009, from http://www.npr.org/news/ specials/healthcare/healthcare_profiles.html.

Organisation for Economic Co-operation and Development. (2009). Retrieved November 10, 2009, from http://stats .oecd.org/Index.aspx?DataSetCode=CSP2009.

Ritzenthaler, B. A. (2009). Healthcare and President Obama's address: Electronic health records are a key element to healthcare reform. Retrieved June 3, 2009, from http://generalmedicine.suite101.com/article.crm/healthcare_ and_president_obamas_address.

Rosenthal, M., Landon, B., Normand, S., Frank, R. G., Ahmad, T. S., & Epstein, A. M. (2007). Employers' use of value-based purchasing strategies. *Journal of the American Medical Association*, 21, 2281–2288.

Rovner, J. (2008). In Switzerland, a health care model for America? Retrived June 2, 2009, from http://www.npr.org/ templates/story/story.php?storyId=92106731.

Shafrin, J. (2008). Health care around the world: Switzerland. Retrieved June 2, 2009, from http://healthcare-economist.com/2008/04/23/health-care-around-the-world-switzerland/.

Shi, L., & Singh, D. (2008). *Delivering health care in America*. Sudbury, MA: Jones and Bartlett.

Sultz, H., & Young, K. (2006). *Health care USA: Understanding its organization and delivery* (5th ed.). Sudbury, MA: Jones and Bartlett.

Tanner, M. (2008). The grass is not always greener—A look at national health care systems around the world. Cato Institute. *Policy analysis*, 613, 1–48.

Turncock, J. (1997). *Public health and how it works*. Gaithersburg, MD: Aspen Publishers, Inc.

NOTES

STUDENT ACTIVITY 13-1

CROSSWORD PUZZLE

Instructions: Please complete the puzzle using the vocabulary words found in the chapter. There may be multiple-word answers. The number in the parenthesis indicates the number of words in the answers.

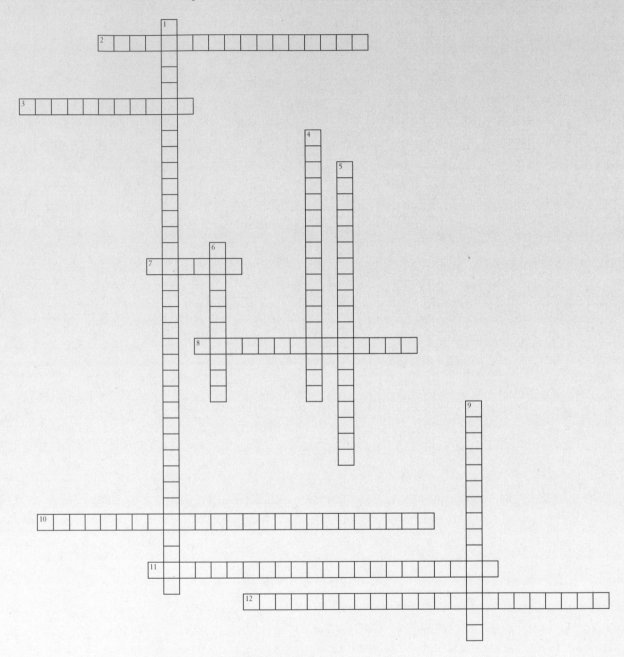

Across

2. This concept describes a healthcare payment system that rewards healthcare providers for efficiency and quality of care. (3 words)

3. This country ranks second to the United States in the cost of their healthcare system. (1 word)

7. This is the term used for the Green House Project inhabitants. (1 word)

8. This technologically advanced procedure enables providers to perform minimally invasive surgery. (2 words)

10. As in Germany, employers and employees are mandated to contribute to not-for-profit insurance companies who pay the healthcare providers for their services. (3 words)

11. This French program is similar to the managed care program in the United States. (3 words)

12. As in Canada, this system is funded by taxes although private providers deliver the care. (3 words)

Down

1. This Massachusetts program requires all adults to purchase healthcare insurance. (4 words)

4. The government pays for all healthcare services in this type of system. (3 words)

5. This city-based program located in California has provided comprehensive healthcare coverage to their uninsured residents. (3 words)

6. This project was developed as an alternative to traditional nursing home living. There are currently 18 of these projects in the United States. (2 words)

9. This occurs when consumers visit many different physicians before selecting their preferred provider. This occurs in France because they traditionally have no restriction on provider choices. (2 words)

STUDENT ACTIVITY 13-2

IN YOUR OWN WORDS

Based on Chapter 13, please provide a description of the following concepts in your own words. DO NOT RECITE the text description.

Commonwealth Health Insurance Connector: _____

_____

_____

Coordinated care pathway: _____

_____

_____

Green House Project: _____

_____

_____

Healthy San Francisco Program: _____

_____

_____

Medical nomadism: _____

_____

_____

National health insurance: _____

_____

_____

National health system: _____

_____

_____

Pay-for-performance (P4P): _____

_____

_____

Single-payer system: _____

_____

_____

Robotic surgery: _____

_____

_____

STUDENT ACTIVITY 13-3

REAL LIFE APPLICATIONS: CASE STUDY

Many experts have indicated that the United States needs some type of healthcare reform. As the special Health Policy Advisor to President Obama, you have been asked to investigate France, Japan, and Switzerland's healthcare systems in order to develop a comparison of other industrialized countries' programs.

ACTIVITY

(1) Analyze the French, Japanese, and Swiss systems, providing both the pros and cons of these systems, and (2) select a system that you feel will be the most effective in the United States. Support your answer.

RESPONSES

STUDENT ACTIVITY 13-4

INTERNET EXERCISES

Write your answers in the space provided.

- Visit each of the Web Sites listed here.
- Name the organization.
- Locate their mission statement or statement of purpose on their Web Site.
- Provide a brief overview of the activities of the organization.
- How do these organizations participate in the US healthcare system?

Web Sites

http://www.healthtransformation.net

Organization Name: _____

Mission Statement:

_____

_____

_____

Overview of Activities:

_____

_____

_____

Importance of organization to US health care:

_____

_____

_____

http://www.drugstorenews.com

Organization Name: _____

Mission Statement:

_____

_____

_____

Overview of Activities:

_____

_____

_____

STUDENT ACTIVITY 13-4

Importance of organization to US health care:

_____
_____
_____

http://www.mahealthconnector.org

Organization Name: _____

Mission Statement:

_____
_____
_____

Overview of Activities:

_____
_____
_____

Importance of organization to US health care:

_____
_____
_____

http://www.ncbcapitalimpact.org

Organization Name: _____

Mission Statement:

_____
_____
_____

Overview of Activities:

_____
_____
_____

Importance of organization to US health care:

_____
_____
_____

STUDENT ACTIVITY 13-4

http://www.iom.gov

Organization Name: _____

Mission Statement:

_____

_____

_____

Overview of Activities:

_____

_____

_____

Importance of organization to US health care:

_____

_____

_____

http://www.kff.org

Organization Name: _____

Mission Statement:

_____

_____

_____

Overview of Activities:

_____

_____

_____

Importance of organization to US health care:

_____

_____

_____

Index

Page numbers followed by t *or* f *indicate material in tables or figures, respectively.*